Sudden Cardiac Death

SUDDEN CARDIAC DEATH

Edited by

Joel Morganroth, M.D.

Director, Sudden Death Prevention Program
Professor of Medicine and Pharmacology
Likoff Cardiovascular Institute of Hahnemann University
Philadelphia, Pennsylvania

Leonard N. Horowitz, M.D.

Professor of Medicine
Director, Clinical Cardiac Electrophysiology Laboratory
Likoff Cardiovascular Institute of Hahnemann University
Philadelphia, Pennsylvania

G&S

Grune & Stratton, Inc.

(Harcourt Brace Jovanovich, Publishers)

Orlando New York San Diego Boston London
San Francisco Tokyo Sydney Toronto

Library of Congress Cataloging-in-Publication Data
Main entry under title:

Sudden cardiac death.

Includes bibliographies.
1. Cardiac arrest. 2. Arrhythmia. 3. Sudden death.
I. Morganroth, Joel. II. Horowitz, Leonard N.
[DNLM: 1. Death, Sudden. 2. Heart Arrest. WG 205 S9412]
RC685.C173S76 1985 616.1'29 85-10015
ISBN 0-8089-1725-0

Grune & Stratton, Inc.
Orlando, FL 32887

Distributed in the United Kingdom by
Grune & Stratton, Ltd.
24/28 Oval Road, London NW 1

Library of Congress Catalog Number 85-10015
International Standard Book Number 0-8089-1725-0

Printed in the United States of America
85 86 87 88 10 9 8 7 6 5 4 3 2 1

CONTENTS

PREFACE

Once every minute a sudden cardiac death occurs in the United States. It is the most common cause of death in people 20–65 years old and the most important public health problem in the industrialized world. Prevention of sudden cardiac death will depend on better understanding of the pathophysiologic mechanisms underlying it, its natural history in various groups of people, advances in models to detect and evaluate high-risk persons, and development of medical, mechanical, and surgical approaches for treating high-risk individuals. *Sudden Cardiac Death* is a collection of up-to-date information available on this topic.

The first four chapters present definitions, general clinical features, risk factors, and natural history in both pediatric and adult populations. While better methods of cardiopulmonary resuscitation and mobile coronary care units have enhanced survival, it is clear that primary prevention of sudden cardiac death will have a far greater impact on survival. Therefore, it becomes critical to identify and treat individuals. Identification of people at high risk by exercise testing, Holter monitoring, and electrophysiology are discussed in Chapters 5 through 8. Medical therapy to prevent sudden cardiac death has had a major advance in the last few years. Greater understanding of the electropharmacology and pharmacodynamics of antiarrhythmic drugs is an extremely important area. This avenue of treatment is comprehensively discussed in Chapters 9 through 13.

Chapter 14 covers the current status of modifiable risk factors. The potential use of mechanical devices (e.g., synchronized, low-energy, transvenous cardioversion) is presented in Chapter 15 as an important development for prevention of sudden cardiac death. While these devices are still in a primarily investigative phase, their use, particularly when adjunctive to pharmacological control, brings great promise in the control of ventricular tachyarrhythmias, which prove to be the acute mechanism of sudden cardiac death in over 80 percent of patients. The role of cardiac surgery for treatment of ventricular arrhythmias, discussed in Chapter 16, provides another avenue to control these few patients with serious ventricular arrhythmias that modern drugs and mechanical devices are unable to effectively manage.

Sudden Cardiac Death will present our current state of knowledge in this area and will provoke questions for further study.

CONTRIBUTORS

J. Thomas Bigger, Jr., M.D. Division of Cardiology, Department of Medicine, Columbia University; The Arrhythmia Control Unit, Columbia Presbyterian Medical Center, New York, New York

Thomas A. Buckingham, M.D. Cardiology Fellow, Division of Cardiology, St. Louis University Medical Center, St. Louis, Missouri

James Coromilas, M.D. Department of Medicine, Columbia University; Arrhythmia Control Unit, Columbia Presbyterian Medical Center, New York, New York

Lawrence M. Friedman, M.D. Chief, Clinical Trials Branch, National Heart, Lung, and Blood Institute, Department of Health and Human Services, National Institute of Health, Bethesda, Maryland

Peter L. Frommer, M.D. Deputy Director, National Heart, Lung, and Blood Institute, Bethesda, Maryland

Curt Furberg, M.D. Associate Director for Clinical Applications and Prevention, Division of Epidemiology and Clinical Applications, National Heart, Lung and Blood Institute, Bethesda, Maryland

Arthur Garson, Jr., M.D. Associate Professor of Pediatrics and Medicine, Baylor College of Medicine, Director of Electrophysiology, Texas Children's Hospital, Houston, Texas

Sidney Goldstein, M.D. Professor of Clinical Medicine, University of Michigan; Head, Division of Cardiovascular Medicine, Henry Ford Hospital, Detroit, Michigan

Allan M. Greenspan, M.D. Associate Professor of Medicine, Associate Director of Clinical Electrophysiology Laboratory, Likoff Cardiovascular Institute, Hahnemann University, Philadelphia, Pennsylvania

James F. Heger, M.D. Associate Professor of Medicine, Department of Medicine, Indiana University School of Medicine; Resident Associate, Krannart Institute of Cardiology

Leonard N. Horowitz, M.D. Professor of Medicine, Director, Clinical Cardiac Electrophysiology Laboratory, Likoff Cardiovascular Institute, Hahnemann University, Philadelphia, Pennsylvania

Abdulmassih S. Iskandrian, M.D. Associate Professor of Medicine, Director, Nuclear Cardiology, Likoff Cardiovascular Institute, Hahnemann University, Philadelphia, Pennsylvania

William B. Kannel, M.D. Professor of Medicine, Chief, Section of Preventive Medicine and Epidemiology, Department of Medicine, Boston University Medical Center, Boston, Massachusetts

Harold R. Kay, M.D. Associate Professor, Department of Cardiothoracic Surgery, Hahnemann University, Philadelphia, Pennsylvania

Harold L. Kennedy, M.D., M.P.H. Professor and Chief, Division of Cardiology, St. Louis University Medical Center, St. Louis, Missouri

Kenneth M. Kessler, M.D. Associate Professor of Medicine, University of Miami School of Medicine; Chief, Section of Cardiology, Veterans Administration Medical Center, Miami, Florida

Morris N. Kotler, M.D. Chief of Cardiology, Division of Cardiovascular Disease, Albert Einstein Medical Center/Northern Division, Philadelphia, Pennsylvania

Daniel L. McGee, Ph.D. Senior Statistician, Agent Orange Project, Centers for Disease Control, Atlanta, Georgia

Joel Morganroth, M.D. Director, Sudden Death Prevention Program, Professor of Medicine and Pharmacology, Likoff Cardiovascular Institute, Hahnemann University, Philadelphia, Pennsylvania

Robert J. Myerberg, M.D. Professor of Medicine and Physiology, Director, Division of Cardiology, University of Miami School of Medicine, Miami, Florida

Pasquale F. Nestico, M.D. Assistant Professor of Medicine, Likoff Cardiovascular Institute, Hahnemann University, Philadelphia, Pennsylvania

Edward L. C. Pritchett, M.D. Associate Professor of Medicine, Division of Cardiology, Duke University Medical Center, Durham, North Carolina

Eric N. Prystowsky, M.D. Associate Professor of Medicine, Indiana University School of Medicine; Resident Associate, Krannart Institute of Cardiology, Indianapolis, Indiana

James A. Reiffel, M.D. Department of Medicine, Columbia University; The Arrhythmia Control Unit, The Columbia Presbyterian Medical Center, New York, New York

Dan M. Roden, M.D. Assistant Professor of Medicine and Pharmacology, Vanderbilt University School of Medicine, Nashville, Tennessee

Linda M. Rolnitsky, M.S. Department of Medicine, Columbia University; The Arrhythmia Control Unit, The Columbia Presbyterian Medical Center, New York, New York

Bernard L. Segal, M.D. Professor of Medicine, Director, Likoff Cardiovascular Institute, Hahnemann University, Philadelphia, Pennsylvania

Victoria L. Vetter, M.D. Associate Cardiologist, Director, Pediatric Electrophysiology Laboratory, The Children's Hospital of Philadelphia; Assistant Professor of Pediatrics, University of Pennsylvania School of Medicine, Philadelphia, Pennsylvania

Francis M. Weld, M.D. Department of Medicine, Columbia University; Arrhythmia Control Unit, Columbia Presbyterian Medical Center, New York, New York

Raymond L. Woosley, M.D., Ph.D. Professor of Medicine and Clinical Pharmacology, Vanderbilt University School of Medicine, Nashville, Tennessee

Daniel P. Zipes, M.D. Professor of Medicine, Indiana University School of Medicine; Senior Resident Associate, Krannert Institute of Cardiology, Indianapolis, Indiana

Sudden Cardiac Death

Bernard L. Segal
Abdulmassih S. Iskandrian
Morris N. Kotler

1

SUDDEN CARDIAC DEATH

Without warning, cardiovascular disease strikes down a sizable portion of the population in industrialized nations and causes prolonged suffering and disability in an even larger number. It is responsible for almost 1 million deaths in the United States each year—well over half of all reported deaths–and about 5 million persons are hospitalized with cardiovascular disease annually. The cost of this disease in terms of human suffering is incalculable, and the money spent each year in caring for these patients exceeds $40 billion dollars.

Sudden cardiac death is a major public health problem, and its prevention depends on a better understanding of the clinical setting in which it occurs, as well as the pathologic and electrophysiologic mechanisms.[1–5] About 20% of all natural deaths in the industrially developed world are sudden cardiac deaths. In the United States each year, 400,000–450,000 persons die of cardiovascular disease. Of more than 700,000 deaths from coronary artery disease every year, 60%–65% are sudden, usually occurring when the victim is engaged in normal, routine activities.

The frustration of failing to identify factors that precipitate sudden cardiac death and to predict the people most likely to die suddenly at a specific time continues to stimulate intense interest. Nothing is more tragic in clinical practice than to hear that an "apparently healthy individual," who had been treated for only minimal nonspecific complaints, was found dead. Nothing is more distressing than to be told that a patient who had survived an acute myocardial infarction, returned to work, and did well for many years, had died suddenly at the office, soon after being given a "clean bill of health" by a physician.

The problem of sudden cardiac death will persist as long as coronary disease is prevalent. Sudden death due to arteriosclerotic heart disease almost always occurs among persons who have severe diffuse coronary atherosclerosis. Even those who were completely asymptomatic before their sudden death ordinarily have extensive coronary artery disease and signs of recent or old myocardial infarction on postmortem examination.[6–17]

SUDDEN CARDIAC DEATH
0-8089-1725-0

Although the death rate attributable to coronary disease is decreasing, it remains the number one killer in the United States. Sudden, unexpected cardiac death is the leading cause of death among middle-aged men. Physicians do not have a highly sensitive and specific way to detect coronary obstructive disease in asymptomatic people except for coronary arteriography. In addition, the specific pathophysiologic mechanism of sudden and unexpected cardiac death is incompletely understood. Practitioners can only describe the culminating event, that is, cardiac arrhythmia or ventricular fibrillation.[18–41]

The incidence of sudden death among those ages 45–54 years is low, 1 in 1000 a year. Even if the risk were increased to 1 in 100 a year by a combination of known major risk factors, a person's chance of dying suddenly of coronary artery disease within 5 years would be only about 5%. This figure is admittedly unacceptable, but 95 of 100 high-risk persons likely to die suddenly within 5 years would defy the odds.

The risk of sudden death for persons who have had prior myocardial infarctions is clearer. For patients who survive the first month, the risk of dying of a heart attack is about 5% each year; about half of these deaths will probably be sudden. Each year, about 1.2 million Americans have acute myocardial infarctions, and more than half of those who die succumb before they reach the hospital. Of those who reach the hospital, 10%–15% die before they are discharged; the mortality in the first year after infarction is estimated at another 5%–10%. The combination of life-threatening cardiac arrhythmias, abnormal left ventricular function, and extensive obstructive coronary artery disease might increase the risk of sudden death several times. The addition of other risk factors such as congestive heart failure, diabetes, recurrent and intractable life-threatening arrhythmias, and severe left ventricular dysfunction increases the risk even more.[42–54]

DEFINITION OF SUDDEN DEATH

There is no consensus as to what constitutes sudden cardiac death. The definitions differ, depending on who is determining the pathophysiologic mechanisms, clinician, epidemologist, or scientist. Sudden death may be natural or unnatural, thus excluding homicide, accidents, poisoning, and suicide from the definition. An essential element is its unanticipated occurrence. Although serious cardiac disease may have been diagnosed, death was not considered imminent.

For general purposes, the definition of sudden death is restricted to a narrow time span, such as instantaneous death, death within 1 hour, 2 hours, 6 hours, and so on, not to exceed 24 hours, or simply prehospitalization death. The definition should include three essential elements: (1) a natural process, (2) an unexpected occurrence, and (3) a rapid development. Aside from these criteria, it is not possible to give a single best definition. A broad definition is that sudden cardiac death is an unexpected, nontraumatic fatality (not self-inflicted) in patients with or without preexisting disease who die within 1–6 hours of onset. In cases of unwitnessed death, the victim was observed to be well within the preceding 24 hours. Such time frames seem rather arbitrary but are consistent with the widely accepted World Health Organization criteria.

TIME INTERVAL FROM ONSET OF SYMPTOMS TO DEATH

The time of death for persons who die outside the hospital is usually approximated by the point of collapse and the cessation of obvious vital signs as observed by a witness who is not a physician.[3] Electrocardiographic (ECG) monitoring shows that many victims of sudden death had ventricular fibrillation or serious cardiac arrhythmias at the time of collapse. Some patients can be saved by a bystander who can perform effective cardiopulmonary resuscitation.

Prodromal symptoms are frequently associated with sudden death.[53] Most are nonspecific, such as fatigue, chest pain, weakness, dyspnea, and palpitations. Many persons who die are later found to have myocardial scars suggestive of old or recent myocardial infarction, but there usually is no relevant clinical history. The relationship of these symptoms to the pathologic condition is still controversial. The validity of symptoms reported by witnesses, relatives, friends, or even from survivors of sudden death is suspect. Retrograde amnesia often limits the utility of this information.

Instantaneous deaths should be separated from other sudden deaths because of differences in the pathologic conditions.[11] People who die instantly rarely show any acute pathologic changes, whereas those who survive for several minutes or even up to 24 hours often have hemorrhage, ruptured atherosclerotic plaque, or acute thrombosis of the coronary artery.

WITNESSING SUDDEN DEATH

Certain studies report that up to one third of all sudden, unexpected deaths are unwitnessed.[4] Persons who live alone and women are more likely to die unwitnessed deaths. The place of onset is also important—sudden deaths at home are more likely to be unwitnessed.[3]

Sudden deaths in a hospital or a similar institution should be differentiated from those which occur in the community. Sudden deaths due to coronary artery disease should be categorized according to a clinical history of heart disease, which can be documented on postmortem examination by the presence of a recent or old myocardial infarction, and acute pathologic disorders in the coronary arteries.

In most community studies, about half of the sudden and unexpected deaths are noted in patients who had a prior history of heart disease. Mortality is extrapolated from the pool of patients with angina pectoris and survivors of myocardial infarctions. Often physicians sign a death certificate without a postmortem examination or even a referral to the medical examiner or coroner's office. Studies of sudden death based on the medical examiner's or coroner's records are thus substantially biased against deaths of patients with a prior history of heart disease. Studies based on review of death certificates are fraught with many inaccuracies. A physician is likely to attribute sudden death to ventricular fibrillation in a patient with a known history of coronary artery disease. Rarely is a postmortem examination complete; if it is performed, it is not necessarily standardized.[3]

RISK FACTORS

The risk factors predisposing to sudden cardiac death are generally the same as for coronary artery disease. Elevated levels of blood lipids, elevated systemic blood pressure, obesity, smoking, and ECG evidence of left ventricular hypertrophy all increase the risk of sudden death. It is widely assumed that all out-of-hospital sudden deaths represent cardiac arrest resulting from an acute electrical event; this is probably a reasonable assumption. Evidence of myocardial ischemia is found in most survivors of out-of-hospital cardiac arrests, as well as in most autopsies of patients who died.

A distinction can be drawn between out-of-hospital and in-hospital cardiac arrests. Whereas out-of-hospital cardiac arrest is almost invariably the result of a sudden lethal arrhythmia (ventricular fibrillation), the in-hospital cardiac arrest is often the terminal event in patients suffering from various severe life-threatening illnesses. The mechanism of cardiac arrest in critically ill patients in the hospital often is ventricular asystole. Additional factors in the inpatient group are respiratory acidosis, progressive shock, and, in approximately one sixth of the patients, adverse drug effects.

A small but significant group of patients with acute myocardial infarction may die suddenly in the absence of arrhythmias. These patients may have acute electromechanical dissociation. Nearly half of these individuals die abruptly or instantaneously, within seconds or minutes of engaging in normal activity. Instantaneous death in this population is almost always due to a catastrophic arrhythmia, usually ventricular tachycardia, which degenerates to ventricular fibrillation. Autopsy examinations of victims of instantaneous death occasionally reveal evidence of acute occlusive coronary thrombosis or recent myocardial infarction (or both), but in most instances, no evidence of acute infarction is found despite the presence of chronic coronary atherosclerosis. These observations support the concept that instantaneous cardiac death is an electrical event, generally resulting from ventricular fibrillation in the absence of acute infarction.

Extensive coronary atherosclerosis is by far the most common pathologic finding in patients who die suddenly.[20–24] The severity and extent of obstructive coronary lesions are far more marked in victims of sudden cardiac death than in comparable individuals who suffer accidental death. In addition to coronary artery disease, such disorders as hypertension, cardiac enlargement, congestive heart failure, ventricular hypertrophy, and chronic obstructive pulmonary disease have been associated with an increased risk of sudden cardiac death.

The frequency with which acute pathologic changes are identified in both the myocardium and coronary arteries appears to be related to the length of survival and the thoroughness of the postmortem examination. Examinations that do not include multiple sectioning of the coronary arteries and the myocardium are unlikely to discern the acute pathologic changes.

A few large community-based studies of sudden and unexpected deaths have shown that the percentage of sudden deaths not due to coronary artery disease is lowest in young people and among blacks and women[5,17] and that the higher percentage of unwitnessed deaths is attributable to other causes. Persons with a previous history of heart disease who die suddenly are generally included in the group dying of coronary disease.[3]

In community studies of sudden and unexpected deaths, there are few or no pathologic findings on postmortem examination of the coronary arteries or myocardium. Many of these deaths are nevertheless certified as due to coronary disease.[3] Few deaths in the United States, it seems, are attributed to "undetermined causes."

Ventricular Premature Beats

The importance of ventricular premature beats (VPBs) as an independent risk factor for sudden cardiac death has been the subject of considerable study and debate in recent years.[55–57] Inconsistencies in interpreting epidemiologic data and in specific recommendations for the treatment of VPBs have resulted in part from the following factors: (1) VPBs are common in middle age; (2) spontaneous occurrence of and variation in VPB frequency may be significant enough to invalidate the ECG sampling techniques employed in many studies, and (3) most epidemiologic studies to date are not directly comparable because of important differences in patient population and study designs.[3] Also, the efficacy of antiarrhythmic drug therapy in preventing sudden cardiac death has not yet been firmly established by well-controlled prospective clinical trials.

Ventricular Ectopic Activity

Simple ventricular ectopic activity may be defined as VPBs that exhibit a single QRS morphology (uniform or unifocal VPBs), occur in an isolated or nonrepetitive pattern rather than in pairs or salvos, and occur beyond the T wave of the preceding QRS complex. Single VPBs are common in the general population and may be observed in 35%–50% of healthy young adults during ambulatory ECG monitoring. Simple VPBs occur in an even greater percentage of individuals between the ages of 40 and 60, and in nearly all individuals over the age of 60. Complex VPBs are rare in young adults or older individuals who do not have apparent heart disease, however.[58–65]

The frequency of ventricular ectopic activity and its significance as a forerunner of fatal ventricular fibrillation associated with acute myocardial ischemia and infarction have been appreciated for many years. The fact that ventricular fibrillation can be initiated by simple VPBs, as well as more complex forms of ventricular ectopy in the presence of an acute myocardial infarction, has been well-established both experimentally and clinically. The dynamic use of antiarrhythmic drugs to abolish ventricular ectopy when it occurs in the coronary care unit has substantially reduced the incidence of in-hospital ventricular fibrillation.[58–65] Recent clinical studies show that primary in-hospital ventricular fibrillation associated with *acute* myocardial infarction is almost totally preventable if vigorous prophylactic therapy with antiarrhythmic drugs is instituted at the time of admission.

Management of Ventricular Premature Beats

The management of VPBs in the absence of acute myocardial ischemia or infarction constitutes a far more complex clinical problem. Some studies suggest that frequent and early VPBs in randomly selected, actively employed middle-aged men correlate with a substantially increased risk of sudden cardiac death. It is not surprising that a close association exists between frequent VPBs and other risk factors for subsequent sudden death such as preexisting coronary artery disease, hypertension, cardiac enlargement, congestive heart failure, and ventricular hypertrophy.[58–65] Despite this association, frequent or early VPBs (or both) appear to increase the risk of subsequent sudden death independently of the other risk factors. The presence of frequent VPBs alone is rarely associated with subsequent sudden death in the absence of other risk factors.

Lown et al.[18–20,24] suggested more than a decade ago that VPBs in ambulatory patients with coronary artery disease are an index of increased risk of sudden cardiac death. Ruberman et al.[66] recently reported a large-scale, prospective, epidemiologic study on ambulatory men who had survived at least one remote myocardial infarction. The study showed that the presence of complex VPBs in a 1-hour ECG recording indicated a substantially higher risk for sudden cardiac death than comparable men whose ECG recordings were free of complex VPBs.

Ventricular Premature Beats Associated with Other Forms of Heart Disease

Ventricular arrhythmias occurring in patients with coronary disease associated with acute myocardial infarction, angina pectoris, bypass surgery, and exercise may have very different implications.[67–71] The clinical significance and prognostic implications of manifest VPBs are intimately related to the abruptness of the myocardial perfusion deficit and the extent of the ischemic, fibrotic, or infarctive process complicating the coronary disease. The frequency and complexity of VPBs recorded in the coronary care unit are not precisely related to the size of the infarction. Furthermore, specific VPB characteristics, when taken alone, are poor indicators (because of low sensitivity and specificity) of impending ventricular fibrillation.

In short, the risk of sudden death is high in survivors of acute myocardial infarction, particularly when the infarction is complicated by ventricular arrhythmias or left ventricular dysfunction, or both. Recurring VPBs (especially the frequent, complex type) indicate a severalfold increase in the risk of sudden death during the first year after infarction.[61,72]

Complex ventricular arrhythmias occurring with a reduced left ventricular ejection fraction present a serious hazard to the patient. Such risk-stratification techniques can accurately identify a subset of postinfarction patients who are at low risk of sudden death and who do not require special therapy. Similarly, patients with expectable death rates of 10%–30% a year can be identified.

Even though complex VPBs and left ventricular dysfunction tend to occur together and may be pathophysiologically related, the presence of complex VPBs has been established as an independent predictor of risk of sudden cardiac death. Furthermore, complex VPBs in the setting of chronic coronary disease may constitute the most sensitive and readily accessible marker of electrical instability now available to the clinician. The validity of VPBs as an index of ventricular vulnerability is limited because of their prevalence, even among persons without demonstrable heart disease.

Ventricular Premature Beats with No Clinical Evidence of Coronary Disease

In the absence of other risk factors or clinical evidence of coronary disease, the risk of sudden cardiac death in patients with VPBs is not known, but from available clinical observations it appears to be low. The role of antiarrhythmic management hinges on this issue. If complex VPBs are indeed a direct manifestation of electrical instability and are causally related to subsequent ventricular fibrillation, antiarrhythmic management of complex VPBs might be expected to protect against sudden cardiac death. If chronic complex VPBs are not a direct manifestation of electrical instability and are not causally related to ventricular fibrillation, antiarrhythmic therapy directed at suppression of VPBs might fail to favorably influence the underlying electrophysiologic abnormality. It may even enhance susceptibility to ventricular arrhythmias under certain circumstances. This unresolved issue—whether antiarrhythmic management directed at surpressing complex VPBs reduces the risk of sudden death—is one of the most important questions confronting medical practitioners.

RISK STRATIFICATION BY INVASIVE TESTING

Electrophysiologic testing by means of programmed electrical stimulation has been proposed for achieving risk stratification.[72–82] Information from a large number of studies suggests that the initiation of ventricular fibrillation or ventricular tachycardia (sustained or nonsustained, lasting more than five complexes) is closely associated with the future clinical course of life-threatening arrhythmias. The studies were conducted with specific and well-delineated stimulation protocols, including single- and double-extra stimuli. More information is needed, however, before the electrophysiologic identification of patients at high risk of sudden death can be recommended for clinical application.

EXERCISE TESTING IN PATIENTS WITH CHRONIC CORONARY ARTERY DISEASE

Interest exists regarding the prognostic implications of ventricular arrhythmias occurring during graded exercise testing, especially in patients with clinically suspect or arteriographically proven coronary artery disease. Exercise-associated VPBs with ischemic ST segment changes in patients with known or suspected cardiac disease indicate a definite risk of subsequent coronary events.[67–71]

SUDDEN CARDIAC DEATH AND CORONARY ARTERY DISEASE

Coronary artery disease accounts for 90% of all sudden cardiac deaths (Table 1-1). The incidence of sudden death from ischemic heart disease in individuals 50–

Table 1-1 *Causes of Sudden Death*

Coronary artery disease
Aortic stenosis
Hypertrophic cardiomyopathy
Cardiomyopathy
Mitral valve prolapse
Prolonged QT syndrome
Wolff-Parkinson-White syndrome
Drug-induced ventricular arrhythmias

60 years old has been estimated to be about 2/1000 each year for white males, 1.3 for black males, 1.1 for black females, and 0.5 for white females.[83–85] In these retrospective studies of sudden death, up to half of those who died had known heart disease, and they are predominantly male. The risk of sudden death increases with age, hypertension, heavy cigarette smoking, and diabetes mellitus.

Severe obstructive coronary artery disease is present in the major epicardial vessels in most patients who die suddenly. Perper, Kuller, and Cooper[86] found that in nearly two thirds of cases, three vessels showed more than 75% luminal obstruction. The arteries involved in victims of sudden cardiac death were the left anterior descending (96%), right coronary (79%), left circumflex (66%), and left coronary (34%) arteries. The vascular obstruction was generally found in both proximal and distal segments of the epicardial coronary arteries.

In nearly 90% of patients who die of acute transmural myocardial infarction, fresh thrombotic lesions are evident in one or more coronary arteries when death is delayed long after onset; this suggests that thrombosis may be the consequence, rather than the cause, of myocardial infarction. More recent studies, however, suggest strongly that the cause of infarction is coronary atherosclerosis, thrombus, or coronary spasm, or a combination of these factors.

The studies of Cobb et al.[81–89] support the view that although coronary artery obstruction is extensive, myocardial infarction is not usual. Only 57 of 305 patients resuscitated from ventricular fibrillation showed sequential ECG changes consistent with acute transmural infarction. Even this low incidence (20%) may be an excessive figure with regard to the precipitation of sudden cardiac death by acute myocardial infarction. In patients with extensive coronary artery disease, cessation of myocardial perfusion during ventricular fibrillation may cause the infarction.

Most survivors have two- or three-vessel disease, and many also have marked left ventricular contraction abnormalities, both of which are strongly associated with subsequent episodes of cardiac arrest. The mechanisms causing ventricular fibrillation are probably multiple. Sudden cardiac arrest may occur during or after vigorous physical exertion; more commonly, it is an unexpected event during sedentary activity.

Weaver, Cobb, and Hallstrom[90] studied 90 ambulatory patients who were previously resuscitated from out-of-hospital ventricular fibrillation. The patients underwent treadmill exercise testing $11\frac{1}{2}$ months (on the average) after the episode. Contrary to what might be expected, there was no evidence from exercise testing that patients with ventricular fibrillation during exertion had a greater incidence of either evoked ischemia or ventricular arrhythmia than in patients who had collapsed at low levels of physical activity. There was a high association between exercise-evoked angina and systolic hypotension and subsequent death, however.

During a 6-year study in Seattle, more than 400 patients with ventricular fibrillation had been resuscitated before admission to the hospital and were ultimately discharged as long-term survivors.[87–89] An important part of this program was the extensive system of public education in cardiopulmonary resuscitation. In about 35% of patients with cardiac arrest, resuscitation was initiated by one of the 125,000 residents who had completed a specialized training program. When resuscitation was initiated by bystanders, the long-term survival rate was double that of resuscitation delayed until special emergency teams arrived.

Cobb et al.[88] reported a very high rate of recurrence of ventricular fibrillation among patients who underwent cardiopulmonary resuscitation. The mortality was 26% at 1 year and 36% at 2 years. Among the 305 patients with ischemic heart disease who were successfully resuscitated, there were 112 deaths; of these 86 (77%) were due to repeated episodes of ventricular fibrillation or sudden cardiac death. When ventricular fibrillation resulted from acute myocardial infarction, the mortality was only 4% at 1 year and 11% at 2 years. This information is consistent with the experience in most coronary care units: ventricular fibrillation at the inception of an ischemic episode or acute myocardial infarction may not affect prognosis.

Two syndromes of sudden cardiac death can be distinguished. A minority of patients experience myocardial infarction with prodromal chest pain during the preceding several weeks, and death is delayed. In the majority of those dying suddenly (about 80%), primary electrical failure occurs, prodromal symptoms are absent, the predisposition to recurrent ventricular fibrillation after successful resuscitation continues, and death is usually instantaneous. The precipitating factors in this latter group remain to be defined. Exercise and undue exertion are not the usual factors; nearly 75% of all sudden deaths occur at home and 8%–12% occur at work. In less than 5% of the victims, sudden cardiac death was preceded by strenuous physical exertion.

RECOGNITION OF THE HIGH-RISK PATIENT WITH UNSTABLE ANGINA PECTORIS

Unstable angina pectoris represents a clinical spectrum between chronic angina pectoris and acute myocardial infarction.[91–96] Early cardiac mortality in hospitalized patients with unstable angina is low, approximately 2%–3%; at 1 year, the late mortality may be as high as 12%–14%. Patients with unstable angina pectoris who are at high risk of sudden cardiac death or nonfatal myocardial infarction can be identified during their stay in the coronary care unit.

High-risk patients with unstable angina pectoris have the following chracteristics, listed in decreasing order of importance: continuing angina pectoris after hospital admission, ECG ischemic changes, positive pyrophosphate scintigrams[97], a long-standing clinical history of coronary artery disease, a prior history of angina pectoris, clinical cardiac failure, and cardiomegaly on chest x-ray examination.

For the high-risk patient with unstable angina pectoris who is likely to die suddenly, the major risk factors include a markedly positive myocardial scintigram, recurrent angina pectoris during hospitalization, significant ST-T abnormalities caused by myocardial ischemia, congestive heart failure, and cardiomegaly on chest x-ray examination.

BETA-BLOCKERS AND SUDDEN CARDIAC DEATH IN SURVIVORS OF MYOCARDIAL INFARCTION

Three major studies of beta-blocking drugs conducted in Norway, Sweden, and the United States showed that management with timolol, metoprolol, and propranolol reduced cardiac mortality by 26%–42% when administered after a myocardial infarction.[98–100]

In the Norwegian study, 1884 patients were chosen at random in a double-blind study to receive either 10 mg of timolol twice a day or a placebo. Treatment was started at a mean of 11 days after myocardial infarction and was continued for 1–3 years. At the end of the trial, the cardiac mortality, assessed according to the intention-to-treat principle in the treated patients, was 8.8% and in the controls it was 15.5%, a reduction in mortality of 42%.

In the Swedish study, 1395 patients were chosen at random for treatment with either metoprolol or a placebo, starting at a mean of 11 hours after the onset of infarction and continuing for 90 days. In contrast to the propranolol and timolol trials, the first dose of drug or placebo in the metoprolol trial was given intravenously. At the end of the 90-day trial, deaths in treated patients were 5.7%, and deaths in patients receiving the placebo were 8.9%, a reduction in mortality of 36%.

In the United States beta-blocker heart attack trial, 3837 patients were selected at random at a mean of 14 days after infarction to receive either propranolol in dosages of 60–80 mg three times daily or a placebo. After about 2 years, the mortality in the treated group was 7%, and in patients receiving placebos the mortality was 9.5%, a reduction in mortality of 26%.

The cardioprotective mechanism for these drugs is not completely known, but the results of the timolol study suggest that mortality was decreased by prevention of reinfarction and possibly by prevention of sudden cardiac death resulting from ventricular fibrillation in the absence of reinfarction. In contrast to standard antiarrhythmic drugs, beta-blockers used in long-term trials apparently prevented ventricular fibrillation, but are less effective as antiarrhythmic drugs when administered intravenously for established arrhythmias.

In patients with chronic coronary artery disease, the mortality for single-, double-, and triple-vessel disease has improved significantly during the past decade. This may be attributed, in part, to the introduction of beta-blockers.

SUDDEN DEATH AND NONCORONARY CONDITIONS

Aortic Stenosis

The association of aortic stenosis with sudden cardiac death has been established in children and in adults of all ages. Syncope and sudden death also have been reported in patients with subvalvular stenosis. Some studies documented a sudden fall in cardiac output, with or without significant arrhythmias. Transient heart block, ventricular tachycardia, ventricular flutter, and fibrillation precede sudden death.

Hypertrophic Cardiomyopathy

The role of atrial and ventricular arrhythmias ending in sudden death in patients with hypertrophic cardiomyopathy has received much attention in the past several years. Atrial fibrillation with sudden loss of atrial filling might cause hypotension and thus ventricular fibrillation. Myocardial ischemia also can be produced by compression of intramural and subendocardial coronary arteries, with sudden death ensuing.

Ventricular arrhythmias are common in patients with either hypertrophic or diffuse cardiomyopathy.[101] VPBs are fairly common in patients with hypertrophic cardiomyopathy, and ventricular tachyarrhythmias may cause the high incidence of sudden death observed in this condition. Ambulatory Holter monitoring has proved to be the most effective means of identifying these arrhythmias. In 1975, Ingham et al.[102] reported preliminary findings in 27 patients with idiopathic hypertrophic subaortic stenosis. VPBs were recorded in 89%, with high-frequency VPBs (greater than 1 in 1000 sinus beats) occurring in 25% of the total number of patients; ventricular tachycardia was present in 7%. Harrison, Fitzgerald, and Winkle[103] commented that Holter monitoring is more sensitive than treadmill exercise testing in uncovering ventricular arrhythmias in these patients. Savage et al.[104] reported on arrhythmias during 24-hour Holter monitoring and exercise testing in 100 patients with hypertrophic cardiomyopathy. More than 50% of the patients in all subgroups had multiform or repetitive VPBs, including 19% who had ventricular tachycardia. Holter monitoring was superior to exercise testing in detecting these arrhythmias.

Sudden death is often the first manifestation of hypertrophic cardiomyopathy in otherwise asymtomatic persons. Each year 3%–5% of these patients die suddenly. The risk of sudden death appears to be unrelated to the severity of symptoms, the degree of outflow-tract obstruction, or other hemodynamic findings. VPBs are common in patients with this condition, and more than half manifest complex arrhythmias, including unsustained ventricular tachycardia. Holter monitoring is more effective for detecting these arrhythmias.

Cardiomyopathy

Cardiomyopathy may be functionally classified as congestive, obliterative, and restrictive, stemming from diverse causes.[105] Common to all these conditions are a deteriorating clinical course, a high rate of ventricular arrhythmias, and a predisposition to sudden death. Sarcoid heart disease is an example of a specific type of cardiomyopathy in which frequent and complex VPBs have been associated with an ominous prognosis.[106] In all likelihood, the manifest VPBs are markers of extensive myocardial involvement by necrotizing and fibrosing granulomas.[107]

Mitral Valve Prolapse

The wide clinical application of echocardiography has shown the incidence of mitral valve prolapse. It is now known that about 6% of young women show ECHO evidence of mitral valve prolapse. Arrhythmias associated with this syndrome include VPBs, ventricular tachycardia, paroxysmal supraventricular tachycardia, and atrial fibrillation.[108–110]

In a study of 20 patients with mitral valve prolapse, Campbell et al.[111] reported that 24-hour ECG monitoring revealed one or more VPBs in 80%, multiform VPBs in 60%, more frequent VPBs than 30 per hour in 45%, and R on T in 35%. Ventricular tachycardia was recorded in three patients, and transient torsades de pointes rhythm with spontaneous conversion to sinus rhythm was observed in one patient. Although the vast majority of patients with mitral valve prolapse had a benign clinical course, a small subset had the malignant variant associated with ventricular tachyarrhythmias.

As a result of a study of 20 patients with mitral valve prolapse who died suddenly or had documented ventricular fibrillation, Jeresaty[108] compiled a clinical profile of the patient at high risk of sudden death.[108] For example:

> A 40-year-old woman with a history of syncope and dyspnea had late systolic murmur preceded by a click or pansystolic murmur with late systolic accentuation. The ECG shows ST-T wave changes in the inferior and left precordial leads and multiple VPBs. The ECHO displays massive mitral valve prolapse with involvement of both leaflets and minimal to moderate mitral insufficiency.

Prolonged QT Syndrome

Prolongation of a QT interval may be associated with ventricular arrhythmias, syncope, and sudden death.[112–121] The delayed repolarization phenomenon has been classified as primary or idiopathic, with and without hereditable features, and acquired forms secondary to electrolyte imbalance, drugs, and cerebrovascular disease.

Wolff-Parkinson-White Syndrome

Accelerated conduction from the atrium to the ventricle, usually engaging accessory pathways that either bridge the atrioventricular groove or merely bypass atrioventricular junctional nodal tissue, is ordinarily a benign congenital disorder. Disabling arrhythmias afflict only a minority of these patients. Sudden death, however, has been reported.[122,123] Extreme tachycardia is a consequence of atrial fibrillation because of inadequate coronary artery flow and can lead to ischemia, cardiac hypoxia, and ventricular fibrillation.

Sudden Death in the Young Athlete

Maron et al.[124] reported sudden and unexpected death in 29 highly conditioned, competitive athletes, ages 13–30 years old. Twenty-two of the 29 died suddenly during or just after severe exertion on the athletic field. Structural cardiovascular abnormalities were identified on postmortem examination of 28 athletes (97%) and were almost certainly the cause of death in 22 (76%). The most common cause of death in this report was hypertrophic cardiomyopathy (in 14 athletes). Other cardiovascular abnormalities noted in more than one athlete were an anomalous origin of the left coronary artery from the right (anterior) sinus of Valsalva, idiopathic concentric left ventricular hypertrophy, coronary artery disease, and a ruptured aorta.

Sudden Death in the Absence of Heart Disease

Sudden death may occur in the absence of evidence of organic heart disease. It is conceivable that life-threatening arrhythmias are caused by neurochemical and electrophysiologic malfunction that cannot be identified by current techniques. It also has been suggested that ventricular fibrillation, triggered by higher neural activity, is responsible for these sudden deaths.[18–20,122]

Drug-Induced Ventricular Arrhythmias
(Torsades de Pointes)

Various drugs may initiate or aggravate ventricular arrhythmias. The significance of generated VPBs relates to the extent of the underlying disease process, the amount of drug administered (even to the degree of toxicity), and the myocardial sensitivity of the patient. In recent years, the bioavailability pharmacokinetics and pharmacodynamics of cardioactive drugs have been closely scrutinized, and blood level measurements have provided reasonable guidelines for therapeutic and toxic ranges. Digitalis, quinidine, procainamide, disopyramide, doxorubicin (Adriamycin), epinephrine, ephedrine, isoproterenol, theophylline, aminophylline, terbutaline, metaproterenol, isoetharine, and psychotropic drugs have all been reported to be probable causes of death in patients who die suddenly.[123–139]

During the past several years, sudden deaths have been reported among persons on liquid protein diets. By 1979, Isner et al.[140] identified 59 documented deaths among users of liquid proteins. Increased ventricular irritability may have caused sudden death in these subjects.

Sudden Cardiac Death and Psychologic Stress

Recurrent ventricular tachycardia and ventricular fibrillation are usually associated with significant underlying organic heart disease. These life-threatening ventricular arrhythmias occasionally occur in the absence of demonstrable heart disease.[141–142] Lown et al. have published detailed studies suggesting that psychologic and neurophysiologic factors play important roles in the precipitation of ventricular arrhythmias.[143–144]

CLINICAL PREVENTION OF SUDDEN CARDIAC DEATH

Essentially two clinical approaches are considered to prevent sudden cardiac death. The first is a community-wide program to teach cardiopulmonary resuscitation. The main limitation of this approach is that the patient is reached only after the event, and even a slight delay in starting cardiopulmonary support procedures or minor errors in technique can spell disaster. In addition, the most successful outcome does not prevent a recurrence, and the victim may not be so fortunate should another arrest occur.

The second approach to prevention of cardiac death is identification of the patient who is susceptible to ventricular fibrillation, followed by initiation of prophylactic antiarrhythmic therapy. Major risk factors should be identified in ambulatory patients who are asymptomatic and persons who have cardiac arrhythmias. Identification of risk factors are important also in patients with angina pectoris, with or without cardiac arrhythmias, and in patients hospitalized with acute myocardial infarctions.

Patients should be encouraged to proceed immediately to a hospital or to call an emergency ambulance service immediately on experiencing sudden chest pain or changes in the severity or duration of angina pectoris. ECG monitoring is required to identify important arrhythmias, and appropriate management with antiarrhythmic drugs may be lifesaving.

CONCLUSIONS

Much remains to be studied in the mechanisms, management, and prevention of sudden cardiac death. Fortunately, the mortality for coronary artery disease has declined in the United States since 1968, about 2% per year. The cause of the decline is multifactorial. In the United States, overall lifestyle changes have been motivated, in part, by awareness of cardiovascular risk factors. Americans have altered their eating habits because of health and nutritional concerns. There are also clear national trends toward reduction of cigarette smoking and serum cholesterol concentrations, and physical activity is on the rise. In addition, the management of patients with uncomplicated myocardial infarction is changing. Early ambulation and return to work are more common, as is a higher level of patient and family counseling regarding infarction and its management. Routine use of beta-blockers and prophylactic antiarrhythmics has increased. Exercise testing and coronary arteriography are more often employed, as is coronary artery bypass grafting. Although it is tempting to assume that changes in medical advice and therapy are largely responsible for declining mortality, we look to more data to support this.

REFERENCES

1. Gillum RF, Feinleib M, Margolis JR, et al: Community surveillance for cardiovascular disease: The Framingham cardiovascular disease survey. J Chronic Dis 29:289, 1976
2. Kuller L, Perper J, Cooper M: Demographic characteristics and trends in arteriosclerotic heart disease mortality: Sudden death and myocardial infarction. Circulation 52(suppl 3):1, 1975
3. Kuller LH: Sudden death—Definition and epidemiologic considerations. Prog Cardiovasc Dis 23(1):1, 1980
4. Kuller LH, Pepper JA, Copper MC: Sudden and unexpected death due to arteriosclerotic heart disease. Mod Trends Cardiol 3:292, 1974
5. Kuller LH, Lilienfeld AM, Fisher R: An epidemiologic study of sudden and unexpected deaths in adults. Medicine 46:341, 1967
6. Reichenbach DD, Moss NS, Meyer E: Pathology of the heart in sudden cardiac death. Am J Cardiol 39:865, 1977
7. Scott FR, Briggs TS: Pathologic findings in prehospital deaths due to coronary artherosclerosis. Am J Cardiol 29:782, 1972
8. Perper JA, Kuller LH, Cooper M: Arteriosclerosis of coronary arteries in sudden, unexpected death. Circulation 51:27, 1975
9. Bashe WJ, Baba N, Keller MD, et al: Pathology of atherosclerotic heart disease in sudden death. II. The significance of myocardial infarction. Circulation 51–52(Suppl 3):63, 1975
10. Kannel WB, Doyle JT, McNamara PM, et al: Precursors of sudden coronary death: Factors related to the incidence of sudden death. Circulation 51:606, 1975
11. Friedman M, Manwaring JH, Rosenman RH, et al: Instantaneous and sudden deaths: Clinical and pathological differentiation in coronary artery disease. JAMA 225:1319, 1973
12. Schwartz CJ, Gerrity RG: Anatomical pathology of sudden unexpected cardiac death. Circulation 51–52(suppl 3):18, 1975
13. Herrick JB: Clinical features of sudden obstruction of the coronary arteries. JAMA 59:2015, 1912
14. Levine SA: Coronary thrombosis: Its various clinical features. Medicine 8:245, 1929
15. Feinleib M, Simon AB, Gillum RF, et al: Prodromal symptoms—Signs of sudden death. Circulation 52:111, 1975
16. Riechenback DD, Moss NS, Meyer E: Pathology of the heart is sudden cardiac death. Am J Cardiol 39:865, 1977
17. Spain DM, Bradess YA, Mohr C: Coronary atherosclerosis as a cause of unexpected and unexplained death. JAMA 174:384, 1966
18. Lown B, Graboys TB: Management of patients with malignant ventricular arrhythmias. Am J Cardiol 39:910, 1977
19. Lown B, Temte JV, Reich P, et al: Basis for recurring ventricular fibrillation in the absence of coronary heart disease and its management. N Engl J Med 294:623, 1976
20. Lown B, Verrier RL: Neural activity and ventricular fibrillation. N Engl J Med 294:1165, 1976
21. Lawrie DM, Higgins MR, Goodman MJ, et al: Ventricular fibrillation complicating acute myocardial infarction. Lancet 2:523, 1968
22. Geddes JS, Adgey AAJ, Pantridge JF: Prognosis after recovery from ventricular fibrillation complicating acute myocardial infarction. Lancet 2:273, 1967
23. Stannard M, Sloman G: Ventricular fibrillation in acute myocardial infarction: Prognosis following successful resuscitation. Am Heart J 77:573, 1969
24. Raizes G, Wagner G, Hackel D: Instantaneous nonarrhythmic cardiac death in acute myocardial infarction. Am J Cardiol 39:1, 1977

25. Bigger JT Jr, Dresdale RJ, Heissenbuttel RH, et al: Ventricular arrhythmias in ischemic heart disease: Mechanism, prevalence, significance and management. Prog Cardiovasc Dis 29:255, 1977
26. Moss A, Schnitzler R, Green R, et al: Ventricular arrhythmias three weeks after acute myocardial infarction. Ann Intern Med 75:837, 1971
27. Moe GK, Abildskov JA, Han J: Factors responsible for the initiation and maintenance of ventricular fibrillation, in Surawicz B, Pellegrino ED (eds): Sudden Cardiac Death. New York, Grune & Stratton, 1964
28. Cranefield PF: The conduction of the cardiac impulse—The slow response and cardiac arrhythmias. New York, Futura Publishing Co, 1975
29. Garrey WE: The nature of fibrillary contraction of the heart. Am J Physiol 33:397, 1914
30. Cranefield PF: Ventricular fibrillation. N Engl J Med 289:732, 1973
31. Wit AL, Cranefield PF, Hoffman BF: Slow conduction and reentry in the ventricular conduction system. II. Single and sustained circus movement in networks of canine and bovine Purkinje fibers. Circ Res 30:11, 1972
32. Wiffers CJ, Wegria R: Ventricular fibrillation due to single, localized induction and condenser shocks applied during the vulnerable phase of ventricular systole. Am J Physiol 128:500, 1975
33. Cranefield P: Action potentials, afterpotentials and arrhythmias. Cir Res 41:415, 1977
34. Moe GK, Jalife J, Mueller WJ: Reciprocation between pacemaker sites: Reentrant parasystole? in Kulbertus HE (ed): Reentrant Arrhythmias: Mechanisms and Treatment. Lancaster, England, MTP Press, 1977, p 271
35. Jalife J, Moe GK: Effect of electrotonic potentials on pacemaker activity of canine Purkinje fibers in relation to parasystole. Cir Res 39:801, 1976
36. Jalife J, Mueller WJ, Moe C. K, et al: A mathematical model of parasystole and its application to clinical examples. Circulation 56:968, 1977
37. Soloff LA: Ventricular premature beats diagnostic of myocardial disease. Am J Med Sci 242:315, 1961
38. Rosenbaum MB: Classification of ventricular extrasystoles according to form. J Electrocardiol 2:289, 1969
39. Dolara A: Early premature ventricular beats with repetitive ventricular fibrillation. Am Heart J 74:332, 1967
40. Julian DG, Valentine PA, Miller GG: Disturbances of rate, rhythm and conduction in acute myocardial infarction. Am J Med 37:915, 1964
41. Schamroth L: Idioventricular tachycardia. J Electrocardiol 1:205, 1967
42. Lown B, Ruberman W: The concept of precoronary care. Mod Concepts Cardiovasc Dis 39:97, 1970
43. Lown B: Sudden death from coronary artery disease, in Waldenstrom J, Larsson T, & Ljungestedt N (eds): Early Phases of Coronary Heart Disease: The Possibility of Prediction. Proceedings of the Skandia International Symposium, Stockholm, Mordiska Bokhandelns Foriag, 1973, p 255
44. Lown B, Vassaux C, Hood WB Jr, et al: Unresolved problems in coronary care. Am J Cardiol 20:294, 1967
45. Lown B, Wolf M: Approaches to sudden death from coronary heart disease. Circulation 44:130, 1971
46. Roberts R, Sobel B: Relationship between infarct size and ventricular arrhythmia. Br Heart J 37:1169, 1975
47. Sharma SD, Ballantyne F, Goldstein S: The relationship of ventricular asynergy in coronary artery disease to ventricular premature beats. Chest 66:358, 1974
48. Schulze RA Jr, Rouleau J, Rigo P, et al: Ventricular arrhythmias in late hospital phase of acute myocardial infarction: Relation to left ventricular function detected by gated cardiac blood pool scanning. Circulation 52:1006, 1975

49. Schulze RA Jr, Humphries JO, Griffith LSC, et al: Left ventricular and coronary angiographic anatomy: Relationship to ventricular irritability in the late hospital phase of acute myocardial infarction. Circulation 55:839, 1977
50. Calvert A, Lown B, Gorlin R: Ventricular premature beats and anatomically defined coronary heart disease. Am J Cardiol 39:627, 1977
51. Weinblatt E, Shapiro S, Frank CW: Changes in personal characteristics of men, over five years, following first diagnosis of coronary heart disease. Am J Public Health 61:831–842, 1971
52. Coronary Drug Project Research Group: Factors influencing long-term prognosis after recovery from myocardial infarction: Three-year findings of the coronary drug project. J Chronic Dis 27:267, 1974
53. Feinleib M, Simon AB, Gillum RF, et al: Prodromal symptoms and signs of sudden death. Circulation 51–52(suppl 3):155, 1975
54. Ruberman W, Weinblatt E, Goldberg J, et al: Ventricular premature beats and mortality after myocardial infarction. N Engl J Med 293:750, 1977
55. Moss AJ, DeCamilla J, Mietlowski W, et al: Prognostic grading and significance of ventricular premature beats after recovery from myocardial infarction. Circulation 51–52(suppl 3):204, 1975
56. Greene HL, Reid PR, Schaeffer AH: The repetitive ventricular response in man: A predictor of sudden death. N Engl J Med 299:729, 1978
57. Winkle RA: Measuring antiarrhythmic drug efficacy by suppression of asymptomatic ventricular arrhythmias. Ann Intern Med 91:480, 1979 (editorial)
58. Kotler M, Tabatznik B, Mower M, et al: Prognostic significance of ventricular ectopic beats with respect to sudden death in the late postinfarction period. Circulation 47:959, 1973
59. Rehnqvist N, Sjogren A: Ventricular arrhythmias prior to discharge and one year after acute myocardial infarction. Eur J Cardiol 5:425, 1977
60. Weinblatt E, Ruberman W, Goldberg J, et al: Relation of education to sudden death after myocardial infarction. N Engl J Med 299:60, 1978
61. Moss AJ, Davis HT, DeCamilla J, et al: Ventricular ectopic beats and their relation to sudden and nonsudden cardiac death after myocardial infarction. Circulation 60:998, 1979
62. Schulze RA Jr, Strauss HW, Pitt B: Sudden death in the year following myocardial infarction: Relation to ventricular premature contractions in the late hospital phase and left ventricular ejection fraction. Am J Med 62:192, 1977
63. Davis HT, DeCamilla J, Bayer LW, et al: Survivorship patterns in the posthospital phase of myocardial infarction. Circulation 60:1252, 1979.
64. Oliver G, Miller J, Kleiger R: Ventricular arrhythmias in the early posthospital phase of myocardial infarction. Circulation 52(suppl 2):223, 1975
65. DeCamilla J, Davis HT, Moss AJ: Frequency and complexity of ventricular ectopic beats in the posthospital phase of myocardial infarction. J Electrocardiol 13:125, 1980
66. Ruberman W, Weinblatt E, Goldberg J, et al: Ventricular premature beats and mortality after myocardial infarction. N Engl J Med 75:837, 1971
67. Therous P, Waters DD, Halphen C, et al: Prognostic value of exercise testing soon after myocardial infarction. N Engl J Med 301:341, 1979
68. DeBusk RF: Early exercise testing after myocardial infarction. Cardiovasc Clin 9:133, 1978
69. Erickson M, Granath A, Ohlsen P, et al: Arrhythmias and symptoms during treadmill testing three weeks after myocardial infarction in 100 patients. Br Heart J 35:787, 1973
70. Ibsen H, Kjotler E, Styperek J, et al: Routine exercise ECG three weeks after acute myocardial infarction. Acta Med Scand 198:463, 1975
71. Markiewicz W, Houston N, DeBusk

R: Exercise testing soon after myocardial infarction. Circulation 56:26, 1977
72. Green HL, Reid PR, Schaeffer HA: The repetitive ventricular response in many: A predictor of sudden death. N Engl J Med 299:729, 1978
73. Akhtar M: The clinical significance of the repetitive ventricular response. Circulation 63:773, 1981
74. Livelli FS, Bigger JT, Reiffel JA, et al: Response to programmed ventricular stimulation: Sensitivity, specificity and relationship to heart disease. Am J Cardiol 50:452, 1982
75. Hamer A, Vohra J, Hunt D, et al: Prediction of sudden death by electrophysiological studies in high-risk patients surviving acute myocardial infarction. Am J Cardiol 50:223, 1982
76. Ruskin JN, DiMarco JP, Garan H: Repetitive responses to single ventricular extrastimuli in patients with serious ventricular arrhythmias: Incidence and clinical significance. Circulation 63:767, 1981
77. VandePol CJ, Farshidi A, Spielman SR, et al: The incidence and clinical significance of induced ventricular tachycardia. Am J Cardiol 45:725, 1980
78. Ruskin JN, DeMarco JP, Garan H: Out-of-hospital cardiac electrophysiologic observations and selection of long-term antiarrhythmic therapy. N Engl J Med 303:607, 1981
79. Josephson ME, Horowitz LN, Spielman SR, et al: Electrophysiologic and hemodynamic studies in patients resuscitated from cardiac arrest. Am J Cardiol 46:948, 1980
80. Horowitz LN, Josephson ME, Kastor JA: Intracardiac electrophysiologic studies as a method for the optimism of drug therapy in chronic ventricular arrhythmia. Prog Cardiovasc Dis 23:81, 1980
81. Graboys TB, Lown B, Podrid PJ, et al: Long-term survival of patients with malignant ventricular arrhythmias treated with antiarrhythmic drugs. Am J Cardiol 50:437, 1982
82. Horowitz LN, Morganroth J: Can we prevent sudden cardiac death? Am J Cardiol 50:535, 1982
83. Kannel WB, Doyle JT, McNamara PM, et al: Precursors of sudden coronary death: Factors related to incidence of sudden death. Circulation 51:608, 1975
84. Kannel WB: Some lessons in cardiovascular epidemiology in Framingham. Am J Cardiol 37:269, 1976
85. Doyle JT, Kannel WB, McNamara RM, et al: Factors related to the suddenness of death from coronary disease: Combined Albany-Framingham studies. Am J Cardiol 37:1073, 1976
86. Perper JA, Kuller LH, Cooper M: Atherosclerosis of coronary arteries in sudden, unexpected deaths. Circulation 52:111, 1975
87. Cobb LA, Werner JA, Trobaugh GB: Sudden cardiac death: A decade's experience with out-of-hospital resuscitation. Mod Concepts Cardiovasc Dis 49:31, 1980
88. Cobb LA, Baum RS, Alvarez HA, et al: Resuscitation from out-of-hospital ventricular fibrillation: Four-year follow-up. Circulation 51–52(suppl 3):223, 1975
89. Weaver WD, Lorch GS, Alverez HA, et al: Angiographic findings and prognostic indicators in patients resuscitated from sudden cardiac death. Circulation 54:895, 1976
90. Weaver WD, Cobb LA, Hallstrom AP: Characteristics of survivors of exertion- and nonexertion-related cardiac arrest: Value of subsequent exercise testing. Am J Cardiol 50:671, 1982
91. Fulton M, Duncan B, Lutz W, et al: Natural history of unstable angina. Lancet 1:860, 1972
92. Gazes PC, Mobley EM Jr, Faris HM, et al: Preinfarctional (unstable) angina—A prospective study—Ten-year follow-up. Circulation 48:331, 1973
93. Krause KR, Hutter AM, DeSanctis RW: Acute coronary insufficiency—

Course and follow-up. Arch Intern Med 129:808, 1972
94. National Cooperative Study Group to Compare Surgical and Medical Therapy: Unstable angina pectoris. Am J Cardiol 42:839, 1978
95. Hultgren HN: Medical versus surgical treatment of unstable angina. Am J Cardiol 38:479, 1976
96. Schroeder JS, Lamb IH, Harrison DC: Patients admitted to the coronary care unit for chest pain: High-risk subgroup for subsequent cardiovascular death. Am J Cardiol 39:829, 1977
97. Olson HG, Lyons KP, Aronow WS, et al: Follow-up technetium^{99m} stannous pyrophosphate myocardial scintigrams after acute myocardial infarction. Circulation 56:181, 1977
98. The Norwegian Multicenter Study Group: Timolol-induced reduction in mortality and reinfarction in patients surviving acute myocardial infarction. N Engl J Med 304:801, 1981
99. Beta-Blocker Heart Attack Trial Research Group: A randomized trial of propranolol in patients with acute myocardial infarction. I. Mortality results. JAMA 247:1707, 1982
100. Hjalmarson A, et al: Effect on mortality of metoprolol in acute myocardial infarction. Lancet 2:823, 1981
101. Herling IM, Kotler MN, Segal BL: Sudden cardiac death in patients with hypertrophic cardiomyopathy. Prac Cardiol 8(10):197, 1982
102. Ingham R, Rossen R, Goodman D, et al: Ambulatory electrocardiographic monitoring in idiopathic hypertrophic subaortic stenosis. Circulation 52(suppl 2):93, 1975
103. Harrison DC, Fitzgerald JW, Winkle RA: Ambulatory electrocardiography for diagnosis and treatment of cardiac arrhythmias. N Engl J Med 294:373, 1976
104. Savage DD, Seides SF, Maron BJ, et al: Prevalence of arrhythmias during 24-hour electrocardiographic monitoring and exercise testing in patients with obstructive and nonobstructive hypertrophic cardiomyopathy. Circulation 59:866, 1979
105. Goodwin JF, Oakley CM: The cardiomyopathies. Br Heart J 34:545, 1972
106. Roberts W, McAllister H, Ferrans V: Sarcoidosis of the heart: A clinicopathologic study of 35 necropsy patients and review of 78 previously described necropsy patients. Am J Med 63:86, 1977
107. Silverman KJ, Hutchins GM, Bulkley BH: Cardiac sarcoid: A clinicopathologic study of 84 unselected patients with systemic sarcoidosis. Circulation 58:1204, 1978
108. Jeresaty RM: Sudden death in the mitral valve prolapse-click syndrome. Am J Cardiol 37:317, 1976
109. Winkle R, Lopes M, Fitzgerald J, et al: Arrhythmias in patients with mitral valve prolapse. Circulation 52:73, 1975
110. DeMaria AN, Amsterdam EA, Vismara LA, et al: Arrhythmias in the mitral valve prolapse syndrome: Prevalence, nature, and frequency. Ann Intern Med 84:656, 1976
111. Campbell RWF, Godman GM, Fiddler GI, et al: Ventricular arrhythmias in syndrome of balloon deformity of mitral valve: Definition of possible high-risk group. Br Heart J 38:1053, 1976
112. Jervell A, Lange-Nielson F: Congenital deaf-mutism, functional heart disease with prolongation of the Q-T interval, and sudden death. Am Heart J 54:59, 1957
113. Romano C, Gemme G, Pongiglione R: Aritmie cardiache rare dell'eta pediatrics. Clin Pediatr 45:656, 1963
114. Ward OC: New familial cardiac syndrome in children. J Ir Med Assoc 54:103, 1964
115. Moss AJ, Schwartz PG: Sudden death and the idiopathic long Q-T syndrome. Am J Med 66:6, 1979
116. Schwartz PJ, Periti M, Malliani A: The long Q-T syndrome. Am Heart J 89:378, 1975
117. Schwartz PF, Malliani A: Electrical

alternation of the T-wave: Clinical and experimental evidence of its relationship with the sympathetic nervous system and with the long Q-T syndrome. Am Heart J 89:45, 1975
118. Wellens HJJ, Vermeulen A, Durber D: Ventricular fibrillation occurring on arousal from sleep by auditory stimuli. Circulation 46:661, 1972
119. Garza LA, Vick RL, Nora JJ, et al: Heritable Q-T prolongation without deafness. Circulation 41:39, 1970
120. Crampton R: Preeminence of the left stellate ganglion in the long Q-T syndrome. Circulation 59:769, 1979
121. James TN, Groggatt P, Atkinson WJ, et al: Observations on the pathophysiology of the long Q-T syndrome with special reference to the neuropathology of the heart. Circulation 57:1221, 1978
122. Dreifus LS, Haiat R, Watanabe Y, et al: Ventricular fibrillation: A possible mechanism of sudden death in patients with Wolff-Parkinson-White syndrome. Circulation 43:520, 1971
123. Kaplan MA, Fohen KL: Ventricular fibrillation in the Wolff-Parkinson-White syndrome. Am J Cardiol 24:259, 1969
124. Maron BJ, Roberts WC, McAllister HA, et al: Sudden death in young athletes. Circulation 62:218, 1980
125. Smith TW, Haber E: Digitalis. N Engl J Med 289:1063, 1973
126. Ejvinsson G: Effect of quinidine on plasma concentrations of digoxin. Br Med J 1:279, 1978
127. Reiffel JA, Leahey EB, Drusin RE, et al: A digoxin/quinidine adverse drug interaction. Am J Cardiol 41:368, 1978
128. Leahey EB Jr, Reiffel JA, Drusin RE, et al: Interaction between quinidine and digoxin. JAMA 240:533, 1978
129. Hooymans PM, Merkus FWHM: Effect of quinidine on plasma concentration of digoxin. Br Med J 2:1022, 1978
130. Hager WD, Fenster P, Mayersohn M, et al: Digoxin-quinidine interaction. N Engl J Med 300:1238, 1979
131. Kelly HG, Fay JE, Laverty SG: Thioridazine hydrochloride (Mellaril): Its effect on the ECG and a report of two fatalities with ECG abnormalities. Can Med Assoc J 89:546, 1963
132. Desautels S, Filteau C, St-Jean A; Ventricular tachycardia associated with administration of thioridazine hydrochloride (Mellaril). Can Med Assoc J 90:1030, 1964
133. Hollister LE, Kosck JC: Sudden death during treatment with phenothiazine derivatives. JAMA 192:1038, 1965
134. Leestma JE, Koenig KL: Sudden death and phenothiazines. Arch Gen Psychiatry 18:137, 1968
135. Giles TD, Modlin RK: Death associated with ventricular arrhythmia and thioridazine hydrochloride. JAMA 204:108, 1968
136. Fowler NO, McCall D, Chou T, et al: Electrocardiographic changes and cardiac arrhythmias in patients receiving psychotropic drugs. Am J Cardiol 37:223, 1976
137. Jefferson J: A review of the cardiovascular effects and toxicity of tricyclic antidepressants. Psychosom Med 37:160, 1975
138. Vohra J, Burrows G, Hunt D, et al: The effect of toxic and therapeutic doses of tricyclic antidepressant drugs on intracardiac conduction. Eur J Cardiol 3:219, 1975
139. Bigger JT, Giardina EGV, Perel JM, et al: Cardiac antiarrhythmic effect of imipramine hydrochloride. N Engl J Med 296:206, 1977
140. Isner JM, Sours HE, Paris AL, et al: Sudden cardiac death on the liquid protein diet: Clinical and morphologic findings in 16 women. Am J Cardiol 43:421, 1979
141. Mackenzie GJ, Pascual S: Paroxysmal ventricular tachycardia. Br Heart J 26:441, 1964
142. Lesch M, Lewis E, Humphries J, et

al: Paroxysmal ventricular tachycardia in the absence of organic heart disease. Ann Intern Med 66:950, 1967
143. Lown B, Temte JV, Reich P, et al: Basis for recurring ventricular fibrillation in the absence of coronary heart disease and its management. N Engl J Med 294:623, 1976
144. Foster PR, Troup PJ, Noble RJ, et al: Ventricular tachycardia/ventricular fibrillation in a young population. Circulation 55–56(suppl 3):156, 1977

Sidney Goldstein

2

CHARACTERISTICS OF SUDDEN DEATH VICTIMS AND THE NATURAL HISTORY OF SURVIVORS OF OUT-OF-HOSPITAL SUDDEN DEATH

The success of emergency medical units has created a unique group of patients who have survived a cardiac arrest outside the hospital. A number of studies indicate that these survivors of out-of-hospital cardiac arrest face an unusually high rate of subsequent death.[1,2] Thousands of individuals have survived the fall over the precipice of death, and a variety of medical and surgical procedures have been proposed to prevent or delay their presumed recurrence of death. In addition to representing a unique clinical entity, these individuals provide information about the setting in which the cardiac arrest event occurs. They also can provide an opportunity to study the natural history of patients at high risk of sudden death. To prevent repeat cardiac arrest in this population and positively affect the mortality in similar patients with coronary artery disease, it is essential that we understand the event itself and the natural history of this population.

Coronary artery disease is the overwhelming cause of sudden death in the adult population in the Western world. Table 2-1 lists the cardiopulmonary causes that appear to be related to cardiac arrest in 167 patients who have been identified in our study of resuscitated sudden death victims.[1] This discussion will focus specifically on cardiac arrest due to coronary artery disease, since it is by far the largest single factor in sudden death. In doing so, we will also enlarge our perspective of the mechanism of death in patients with coronary artery disease.

Supported in part by NHLBI No.R01-HL18800-07.

SUDDEN CARDIAC DEATH
0-8089-1725-0

Table 2-1 *Cardiopulmonary Causes of Sudden Death As Observed in Survivors of Out-of-Hospital Cardiac Arrest*

Cause	Number Patients
Coronary artery disease	143
Cardiomyopathy	10
Primary arrhythmia	6
Valvular heart disease	5
Congenital heart disease	2
Pulmonary embolism	1
Total	167

THE MECHANISM OF SUDDEN DEATH

Ventricular fibrillation is the dominant electrophysiologic mechanism of sudden death, although in a significant but small group of individuals severe sinus bradycardia, atrial arrest, or heart block has been the observed mechanism.[3,4] The extent of ischemia and infarction associated with the arrest is quite variable and relates to long-term survival. The variability of the extent of disease in the cardiac arrest victim, however, is characteristic of the presentation of coronary artery disease itself. Liberthson et al.[5] observed that 37% of their patients who had cardiac arrest experienced an acute myocardial infarction, and 34% had evidence of acute myocardial ischemia. Postmortem studies have shown a 26% incidence of acute infarction and a 51% incidence of early infarction in the victims examined.[6] Baum, Alvarez, and Cobb[2] reported a 19% incidence of acute myocardial infarction with an additional 38% having evidence of ischemia on the basis of serum lactic dehydrogenase elevation. Our data, shown in Table 2-2, indicate that acute myocardial infarction and ischemia were associated with cardiac arrest in 78% of the resuscitated patients. Myocardial infarction in our study was defined as the development of new Q waves, and myocardial ischemia was defined as significant serum enzyme elevation occurring with the event.[1] Sudden death was ascribed to a primary arrhythmic event in the setting of chronic coronary artery disease in 22% of the victims if there was no evidence of either acute myocardial infarction or ischemia. From these data and that of other investigators it is clear that myocardial ischemia or infarction is commonly associated with the arrest.

Although ventricular fibrillation is the predominant electrophysiologic mechanism, the precipitating cause of the electrical event in coronary artery disease remains controversial. Arrest occurs frequently without prior symptoms, and in a few patients cardiac arrest may be the first evidence of coronary artery disease.

Table 2-2 *Classification of Cardiac Arrest Events*

Event	Number of Patients
Acute myocardial infarction	62 (44%)
Ischemic events	49 (34%)
Primary arrhythmic events	31 (22%)
Total	143

Whether or not the arrhythmic event is primary or secondary has been the subject of a number of studies. Although cardiac arrest may well be a primary arrhythmic event without ischemic background, most of the events are associated with infarction or ischemia.

Predictors of Sudden Death

A number of investigators[1,2,5] have observed that survivors of out-of-hospital cardiac arrest frequently have a history of cardiac disease, particularly myocardial infarction. Figure 2-1 lists the frequency of prior cardiac disease relative to the clinical arrest event observed in the 143 resuscitated cardiac arrest victims in our series on heart disease.[1] Evidence of prior cardiac disease is present in over three fourths of these individuals. (Table 2-3) Although cardiac arrest is sudden, it usually is associated with previous heart disease and is therefore not entirely

Table 2-3 *Prior Clinical Characteristics of Out-of-Hospital Cardiac Arrest Victims*

Clinical History	Number of Patients
Prior History	111 (78%)
Angina pectoris	75
Hypertension	61
Digitalis therapy	38
Myocardial infarction	66
No history	32 (22%)
Total	143

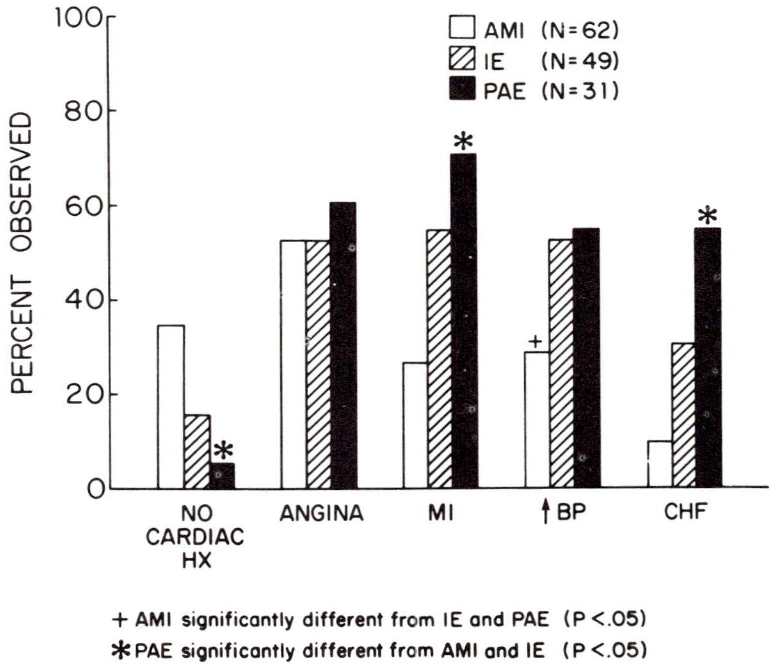

Fig. 2-1. Entry events due to coronary heart disease are *AMI,* acute myocardial infarction; *IE,* ischemic events; and *PAE,* primary arrhythmic events. The prior history (HX) includes *MI,* myocardial infarction; ↑*BP,* hypertension; and *CHF,* congestive heart failure. *ure.*

unexpected. The frequency of prior disease varies with the clinical event associated with the cardiac arrest. In the individual in whom arrest was associated with acute myocardial infarction, 35% occurred without prior cardiac symptoms. In the remaining patients in whom the arrest was associated with an ischemic event, particularly, a primary arrhythmic event, a history of cardiac disease was common.

Although many risk factors have been examined, including hypertension, lipid abnormalities, age, and sex, none of these factors identify the sudden from the nonsudden death victim with coronary artery disease. The only characteristic that does identify the sudden from, the nonsudden death victim is the presence of ventricular premature beats (VPBs). VPB frequency has been identified as a predictor of sudden cardiac death by Hinkle, Carver, and Argyros[7] in healthy middle-aged men and more recently by Ruberman et al.[8–10] in patients who had previously experienced an acute myocardial infarction and angina pectoris. They observed an almost twofold increase in the occurrence of sudden death in patients with complex VPBs present on a 1-hour tape recording. Both the Coronary Drug Project[11] and Aspirin Myocardial Infarction Study[12] also reported that VPBs observed on a standard 12-lead ECG predicted sudden death from nonsudden death victims. In a study of postmyocardial infarction patients Moss et al.[13] concluded that complex VPBs identified individuals at increased risk of death, but did not discriminate between sudden and nonsudden death.

The relationship of the specific coronary angiographic abnormalities that antedate the development of sudden death has been studied by Steinbrunn, Kappenberger, and Lichtlen.[4] In a coronary angiographic study of 229 patients they observed that sudden cardiac death represented 68% of all cardiac deaths. Sudden death occurred in 74% of patients with triple-vessel disease, 83% of patients with left main coronary artery disease, 81% of patients with ejection fractions over 0.50, and 75% of patients with ejection fractions under 0.36. They concluded that sudden cardiac death was likely to occur as frequently with normal ejection fractions as with severely reduced ejection fractions.

We studied the coronary angiograms of patients who experienced out-of-hospital cardiac arrest with coronary artery disease. In 17 patients coronary angiograms were performed before arrest and 5 before and after arrest. Patients with acute myocardial infarction as the arrest event usually have less left ventricular impairment before the arrest, but tend to end up with an equal amount of left ventricular dysfunction after the arrest. In those individuals in whom angiography was available before and after the arrest the cardiac arrest event was always associated with progression of coronary artery disease and left ventricular dysfunction.

Why some individuals sustain an acute myocardial infarction and develop ventricular fibrillation and die and others survive remains unclear. Investigations in behavioral and neurosciences have attempted to ascertain whether or not there are unique personality characteristics of sudden death victims. Greene, Goldstein, and Moss[15] compared sudden death victims with patients who had survived an acute myocardial infarction by interviewing next of kin. They observed a greater degree of emotional instability and depression in the sudden death victim. Skinner[16] has suggested that certain central nervous system control mechanisms may be related to ventricular fibrillation in the setting of acute ischemia and infarction. The interrelationship between the ischemic event and the central nervous system still requires further examination.

NATURAL HISTORY OF SURVIVORS

Some studies[1,17] have explored the natural history of survivors of out-of-hospital cardiac arrest in an attempt to understand the risks of subsequent death. The survival experience of all 142 patients in our study, as a group, shows a 1-year mortality of 18% and a 2-year mortality of 34%. When one further analyzes this population, however, two clearly defined risk groups emerge (*Figure 2-2*). The low-risk population is characterized by those who have evidence of infarction or ischemia at the time of arrest. The high-risk group is characterized as having a primary arrhythmic event and evidence of left ventricular dysfunction and congestive heart failure prior to and associated with their arrest. The patients with acute myocardial infarction and ischemia have a 1- and 2-year mortality risk of 15% and 31%, respectively. The high-risk group has a 1-year mortality risk of 31% and a 2-year risk of 45% ($P<.05$). The low-risk group has a 1-year survival rate similar to that of patients who experience an acute myocardial infarction as seen in the placebo population in the Norwegian timolol trial.[18] The improved survivorship of patients with acute myocardial infarction and cardiac arrest also has been noted

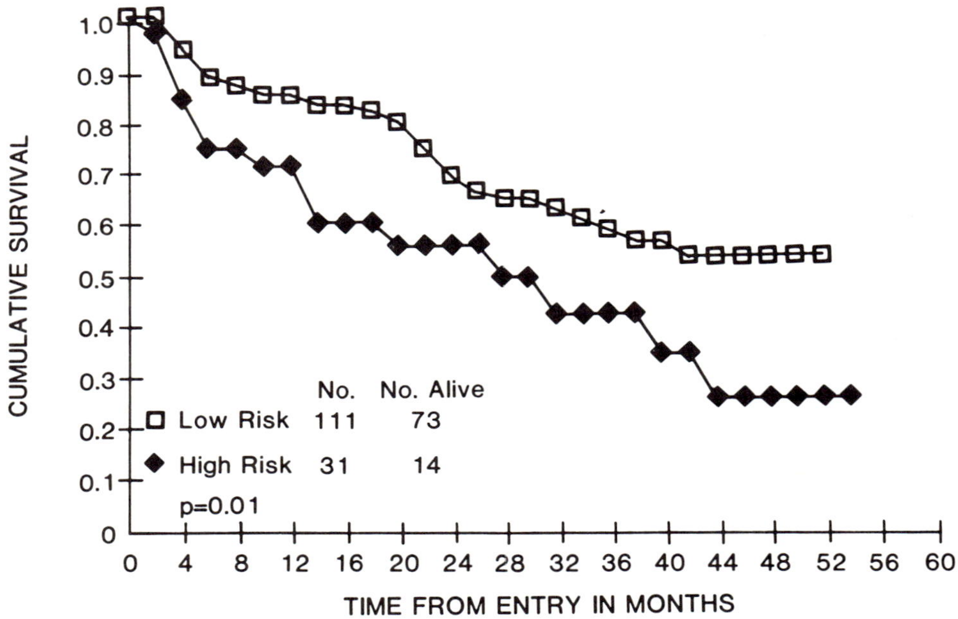

Fig. 2-2. Cumulative survival of resuscitated sudden death victims related to high- and low-risk entry classification. From Goldstein S, Landis J, Leighton R, et al: Characteristics of resuscitated out-of-hospital cardiac arrest victims with coronary heart disease. Circulation 64:977, 1981. With permission.

by Baum, Alvarez, and Cobb.[2] Eisenberg, Hallstrom, and Bergner.[19] observed that long-term survival was also related to age at the time of arrest and the duration of time before defibrillation was administered to the patient.

Angiographic Abnormalities

Coronary angiography performed in the resuscitated population indicates that the extent of left ventricular dysfunction and coronary artery disease is relatively uniform.[20,21] In a study by Tresch et al.[20] of 57 survivors of out-of-hospital cardiac arrest, severe left ventricular dysfunction with multiple-vessel coronary artery disease was common. Patients who experienced acute myocardial infarction as the cause of sudden death had less extensive coronary artery disease and left ventricular dysfunction when compared to those who died suddenly of arrhythmia without myocardial infarction. Weaver et al.[21] observed that patients who had recurrent sudden death had more extensive triple-vessel disease and lower ejection fractions than those who did not. In general, however, patients who survived out-of-hospital cardiac sudden death usually had extensive triple-vessel disease, and 70% had significant ventricular wall contraction abnormalities.

In our study, 37 patients had angiography performed after arrest. The extent of coronary artery disease and left ventricular dysfunction was similar regardless of the nature of the cardiac arrest event during the subsequent follow-up. Of those patients in whom myocardial infarction was the arrest event, 18.8% have died; 28.6% of the ischemic event group and 85.7% of the primary arrhythmic event group died during follow-up. All of the deaths were confined to those with moderate to severe left ventricular dysfunction. Subsequent death therefore was related not only to the extent of coronary artery disease and left ventricular dysfunction but also to the nature of the arrest.

In addition to the angiographic abnormalities, radionuclide angiography[22] suggests that the left ventricular ejection fraction is significantly lower in those who died during acute hospitalization. These observations, of course, are not unique to sudden death victims, but are characteristic of all patients with coronary artery disease.

Electrocardiographic Abnormalities

ECG studies, particularly ambulatory ECG assessment of rhythm disturbances, add a further dimension to risk stratification. Weaver, Cobb, and Hallstrom[23] noted that complex VPBs were observed in two thirds of resuscitated patients during a 24-hour ambulatory recording. This was seen in 56% of those who experienced recurrent sudden death and in 28% of the survivors. Other characteristics of VPBs were more sensitive predictors of death but less specific and were usually associated with clinical features of congestive heart failure. Our studies[24] indicate that VPB complexity was predictive of recurrent death but not sudden death. Examination of other factors, including VPB frequency, ventricular tachycardia, and other individual characteristics of complexity, failed to identify a high-risk group.

Changes in the standard ECG also have been evaluated in patients who had had cardiac arrest. The occurrence of repolarization abnormalities such as ST segment and T wave changes and QT prolongation have been studied by Haynes, Hallstrom, and Cobb.[25] They suggested that when arrest victims were compared to patients with myocardial infarction, repolarization abnormalities were more frequent in sudden death survivors. This study, however, was contaminated by the administration of antiarrhythmic and cardiac drugs and is difficult to assess.

Electrophysiologic studies in these patients indicate that there is a high frequency of artificially produced reentrant ventricular arrhythmias. Myerberg et al.[26] produced ventricular tachycardia in 26% of the patients using a single extra stimulus. Other investigators[27-29] induced ventricular tachycardia in two thirds to three fourths of the out-of-hospital cardiac arrest victims using multiple extra stimuli. In addition to stimulating the right ventricle, they also explored areas in the left ventricle. From these studies, it appears that electrophysiologically inducible reentrant rhythm disturbances can be produced in a significant number of these patients. For those patients in whom it was possible to induce ventricular tachycardia, the subsequent mortality is increased.[29] It appears that the ability to induce ventricular arrhythmias by electrical stimulation techniques represents a poor prognosis. These electrophysiologic characteristics, including the presence of VPBs as a predictor of recurrent death, again are not unique to this population, but are characteristic of many patients with coronary artery disease.

ANTI-ARRYTHMIC THERAPY

Because of the high-risk characteristics of the arrest victim, a number of interventions have been administered to suppress these inducible arrhythmias. The use of antiarrhythmic agents is associated with a good prognosis,[29] and variable success in suppressing induced rhythms using procainamide and quinidine has been shown. Recently, Morady et al.[27] indicated that perhaps the most reasonable pharmacologic approach is to administer amiodarone to all the patients who have inducible rhythm disturbances. Clinical studies in this area by a number of investigators indicate that a salutary effect may occur in high-risk populations similar to the out-of-hospital cardiac arrest patients using this drug. A number of surgical interventions have been proposed in addition to the use of automatic internal defibrillation. Selection of the appropriate intervention for individual patients is currently open to extensive investigation.

SUMMARY AND CONCLUSIONS

From these studies it is clear that the out-of-hospital cardiac arrest patient is a reflection of patients with heart disease in general. The variety of presentation and extent of coronary artery disease and left ventricular dysfunction that occur in heart disease occur in the out-of-hospital cardiac arrest population also. The fatal rhythm disturbances are either a primary or secondary manifestation of acute ischemia. The major pathologic mechanism associated with sudden death, however, is myocardial infarction or ischemia. It has been difficult to identify patients with coronary artery disease who are prone to sudden cardiac death except for the presence of VPBs. With this exception, the patients appear similar in all respects to patients who will die of coronary artery disease, whether they died suddenly or nonsuddenly. Why some individuals die suddenly and others experience an acute myocardial infarction and survive is not clear. Nevertheless, sudden death should not be viewed as a unique syndrome, but as an intimate expression of coronary heart disease and its ischemic outcome.

REFERENCES

1. Goldstein S, Landis J, Leighton R, et al: Characteristics of resuscitated out-of-hospital cardiac arrest victims with coronary heart disease. Circulation 64:977, 1981
2. Baum R, Alvarez H, Cobb L: Survival after resuscitation from out-of-hospital ventricular fibrillation. Circulation 50:1231, 1974
3. Nikolic G, Bishop R, Singh J: Sudden death recorded during Holter monitoring. Circulation 66:218, 1982
4. Iseri L, Humphrey S, Siner E: Prehos-

pital brady-asystolic cardiac arrest. Ann Intern Med 88:741, 1978

5. Liberthson R, Nagel E, Hirschman J, et al: Prehospital ventricular defibrillation. N Engl J Med 291:317, 1974
6. Rissanen M, Romo M, Siltanen P: Prehospital sudden death from ischemic heart disease: A postmortem study. Br Heart J 40:1025, 1978
7. Hinkle L, Carver S, Argyros D: The prognostic significance of ventricular premature contractions in healthy people and in people with coronary heart disease. Acta Cardiol 18:5, 1974
8. Ruberman W, Weinblatt E, Goldberg J, et al: Ventricular premature complexes and sudden death after myocardial infarction. Circulation 64:297, 1981
9. Ruberman W, Weinblatt E, Goldberg J, et al: Ventricular premature beats and mortality after myocardial infarction. N Engl J Med 297:750, 1977
10. Ruberman, W, Weinblatt E, Goldberg J, et al: Ventricular premature complexes in prognosis of angina. Circulation 61:1172, 1980
11. The Coronary Drug Project Research Group: Prognostic importance of premature heart beats following myocardial infarction: Experience in the Coronary Drug Project. JAMA 223:1116, 1973
12. Goldstein S, Romhilt D, Hutchinson R, et al: The timing and mechanism of witnessed coronary heart disease death. Am J Cardiol 49:1007, 1982
13. Moss A, Davis H, DeCamilla J, et al: Ventricular ectopic beats and their relation to sudden and nonsudden cardiac death after myocardial infarction. Circulation 60:998, 1979
14. Steinbrunn W, Kappenberger L, Lichtlen P: Die Hufigkeit des plotzlichen Herztodes bei der koronaren herzkrankheit. Schweiz Med Wochenschr 3:1697, 1981
15. Greene W, Goldstein S, Moss A: Psychosocial aspects of sudden death. Arch Intern Med 129:725, 1972
16. Skinner J: Regulation of cardiac vulnerability by the cerebral defense system, in Sobel E, Dingell J, Mock M (eds): Electrophysiological Mechanisms Underlying Sudden Cardiac Death. Futura Publishing Co, New York, 1982, p 131
17. Cobb L, Hallstrom A, Weaver W, et al: Prognostic factor in patients resuscitated from sudden cardiac death, in Wilhelmsen L, Hjalmarson A (eds): Acute and Long-Term Management of Myocardial Ischemia. Lindgren Sooner AB, Mondal, Sweden, 1978
18. The Norwegian Multicenter Study Group: Timolol-induced reduction in mortality and reinfarction in patients surviving acute myocardial infarction. N Engl J Med 304:801, 1981
19. Eisenberg M, Hallstrom A, Bergner L: Long-term survival after out-of-hospital cardiac arrest. N Engl J Med 306:1338, 1982
20. Tresch D, Grove R, Siegal R, et al: Survivors of prehospital sudden death. Arch Intern Med 141:1154, 1981
21. Weaver W, Lorch G, Alvarez H, et al: Angiographic findings and prognostic indicators in patients resuscitated from sudden cardiac death. Circulation 54:895, 1976
22. Trobaugh G, Gross B, Werner J, et al: Radionuclide ventriculography following resuscitation from out-of-hospital ventricular fibrillation. Am J Cardiol 47:474, 1981
23. Weaver W, Cobb L, Hallstrom A: Ambulatory arrhythmias in resuscitated victims of cardiac arrest. Circulation 66:212, 1982
24. Temesy-Armos P, Goldstein S, Landis J, et al: Complex ventricular premature depolarizations as a predictor of mortality in survivors of out-of-hospital cardiac arrest. Am J Cardiol 49:928, 1981
25. Haynes R, Hallstrom A, Cobb L: Repolarization abnormalities in survivors of out-of-hospital ventricular fibrillation. Circulation 57:654, 1977
26. Myerburg R, Conde C, Sung R, et al: Clinical, electrophysiologic and hemodynamic profile of patients resusci-

tated from prehospital cardiac arrest. Am J Med 68:568, 1980

27. Morady F, Scheinman M, Hess D, et al: Electrophysiologic testing in the management of survivors of out-of-hospital cardiac arrest. Am J Cardiol 51:85, 1983
28. Josephson M, Horowitz L, Spielman S, et al: Electrophysiologic and hemodynamic studies in patients resuscitated from cardiac arrest. Am J Cardiol 46:948, 1980
29. Ruskin J, DiMarco J, Garan H: Out-of-hospital cardiac arrest: Electrophysiologic observations and selection of long-term antiarrhythmic therapy. N Engl J Med 303:607, 1980

Victoria L. Vetter

3

SUDDEN DEATH IN CHILDREN AND ADOLESCENTS

Sudden death is generally considered to be a problem of adults with advanced coronary artery disease. The sudden and unexpected death of a young person is considered to be especially tragic. Fortunately, sudden unexpected death is rare in children. The leading causes of death in childhood include accidents, malignancies, congenital anomalies, and infectious diseases.[1] Cardiac diseases rank fifth as the cause of death among children 1–14 years of age in the United States. Sudden unexpected cardiac death is becoming a significant problem for pediatric cardiologists. Because many of these deaths may be preventable, a discussion of the problem is especially pertinent. The definition of "sudden unexpected (natural) death as death occurring instantaneously or within an estimated 24 hours of the onset of acute symptoms or signs" as used by adult cardiologists will be used for the purposes of this discussion.[2]

As in adult patients, the majority of sudden unexpected deaths in children are of cardiac origin.[3] Other causes include pulmonary problems that produce acute airway obstruction, vascular problems resulting in intracranial or other exsanguinating hemorrhage, infectious diseases, or chronic diseases such as epilepsy and diabetes.

There are few studies of sudden death in children. One recent study from Sweden describes the sudden deaths of 31 children ages 1–20 years.[4] Seven were known to have underlying diseases: epilepsy, asthma, diabetes, and cardiomyopathy. Fourteen were known to have "trivial" disorders or short duration, such as pneumonia, peritonitis, mononucleosis, meningitis, epiglottitis, upper respiratory tract infections, and myocarditis. The remaining 10 individuals died suddenly with no known preceding illnesses. Of these 10 patients, 6 had cardiac problems: 3 had myocarditis, 1 had myocardial fibrosis, 1 had Wolf-Parkinson-White syndrome and an enlarged heart, and 1 had coronary artery stenosis with myocardial infarction. Two deaths in this group were related to infectious diseases, one to adrenal failure, and one was unexplained.

Of these, 73% had no previous surgery and were described as medical deaths. Four medical conditions accounted for two thirds of these "medical" deaths:

SUDDEN CARDIAC DEATH
0-8089-1725-0

congenital aortic stenosis, cardiomyopathies, Eisenmenger's syndrome, and cyanotic heart disease with pulmonary stenosis or atresia. Thirty-three different types of cardiac disease were present with the diagnosis known or suspected in 95% of these patients. Of the 254 patients studied, 27% had previous cardiac surgery. The authors stated that approximately one third of these postoperative deaths were presumed to be secondary to arrhythmias. Of 39 sudden death patients who had undergone previous open heart surgery and who had later sudden death, 25 deaths (64%) were presumed to be secondary to arrhythmias. The other postoperative sudden deaths occurred in patients who underwent palliative or closed procedures. The precise circumstances surrounding these deaths were not discussed.

Other lesions associated with sudden unexpected cardiac death in children include congenital coronary artery anomalies,[6,7] atherosclerotic coronary artery disease,[8,9] myocarditis,[10] cardiac tumors, [11,12] mitral valve prolapse, [13,14] aneurysm of aortic cusps with thrombus formation, [15] cardiomyopathies associated with muscular dystrophy and Friedreich's ataxia,[16] obstructive cardiomyopathies,[3,6,17] long QT syndromes of Jervell and Lange-Nielsen and Romano-Ward,[18,19] aortic rupture or dissection associated with coarctation or Marfan's syndrome,[20] endocardial fibroelastosis and congestive cardiomyopathies,[5] familial conduction system anomalies,[21] and other primary arrhythmias.[22]

AORTIC STENOSIS

The incidence of sudden death in children with valvular aortic stenosis has been reported to be approximately 1%[23,24] The patients at highest risk for sudden death appear to be those with severe left ventricular outflow tract obstruction, left ventricular hypertrophy with a strain pattern, syncope, dyspnea, or chest pain.[25,26] Unfortunately, valvulotomy does not obliterate the risk of sudden death, since sudden death is a common cause of death postoperatively. The postoperative risk has been calculated to be 0.29% each year.[25] The sudden death in patients with aortic stenosis is presumed to be secondary to diminished coronary artery blood flow. The predisposing factors appear to be left ventricular enlargement, a critical reduction in valve area with a large gradient across the outflow tract, and replacement of the myocardium by fibrosis. In adults, near syncope has been shown to be related to a fall in cardiac output without associated arrhythmias.[27] More prolonged syncopal episodes have been shown to be associated with cardiac arrhythmias, specifically, cardiac standstill and ventricular flutter or fibrillation.[26] Although children may have less myocardial fibrosis, it seems reasonable to presume that the mechanism of sudden death associated with aortic stenosis would be similar to that seen in adults. Patients with supravalvar and subvalvar aortic stenosis also have been noted to be at risk for sudden death.

CARDIOMYOPATHIES

Idiopathic hypertrophic subaortic stenosis is frequently mentioned in studies of sudden death in children and account for 9% of the sudden deaths in Lambert's series.[5] One study has shown a 31% incidence of sudden death in children with idiopathic hypertrophic subaortic stenosis treated medically.[28] Other studies have confirmed a higher incidence of sudden death in children with this lesion as compared to adults.[29,30]

Almost half of the sudden deaths in young athletes reported by Maron et al.[6] had idiopathic hypertrophic subaortic stenosis. In most of these cases, cardiac disease was not suspected during life. Many other reports substantiate the presence of idiopathic hypertrophic subaortic stenosis in patients who die during exertion.[3,5,17] In many patients, sudden death is the first manifestation of disease. Sudden death in idiopathic hypertrophic subaortic stenosis is associated with youth,[30] family history of sudden death,[31] and ventricular arrhythmias on 24-hour ECGs.[30,32] Sudden death is more commonly seen in patients with abnormal ECGs and a moderately to severely thickened ventricular septum.[32] It is disputed whether preceding syncope increases the risk of sudden death or not. It is speculated that ventricular arrhythmias are the cause of sudden death.[33-35] In the study by McKenna et al.[30] sudden death in young patients was unrelated to severe functional limitation, elevated filling pressure, or the presence of a left ventricular outflow tract gradient.

Although surgical myectomy may be effective in relieving obstruction, late postoperative sudden death remains significant, as high as 8%–11%.[37,38] This is a lower incidence than the medically treated patients but remains significant.

In the study by Fiddler et al.[37] young patients treated with propranolol fared better than patients receiving no treatment. Other studies have shown that propranolol does not prevent sudden death.[28]

There are reports in the literature of familial or other nonobstructive cardiomyopathies associated with sudden death.[38] Infants and children with endocardial fibroelastosis also have shown a significant incidence of sudden death.[5,39] The presence of complex or high-grade ventricular arrhythmias in these patients seems to be associated with sudden death.

PRIMARY PULMONARY HYPERTENSION AND EISENMENGER'S SYNDROME

Primary pulmonary hypertension and Eisenmenger's syndrome represent 17% of the sudden deaths in medically treated patients described by Lambert et al.[5] Presumably, either a bradyarrhythmia or a tachyarrhythmia is the leading cause of death in these patients.[40]

Sudden death has been reported in 14%–47% of patients with Eisenmenger's syndrome.[41-43] More of these deaths occur in the second decade of life than the first.

Sudden death has been noted frequently in patients with primary pulmonary hypertension.[44] Frequent syncopal episodes may occur before sudden death.[45,46] Death associated with cardiac catheterization in these patients has been related to both bradycardia and ventricular fibrillation.[47]

CYANOTIC CONGENITAL HEART DISEASE WITH PULMONIC STENOSIS OR PULMONARY ATRESIA

In the study by Lambert et al.[5] 10% of the medical sudden deaths occurred in patients with inadequate pulmonary blood flow from pulmonary stenosis or atresia. It has been presumed that the children die from a hypoxic spell, and it is possible that severe hypoxia triggers the arrhythmias that lead to sudden death. Sudden death was also relatively common in those patients who had palliative surgery for cyanotic defects, although the effectiveness of the palliation at the time of death is not discussed.

POSTOPERATIVE CONGENITAL HEART DEFECTS

There is a significant incidence of sudden death in patients who have undergone operative repair of congenital heart defects. The risk of sudden death is greatest in patients who have repair of certain lesions, including tetralogy of Fallot, ventricular septal defect,[5] complete atrioventricular canal,[48] and transposition of the great arteries. Sudden death is stated to occur in 2%–5% of patients with repair of tetralogy of Fallot[49,50] and 2%–8% of patients with repair of transposition of the great arteries.[51,52] A lower incidence has been noted after repair of atrial septal defects.[5] A recent report noted a 5% incidence of sudden death after intracardiac conduit repair of congenital cardiac defects[53]; the deaths were presumed to be secondary to arrhythmias.

In patients with tetralogy of Fallot, sudden death was attributed to conduction disturbances such as right bundle branch block or left anterior hemiblock with presumed progression to complete heart block.[49] Recent reports suggest that ventricular arrhythmias may be equally or more important as a cause of sudden death. An incidence of sudden death of 30%–38% has been noted in tetralogy of Fallot patients who have PVCs on the resting, stress, or ambulatory ECG.[50,54,55] Recently, the electrophysiologic study has been used to induce ventricular tachycardia in these patients in an attempt to identify and pretreat those patients at risk for sudden death.[56-59] Patients with both hemodynamic and electrophysiologic aberrations seem to be at greatest risk for sudden death.[57]

In patients with transposition of the great arteries after the Mustard operation, sudden death has been postulated to be secondary to sick sinus syndrome.[60-62] Sudden death is not an uncommon occurrence in these postoperative patients who also have atrial flutter.[63]

The current postoperative incidence of complete heart block is less than 1%.[64] It has been reported to occur as late as 14 years postoperatively and is most frequently associated with repairs of ventricular septal defects, tetralogy of Fallot, or complete atrioventricular canal defects.[65] Patients known to have postoperative heart block who are not treated with pacemakers have a postoperative death rate of approximately 60%–80%.[64,66,67] Survival rates are quite good after pacemaker placement in this group of patients.[67-69]

MITRAL VALVE PROLAPSE

Sudden cardiac death has been reported in children with mitral valve prolapse,[13] including several reports of sudden death in athletes.[6] This sudden death has been postulated to be secondary to lethal arrhythmias.[70] Although the incidence of sudden death in adults with mitral valve prolapse has been reported to be 1.4%,[71] the precise incidence in children and adolescents is not known. Sudden death appears to be associated with the presence of ventricular arrhythmias, previous syncope, and a family history of sudden death.[71,72] Postmortem studies have shown associated involvement of the conduction system that could explain sudden death.[73]

CORONARY ARTERY ANOMALIES

Coronary artery anomalies may present as sudden death.[74-76] One type is an anomalous origin of the left main coronary artery from the right sinus of Valsalva. In this condition, the anomalous coronary artery courses between the aorta and pulmonary artery where it may be compressed. These patients are usually asymptomatic and may not be diagnosed until a postmortem examination after sudden death. These sudden deaths are frequently associated with physical exertion.

Another coronary artery anomaly associated with sudden death is coronary artery isolation by aortic valve adhesion.[77] In addition, ostial stenosis has been associated with sudden death in adolescents.[78] Anomalous origin of the left coronary artery from the pulmonary artery may also predispose to sudden death. Presumably, the mechanism of sudden death is similar in all the patients and is secondary to coronary insufficiency with subsequent ventricular arrhythmias.

Acquired coronary artery lesions may result in sudden death. Of increasing significance are those coronary lesions associated with Kawasaki's disease, the mucocutaneous lymph node syndrome.[79-81] The incidence of sudden death in this syndrome is reported to be approximately 2%.[80] Acquired coronary artery disease from progressive systemic sclerosis has been postulated to cause functional coronary artery involvment and sudden death in children.[82]

ANOMALIES OF THE AORTA

Sudden death has been reported in patients after repair of coarctation of the aorta.[23,83] Many of these deaths have been shown to be secondary to dissection or rupture of the ascending aorta. Many patients with Marfan's disease who have died suddenly have had rupture of aortic aneurysms[5] and cardiac arrhythmias.[17] It is not known whether these arrhythmias occur more frequently in those patients with significant mitral valve prolapse.

MYOCARDITIS

Most series concerning sudden death include cases of acute myocarditis as an important etiology. In one study from Canada, 6% of the patients who had sudden unexpected "natural" deaths were found to have myocarditis.[10] Lambert et al.[5] reported that 5% of the medical deaths were secondary to myocarditis.

Arrhythmias associated with myocarditis that might result in sudden death include both abnormalities of conduction that produce complete heart block and ventricular arrhythmias such as ventricular tachycardia or ventricular fibrillation.

EBSTEIN'S ANOMALY

The study on sudden death by Lambert et al.[5] indicates that 6% of the patients who had no surgery had Ebstein's anomaly of the tricuspid valve. If only patients with Ebstein's anomaly are discussed, it would appear that sudden death occurs in at least 20% of these patients over 1 year of age.[84] These patients are known to have a high incidence of cardiac arrhythmias, including paroxysmal supraventricular arrhythmias, atrioventricular nodal reentry, and supraventricular tachycardia associated with the Wolff-Parkinson-White syndrome. Atrial fibrillation and and ventricular arrhythmias are also seen.[85] These rhythm disturbances may be responsible for the high incidence of deaths associated with cardiac catheterization and surgical repairs.

CORRECTED TRANSPOSITION OF THE GREAT ARTERIES

Corrected transposition of the great arteries was noted in only one patient in the international study by Lambert et al.[5] Other reports[86-88] of patients with corrected transposition do relate a significant incidence of sudden death. This is presumed to be secondary to the arrhythmias associated with corrected transposition, which include the Wolff-Parkinson-White syndrome, paroxysmal supraventricular arrhythmias, and complete heart block.

ARRHYTHMIAS

Although arrhythmias are uncommon in children, they may occur with congenital heart defects pre-operatively or postoperatively, acquired cardiac problems, or normal hearts. The problem of sudden death as associated with specific arrhythmias will be discussed.

Long QT Syndrome

Two hereditary syndromes that have prolongation of the QT interval have been described in children. These include the Jervell and Lange-Nielsen syndrome associated with congenital deafness[89] and the Romano-Ward syndrome without deafness.[90,91] Asymmetric activation of the sympathetic nervous system is seen in this syndrome. Both are associated with a very high incidence of sudden death with a mortality of 73% in untreated patients. Medical or surgical treatment has markedly lessened the incidence of sudden death but has not abolished it.[92] The sudden death is presumed to be secondary to ventricular arrhythmias.[19]

Sudden death is also associated with prolongation of the QT interval secondary to certain drugs such as procainamide, quinidine, and phenothiazines.[3]

Complete Heart Block

Complete heart block in children may be congenital or acquired. The incidence of sudden death in congenital complete heart block not treated with a pacemaker is as high as 2%–3%.[93] Acquired cases occur most frequently with specific lesions. For example, patients with corrected transposition of the great arteries have a 30%–60% incidence of developing complete heart block.[86,94] Complete heart block also may be acquired with myocarditis or may occur postoperatively, as previously discussed.

Sick Sinus Syndrome

Sick sinus syndrome is uncommon as a primary arrhythmia in children, being most commonly associated with repair of congenital heart defects such as transposition of the great arteries by the Mustard operation or closure of a sinus venosus atrial septal defect.[95] It is also seen with acquired heart disease such as myocarditis.[95] Although it is rare, severe sinus node dysfunction may cause sudden death in children.[96,97]

Preexisting Syndromes

The Wolff-Parkinson-White syndrome is commonly associated with congenital heart defects, especially Ebstein's anomaly of the tricuspid valve and corrected transposition of the great arteries.[98] It also may be seen in the absence of a congenital heart defect. Sudden death has been noted in children with the Wolff-Parkinson-White syndrome. It is presumed to be secondary to ventricular fibrillation induced either by early depolarization of the ventricle from a rapidly conducted premature atrial depolarization or from 1:1 atrioventricular conduction of a rapid supraventricular tachycardia that degenerates to ventricular fibrillation.[98] Digoxin may facilitate conduction in the bypass tract and increase the chances of a life-threatening arrhythmia, although this correlation has not been substantiated to date in children. In one study of eleven young patients who had experienced cardiac arrest, two were found to have previously undiagnosed bypass tracts.[99]

Ventricular Tachycardia

In the study by Benson et al.[99] of eleven young patients who had experienced cardiac arrest, with documented ventricular tachycardia or ventricular fibrillation, ventricular tachycardia could be induced in six patients. Ventricular arrhythmias appear to increase the risk of sudden death, especially in the presence of underlying heart disease such as mitral valve prolapse, cardiomyopathies, idiopathic hypertrophic subaortic stenosis, and myocarditis.[100] Sudden death rarely has been reported in the presence of normal hearts when ventricular arrhythmias were present.[101] Familial ventricular arrhythmias associated with sudden death have been reported.[21]

CLINICAL CHARACTERISTICS OF SUDDEN DEATH PATIENTS

The conditions surrounding sudden death in children differ somewhat from adults. Death is usually instantaneous. Warning syncope occurs in only 16%. Most patients are relatively inactive at the time of death, with only a small percentage engaged in active sports.[5] The cardiac abnormalities most commonly seen in athletes or those who die when active include hypertrophic cardiomyopathies, mitral valve prolapse, coronary artery abnormalities, or a ruptured aorta.[6,7] Patients with severe aortic stenosis are also at risk for sudden death during strenuous exercise,[3] as are patients with the long QT syndrome, myocarditis, cyanotic congenital cardiac defects, and pulmonary hypertension.

Endocardial fibroelastosis and other nonobstructive cardiomyopathies, myocarditis, congenital complete heart block, and cyanotic heart disease with pulmonic stenosis result in death at younger ages. Patients with aortic stenosis and idiopathic hypertrophic subaortic stenosis tend to experience sudden death at older ages. Overall, more sudden deaths occur during the second decade of life than the first.[5]

MECHANISMS OF SUDDEN DEATH

The usual mechanism of sudden cardiac death is considered to be an arrhythmia, generally, ventricular fibrillation. Bradycardic cardiac arrest has been documented, especially in young children.[102] In a study on terminal cardiac electrical activity, patients with congenital heart disease were more likely to have ventricular fibrillation as the terminal event. Hypoxia and coronary insufficiency have been suggested as mechanisms of sudden death in children with congenital heart disease, but ventricular arrhythmias secondary to these factors are most likely to be responsible for the deaths.

Hemorrhage associated with a ruptured aorta in Marfan's syndrome and hemorrhage associated with ruptured berry aneurysms in children with coarctation of the aorta have been responsible for sudden death in these patients.

Patients with severe congestive heart failure die suddenly, possible secondary to an arrhythmia induced by low cardiac output, hypoxia, and acidosis.

PREVENTION OF SUDDEN DEATH

It is hoped that identification of high-risk patients with subsequent appropriate intervention and treatment will lead to the prevention of sudden death in children. For example, early or appropriately timed surgical intervention in children with lesions that produce cyanosis or predispose the patient to pulmonary hypertension should be effective in preventing sudden death.

Treatment of arrhythmias in patients with idiopathic hypertrophic subaortic stenosis or other cardiomyopathies may lower the incidence of sudden death. The same intervention in patients with mitral valve prolapse should be effective. Restriction of strenuous physical activity in patients prone to develop sudden death with activity (idiopathic hypertrophic subaortic stenosis, mitral valve prolapse, long QT syndrome) should lower the risk in this group.

With regard to postoperative sudden death, it is hoped that treatment of arrhythmias after repair of tetralogy of Fallot and transposition of the great arteries will lessen the incidence of sudden death. Identification of high-risk patients using electrophysiologic studies may be helpful. Pacemaker placement in patients with congenital or acquired heart block or sick sinus syndrome should prevent sudden death in many of these patients.

Medical treatment of patients with cardiac arrhythmias, including ventricular arrhythmias, the long QT syndrome, or preexcitation, should lower the risks in these groups. Some patients with preexcitation may benefit from surgical interruption of the bypass tract.

Obviously, a better understanding of the mechanisms of sudden death will allow more appropriate and timely treatment of all of the conditions discussed in this chapter.

SUMMARY

Sudden death in children and adolescents is usually associated with cardiac disease. The major congenital lesions associated with sudden death include aortic stenosis, cardiomyopathies, idiopathic hypertrophic subaortic stenosis, Eisenmenger's syndrome, and cyanotic congenital defects with pulmonary stenosis or atresia. An especially high incidence of postoperative sudden death is associated with repair of tetralogy of Fallot and transposition of the great arteries. Cardiac arrhythmias, including the long QT syndrome, sick sinus syndrome, complete heart block, ventricular tachycardia, and preexcitation are associated with sudden death.

It is hoped that identification of high-risk patients along with appropriate intervention and treatment may significantly lower or prevent sudden death in children.

REFERENCES

1. Monthly Vital Statistics Report 28(13):23, 1980
2. Oglesby P, Schatz M: On sudden death. Circulation 43:7, 1971 (editorial)
3. Manning JA: Sudden unexpected

death in children. Am J Dis Child 13:1201, 1977
4. Molander N: Sudden natural death in later childhood and adolescence. Arch Dis Child 57:572, 1982
5. Lambert EC, Menon VA, Wagner HR, et al: Sudden unexpected death from cardiovascular disease in children: A cooperative international study. Am J Cardiol 34:89, 1974
6. Maron BJ, Roberts WC, McAllister HA, et al: Sudden death in young athletes. Circulation 62;218, 1980
7. Tsung SH, Huang TY, Chang HH: Sudden death in young athletes. Arch Pathol Lab Med 106:168, 1982
8. Berkheiser SW: Cardiovascular disease in the younger age group. Aerospace Med 41:1307, 1970
9. Johnson WD, Strong TJ, Oalmann MC et al: Sudden death from coronary disease in young men. Arch Pathol Lab Med 105:227, 1981
10. Wentworth P, Jentz LA, Croal AE: Analysis of sudden unexpected death in southern Ontario with emphasis on myocarditis. Can Med Assoc J 120:676, 1979
11. James TN, Derek JL, Carson DJL, et al: De subitaneis mortibus. I. Fibroma compressing the His bundle. Circulation 48:428, 1973
12. Jolk E: Exercise and cardiac death. JAMA 218:1707, 1971
13. Anderson RC: Idiopathic mitral valve prolapse and sudden death. Am Heart J 100:941, 1980
14. Cooper MJ, Abinader EG: Family history in assessing the risk for progression of mitral valve prolapse. Am J Dis Child 135:647, 1981
15. Mant AK: Sudden death due to unusual cardiac pathology. Forensic Sci 8:7, 1976
16. James TN, Marshall TK: De subitaneis mortibus. XVIII. Persistent fetal dispersion of the atrioventricular node and His bundle within the central fibrous body. Circulation 53:1026, 1976
17. Luckstead EF: Sudden death in sports. Pediatr Clin North Am 29:1355, 1982
18. Park MK, Gunteroth WG: Long Q-T syndrome: A preventable form of sudden death. J Fam Pract 5:945, 1978
19. James TN: QT prolongation and sudden death. Mod Concepts Cardiovasc Dis 38:35, 1969
20. Forfang K, Rostad H, Sorland S, et al: Late sudden death after surgical correction of coarctation of the aorta. Acta Med Scand 206:375, 1979
21. James TN, MacLean WAH: Paroxysmal ventricular arrhythmias and familial sudden death associated with neural lesions in the heart. Chest 78:24, 1980
22. James TN, Puech P: De subitaneis mortibus. X. Type A Wolff-Parkinson-White syndrome. Circulation 50:1276, 1974
23. Thornbach P, Fowler RS: Sudden death in children with congenital heart disease. Paper presented at the Canadian Pediatric Society Meeting, July 1972
24. Campbell M: The natural history of congenital aortic stenosis. Br Heart J 30:514, 1968
25. Stewart JR, Paton BC, Blount SG Jr, et al: Congenital aortic stenosis: 10 to 22 years after valvulotomy. Arch Surg 113:1248, 1978
26. Schwartz LS, Goldfischer J, Sprague GJ, et al: Syncope and sudden death in aortic stenosis. Am J Cardiol 23:647, 1969
27. Flann MD, Braniff BA, Kimball R, et al: Mechanism of effort syncope in aortic stenosis. Circulation 26:11, 1967
28. Maron BJ, Henry WL, Clark CE, et al: Asymmetric septal hypertrophy in childhood. Circulation 53:9, 1976
29. Maron BJ, Roberts WC, Epstein SE: Sudden death in hypertrophic cardiomyopathy: A profile of 78 patients. Circulation 65:1388, 1982
30. McKenna W, Deanfield J, Faruqui A, et al: Prognosis in hypertrophic cardiomyopathy: Role of age and clinical, electrocardiographic and hemodynamic features. Am J Cardiol 47:532, 1981

31. Maron BJ, Lipson LC, Roberts WC, et al: "Malignant" hypertrophic cardiomyopathy: Identification of a subgroup of families with frequent premature death. Am J Cardiol 41:1133, 1978
32. Maron BJ, Roberts WC, Edwards JE, et al: Sudden death in patients with hypertrophic cardiomyopathy: Characterization of 26 patients without functional limitation. Am J Cardiol 41:803, 1978
33. McKenna WJ, England D, Doi YL, et al: Arrhythmia in hypertrophic cardiomyopathy. I. Influence on prognosis. Br Heart J 46:168, 1981
34. Maron BJ, Savage DD, Wolfson JK, et al: Prognostic significance of 24-hour ambulatory electrocardiographic monitoring in patients with hypertrophic cardiomyopathy: A prospective study. Am J Cardiol 48:252, 1981
35. Anderson KP, Stinson EB, Derby GC, et al: Vulnerability of patients with obstructive hypertrophic cardiomyopathy to ventricular arrhythmia induction in the operating room. Am J Cardiol 51:811, 1983
36. Bearhs MM, Tajik AJ, Seward JB, et al: Hypertrophic obstructive cardiomyopathy: 10- to 21-year follow-up after partial septal myectomy, Am J Cardiol 51:1160, 1983
37. Fiddler GI, Tajik AJ, Weidman WH, et al: Idiopathic hypertrophic subaortic stenosis in the young. Am J Cardiol 42:793, 1978
38. Ross RS, Buckley BH, Hutchins GM, et al: Idiopathic famiail myocardiopathy in three generations: A clinical and pathologic study. Am Heart J 96:170, 1978
39. Fisher JH: Primary endocardial fibroelastosis: A review of 15 cases. Can Med Assoc J 87:105, 1962
40. Graham TP Jr: The Eisenmenger reaction and its management, in Roberts WC (ed): Congenital Heart Disease in Adults. Philadelphia, FA Davis Co, 1979, p 531
41. Clarkson PM, Frye RL, DuShane JW, et al: Prognosis for patients with ventricular septal defect and severe pulmonary vascular obstructive disease. Circulation 38:129, 1968
42. Young D, Mark H: Fate of the patient with Eisenmenger syndrome. Am J Cardiol 28:658, 1971
43. Wood P: The Eisenmenger syndrome. Br Med J 2:701, 1958
44. Perloff JK: Primary pulmonary hypertension, in Perloff JK: The clinical Recognition of Congenital Heart Disease. Philadelphia, WB Saunders Co, 1970, p 201
45. Sleeper JC, Orgain ES, McIntosh HD: Primary pulmonary hypertension: Review of clinical features. Circulation 26:1358, 1962
46. Thilenius OG, Nadas AS, Jockin H: Primary pulmonary vascular obstruction in children. Pediatrics 36:75, 1965
47. Keane JF, Fyler DC: Hazards of cardiac catheterisation in children with primary pulmonary vascular obstruction. Lancet 1:863, 1977
48. Goldfaden DM, Jones M, Morrow AG: Long-term results of repair of incomplete persistent atrioventricular canal. J Thorac Cardiovasc Surg 82:669, 1981
49. Wolff GS, Rowland TW, Ellison RC: Surgically induced right bundle branch block with left anterior hemiblock. Circulation 46: 587, 1972
50. Quattlebaum TG, Varghese PJ, Neill CA, et al: Sudden death among post-operative patients with tetralogy of Fallot. Circulation 54:289, 1976
51. Saalouke MG, Rios J, Perry LW, et al: Electrophysiologic studies after Mustard's operation for *d*-transposition of the great vessels. Am J Cardiol 41:1104, 1978
52. Champsaur GL, Sokol DM, Trusler GA, et al: Repair of transposition of the great arteries in 123 pediatric patients. Circulation 47:1032, 1973
53. McGoon DC, Danielson GK, Puga FJ, et al: Late results after extracardiac conduit repair for congenital cardial defects. Am J Cardiol 49:1741, 1982
54. Gillette PC, Yeoman MA, Mullins

CE, et al: Sudden death after repair of tetralogy of Fallot. Circulation 56:566, 1977

55. James FW, Kaplan S, Chou T: Unexpected cardiac arrest in patients after surgical correction of tetralogy of Fallot. Circulation 52:691, 1975
56. Horowitz LN, Vetter VL, Harken AH, et al: Electrophysiologic characteristics of sustained ventricular tachycardia occurring after repair of tetralogy of Fallot. Am J Cardiol 46:446, 1980
57. Garson A, Porter C, Gillette PC, et al: Induction of ventricular tachycardia during electrophysiologic study after repair of tetralogy of Fallot. J Am Coll Cardiol 1:1492, 1983
58. Kugler JD, Mooring PH, Pinsky WW, et al: Sustained ventricular tachycardia following repair of tetralogy of Fallot: New electrophysiologic findings. Am J Cardiol 49:998, 1982
59. Vetter VL, Horowtiz LN: Electrophysiologic results of repair of tetralogy of Fallot. Am J Cardiol 49:999, 1982
60. Gillette PC, El-Said GM, Silvarjan N, et al: Electrophysiological abnormalities after Mustard operation for transposition of the great arteries. Br Heart J 36:186, 1974
61. Gillette PC, Kugler JD, Garson A, et al: Mechanisms of cardiac arrhythmias after the Mustard operation for transposition of the great arteries. Am J Cardiol 45:1225, 1980
62. Bharati S, Molthan ME, Veasy G, et al: Conduction system in two cases of sudden death two years after the Mustard procedure. J Thorac Cardiovasc Surg 77:101, 1979
63. Postoperative Atrial Flutter. Paper presented at the Pediatric Dysrhythmia Conference, Fifty-Fifth Scientific Session of the American Heart Association, Dallas, November 1982
64. Lillehei CW, Sellers RD, Bonnabeau RC et al: Chronic postsurgical complete heart block. J Thorac Cardiovasc Surg 46:436, 1963
65. Godman MJ, Roberts NK, Izukawa T: Late postoperative conduction disturbances after repair of ventricular septal defect and tetralogy of Fallot. Circulation 49:214, 1974
66. Levy MJ, Cuello L, Tuna N et al: Atrioventricularis communis. Am J Cardiol 14:587, 1964
67. Stanton RE, Lindesmith GG, Meyer BW: Pacemaker therapy in children with complete heart block. Am J Dis Child 129:484, 1975
68. Benrey J, Gillette PC, Nasrallah AT, et al: Permanent pacemaker implantation in infants, children and adolescents. Circulation 53:245, 1976
69. Hofschire PJ, Nicoloff DM, Moller JH: Postoperative complete heart block in 64 children treated with and without cardiac pacing. Am J Cardiol 39:559, 1977
70. Swartz MH, Teichholz LE, Donoso E: Mitral valve prolapse: A review of associated arrhythmias. Am J Med 62:377, 1977
71. Jeresaty RM: Sudden death in the mitral valve prolapse click syndrome. Am J Cardiol 37:317, 1976
72. Shappel SD, Marshall CE, Brown RE: Sudden death and the familial occurrence of midsystolic click, late systolic murmur syndrome. Circulation 48:1128, 1973
73. Bharati S, Bauernfeind R, Miller LB, et al: Sudden death in three teenagers: Conduction system studies. J Am Coll Cardiol 1:879, 1983
74. Liberthson RR, Dinsmore RE, Fallon JT: Aberrant coronary artery origin from the aorta. Circulation 59:748, 1979
75. Cheitlin MD, DeCastro CM, McAllister HA: Sudden death as a complication of anomalous left coronary origin from the anterior sinus of Valsalva: A not so minor congenital anomaly. Circulation 50:780, 1974
76. Kimbiris D, Iskandrian AS, Segal BL, et al: Anomalous aortic origin of coronary arteries. Circulation 58:606, 1978
77. Kurosawa H, Wagenaar SS, Becker

AE: Sudden death in a youth: A case of quadicuspid aortic valve with isolation of origin of left coronary artery. Br Heart J 59:748, 1981
78. Koskenvuo K, Karvonen MJ, Rissanen V: Death from ischemic heart disease in young Finns aged 15 to 24 years. Am J Cardiol 42:114, 1978
79. Fujiwara H, Hamashima Y: Pathology of the heart in Kawasaki disease. Pediatrics 61:100, 1978
80. Morens DM, Anderson LJ, Hurwitz ES: National surveillance of Kawasaki disease. Pediatrics 65:21, 1980
81. Kato H, Koike S, Yamamoto M, et al: Coronary aneurysms in infants and young children with acute febrile mucocutaneous lymph node syndrome. J Pediatr 86:892, 1975
82. Bukley BH, Klacsmann PG, Hutchins GM: Angina pectoris, myocardial infarction and sudden cardiac death with normal coronary arteries: A clinicopathologic study of 9 patients with progressive systemic sclerosis. Am Heart 95:563, 1978
83. Reifenstein GH, Levine SA, Gross RE: Coarctation of the aorta: A review of 104 autopsied cases of the "adult type," 2 years of age or older. Am Heart J 33:146, 1947
84. Watson H: Natural history of Ebstein's anomaly of tricuspid valve in childhood and adolescence: An international cooperative study of 505 cases. Br Heart J 36:417, 1974
85. Bialostozky D, Horwitz S, Espino-Vela J: Ebstein's malformation of the tricuspid valve: A review of 65 cases. Am J Cardiol 29:826, 1972
86. Friedberg DZ, Nadas AS: Clinical profile of patients with congenital corrected transposition of the great vessels. N Engl J Med 282:1053, 1970
87. Foster JR, Damato, AN, Kline LE, et al: Congenitally corrected transposition of the great vessels: Localization of the site of complete atrioventricular block using His Bundle electrograms. Am J Cardiol 38:383, 1976
88. Gillette PC, Busch U, Mullins CE et al: Electrophysiologic studies in patients with ventricular inversion and "corrected transposition." Circulation 60:939, 1979
89. Jervell A, Lange-Nielsen F: Congenital deaf-mutism, functional heart disease with prolongation of Q-T interval and sudden death. Am Heart J 54:59, 1957
90. Romano C, Gemme G, Pongiglione R: Aritmie cardiche rare dell'eta pediatrica. La Clinic Paed 45:656, 1963
91. Ward OC: A new familial cardiac syndrome in children. J Ir Med Assoc 54:103, 1964
92. Schwartz PJ, Periti M, Malliani A: The long QT syndrome. Am Heart J 89:378, 1975
93. Michaelsson M, Engle MA: Congenital complete heart block: An international study of the natural history, in Engle MA (ed): Pediatric Cardiology. Philadelphia, FA Davis Co, 1972, p 85
94. Walker WJ, Cooley DA, McNamara DG, et al: Corrected transposition of the great vessels, atrioventricular heart block and ventricular septal defect: A clinical triad. Circulation 17:249, 1958
95. Varghese PJ: Sinus node disorders, in Roberts NK, Gelband H (eds): Cardiac Arrhythmias in the Neonate, Infant and Child. New York, Appleton-Century-Crofts, 1977 p 159
96. James TN, Froggatt P, Marshall TK: Sudden death in young athletes. Ann Intern Med 67:1013, 1967
97. Roland J-M, Varghese PJ, Shematek J, et al: Sinus node dysfunction in young athletes: A possible cause of sudden death. Circulation 52 (suppl 2):233, 1975
98. Gillette PC: The preexcitation syndromes, in Gillette PC, Garson A (eds): Pediatric Cardiac Dysrhythmias. New York, Grune & Stratton, 1981, p 153
99. Benson DW, Benditt DG, Anderson RW, et al: Cardiac arrest in young, ostensibly healthy patients: Clinical, hemodynamic, and electrophys-

iologic findings. Am J Cardiol 52:65, 1983

100. Pedersen DH, Zipes DP, Foster PR, et al: Ventricular tachycardia and ventricular fibrillation in a young population. Circulation 60:988, 1979

101. James TN, Marilley RJ, Marriott HJL: De subitaneis mortibus. XI. Young girl with palpitations. Circulation 51:734, 1975

102. Walsh CK, Krongrad E: Terminal cardiac electrical activity in pediatric patients. Am J Cardiol 51:557, 1983

Arthur Garson, Jr., M.D.

4

SUDDEN DEATH IN A PEDIATRIC CARDIOLOGY POPULATION, 1958–1983

A study was carried out in the Section of Pediatric Cardiology at Texas Children's Hospital to obtain current data on sudden death in pediatric patients with cardiac disease.[1] The study covered the 25-year period between 1958 and 1983. A review of the charts of patients who died suddenly during this period allowed us to examine the factors present in this population, particularly chronic dysrhythmias.

MATERIAL AND METHODS

Patients were included in the study if they had sudden death that met the following criteria: (1) age over 1 year at the time of death, (2) the sudden event rendered the patient unconscious until death, (3) the sudden event occurred outside the hospital, and (4) absence of acute illness shortly before sudden death. Patients were excluded from this study if they had had cardiac catheterization or cardiac surgery within 1 month before death.

We used the New York Heart Association criteria for clinical status as the basis for gathering data. Cardiac catheterization hemodynamic findings were classified as (1) excellent—normal hemodynamics; (2) fair—unoperated or postoperative patients that do not require medical or surgical treatment; (3) causes of poor—hemodynamics that require eventual operative intervention, or, if inoperable, a subpulmonary ventricular pressure that is two thirds the systemic blood pressure or end diastolic pressures greater than 1.5 times normal; and (4) pulmonary hypertension— pulmonary artery systolic pressure beyond any stenoses of at least two thirds the systemic blood pressure. A review of routine resting ECGs taken during two time periods, 1 week to 1 year before sudden death and 1–2 years before sudden death, verified the presence of dyrhythmias. We did not use 24-hour ECGs, since there were insufficient data on these patients to permit

SUDDEN CARDIAC DEATH
0-8089-1725-0

adequate comparison. A "probable dysrhythmia" was identified as the cause of death if an ECG was obtained at the time of the sudden event or if the patient had a previous episode of a documented dysrhythmia causing syncope and the event leading to sudden death had a similar history. A "possible dysrhthmia" was said to be present in a high-risk patient with a prior history of dysrhythmia in whom the exact dysrhythmia at the time of death was unknown, for example, a patient with postoperative tetralogy of Fallot who had a prior ventricular dysrhythmia or a patient who had undergone a Mustard operation and had a history of bradydysrhythmia.

RESULTS

Patient Profile Associated With Sudden Death

Diagnostic Categories

Of the 981 patients seen in the Section of Pediatric Cardiology at Texas Children's Hospital who died in the last 25 years, 101 (9%) died suddenly. We have divided the diagnoses of these 101 patients into five categories (Table 4-1). The largest two categories were unoperated congenital heart disease and postoperative repair of congenital heart disease, followed by palliated congenital heart disease, unoperated acquired heart disease, and a prolonged QT interval. None of the patients who died suddenly had a normal heart. Each was seen in a pediatric cardiology clinic at least once and was believed to have heart disease. No patient discharged from the clinic with a normal heart later died suddenly.

Clinical Information

The ratio of males to females was 1.5:1 (62 male, 39 female). Although this indicated a trend, it did not achieve statistical significance. Of the 101 patients, 86% had been seen in the Pediatric Cardiology Clinic within 1 year before death. The clinical status, based on New York Heart Association criteria, broke down as follows: classes I and II, 28%; class III, 49%, and class IV, 23%. Therefore, 72% of the patients were believed to be in fair or poor condition at the time of their last clinic visit. Chest radiography at the last visit showed that 87% had cardiac enlargement.

Hemodynamic assessment took place at cardiac catheterization in 75 of the patients an average of 2.3 years before death; 89% of the patients were catheterized less than 5 years before death. The hemodynamics were excellent in 6%, fair in 5%, poor in 46%, and pulmonary hypertension in 43%. A severe hemodynamic abnormality was present in 89% of the patients. Over three quarters of the patients who died suddenly in this study were either severely symptomatic, had an abnormal chest x-ray film, or had poor hemodynamics at cardiac catheterization.

Table 4-1. *Sudden Death in Cardiovascular Patients at Texas Children's Hospital from 1959 to 1983*

Diagnosis*	Number of Patients
Unoperated congenital heart disease (36)	
Left-to-right shunt with pulmonary hypertension	11
Tetralogy of Fallot/pulmonary atresia/ventricular septal defect	7
Cardiomyopathy	5
Aortic insufficiency	3
Hypertrophic obstructive cardiomyopathy	3
L-transposition of great arteries	2
Aortic stenosis	2
Aortic aneurysm	1
Hypoplastic coronary arteries	1
Myxomatous mitral and tricuspid valves	1
Unoperated acquired heart disease (7)	
Primary pulmonary hypertension	4
Acquired cardiomyopathy	3
Prolonged QT interval (5)	
No congenital heart disease	4
With congenital heart disease	1
Palliated congenital heart disease (17)	
Right-to-left shunt with postoperative aorticopulmonary anastomosis	12
Transposition Postoperative Blalock-Hanlon Operation	12
Left-to-right shunt, postoperative banding	1
Postoperative repair of congenital heart disease (36)	
Tetralogy of Fallot/pulmonary atresia/ventricular septal defect	11
Atrioventricular canal/ventricular septal defect	5
Transposition postoperative Mustard operation	5
Transposition and ventricular septal defect - postoperative Mustard procedure and ventricular septal defect closure	4
Aortic valve replacement	4
Mitral valve replacement	3
Tricuspid valve replacement	1
Atrial septal defect/ostium primum	1
Hypertrophic obstructive cardiomyopathy/postoperative myotomy	1
Patent ductus arteriosus (with complete atrioventricular block)	1
Total	101

Table 4-2 *ECG Dysrhythmias 1 week to 1 year before Death*

Dysrhythmia*	Percentage (%)
PVBs	20
AFL	8
Sinus bradycardia	7
Junctional rhythm	7
CAVB	6
CAVB with pacemaker	5
JR and PVC	5
CAVB, PM, and PVC	2
AFL and PVC	2
SVT	1
VT	1
Any dysrhythmia	57
No dysrhythmia	43

* *AFL,* Atrial flutter; *AV block,* atrioventricular block; *CAVB,* complete AV block; *JR,* junctional rhythm; *PM,* pacemaker; *PVBs,* premature ventricular beats; *SVT,* supraventricular tachycardia; *VT,* ventricular tachycardia.

Electrocardiographic Findings

DYSRHYTHMIAS. A routine ECG taken between 1 week and 1 year before the patient's death was available in 86 patients. Of these patients, 57% had a dysrhythmia and 43% had no dysrhythmia (Table 4-2).

The study compared dysrhythmias present within 2 years before death with those present within 1 year before death. In the ECGs taken 2 years before death, only 42% of the patients had dysrhythmias. A significantly higher ($P < .05$) proportion of patients had dysrhythmias in the year before death than 2 years before death. The reason for the change in dysrhythmia was that an operation occurred in the year before death. It appears that in a certain number of patients, dysrhythmias develop in the year before sudden death. This does not necessarily imply that the dysrhythmia caused the death, only that the development of a dysrhythmia was associated with later sudden death.

OTHER ELECTROCARDIOGRAPHIC FINDINGS. In ECGs taken less than 1 year before death, 9 patients without dysrhythmias had other severe abnormalities: 3 had prolonged QT intervals, 3 had old myocardial infarctions, 1 had left ventricular strain in hypertrophic cardiomyopathy, 1 had left ventricular strain after aortic valve replacement, and 1 had complete right bundle branch block after a left septal myotomy for hypertrophic obstructive cardiomyopathy. If these 9 patients are added to the 49 who had dysrhythmias before sudden death, 67% had an ECG abnormality other than that which usually might be expected for the underlying lesion (e.g., the usual abnormality for tetralogy of Fellot is right ventricular hypertrophy; this was not included).

Treatment

Drug treatment at the time of death included digoxin (79%), diuretic (49%), quinidine (7%), propranolol (3%), mexiletine (1%), isoproterenol (2%), and belladonna (1%). Three patients being treated with quinidine for atrial flutter were noted to have a slow heart rate at the time of their sudden episode; one had a high-grade atrioventricular block and the other two had slow junctional rhythms. An additional patient with junctional rhythm and PVBs who was being treated with quinidine was found to have extremely slow junctional rhythm at the time of his death. Propranolol had been prescribed for three patients. In one, the drug had been prescribed for atrial flutter and was ineffective. The other two patients had a prolonged QT interval and were known to be noncomplaint in taking the propranolol. Only one patient had been prescribed phenytoin at the time of death. This drug had been effective in treating PVBs, but the patient was noncompliant. The one patient who had been prescribed mexiletine was also noncompliant. Isoproterenol had been given to two patients with complete atrioventricular block who died suddenly, and belladonna had been given to one patient with junctional rhythm. In three of these patients, ventricular dysrhythmias were also documented. Medical treatment had been prescribed for only a small number of the patients who had died suddenly.

Circumstances of Death

The patient's activity immediately preceding death was known in 46 of the 101 cases. Sudden death occurred during sports in 22%, with the patient awake but not active in 50%, and with the patient asleep in 28%. The mean age at death was 12.4 years (1–30 years). In postoperative patients, sudden death occurred an average of 4.5 years after surgery (2 months to 18 years). A presumed cause of death was known in 53 of the 101 patients (Table 4-3).

Diagnostic Class

Among the five diagnostic classes, unoperated congenital heart disease, unoperated acquired heart disease, palliated congenital heart disease, postoperative congenital heart disease, and a long QT interval, the clinical findings differed in four major areas. With respect to clinical status, the unoperated patients were more limited than those with palliated disease or postoperative congenital heart disease patients: 95% of the unoperated patients were in classes III to IV compared with 62% of those with congenital heart disease who had been palliated or repaired ($P < .001$).

Table 4-3 *"Cause" of Death*

Diagnosis*		Percentage (%)
Dysrhythmia		62
Probable	32	
Possible	21	
Pacemaker	9	
SBE		11
CVA		9
Pulmonary embolus		8
Aspiration		4
Penicillin anaphylaxis		2
Hemoptysis		2
Aortic aneurysm dissection		2
		100

* *CVA*, Cerebrovascular accident; *SBE*, subacute bacterial endocarditis.

There was a marked difference in the presence of preceding dysrhythmias. A dsrhythmia was present in the year before sudden death in 88% of those who had undergone repair of congenital heart disease compared with 35% of the unoperated or palliated group ($P < .0001$). PVBs in the year preceding sudden death was significantly higher in the postoperative repair group (34%) than the untreated group (8%) ($P < .01$).

The activity preceding death varied with the group. Those patients who died during sports were in the following three groups: (1) unoperated congenital heart disease, (2) prolonged QT interval, and (3) postoperative congenital heart disease. None of the patients with palliated congenital heart disease died during sports. Perhaps this is because these patients were not physically capable of participating in vigorous sports. Finally, death occurred during sleep in all of the groups except the patients with a prolonged QT interval.

With respect to the cause of death, patients who underwent repair of congenital heart disease had significantly more known or suspected dysrhythmias (78%) compared with patients who did not undergo surgery or palliative treatment (31%) ($P < .001$).

The Eight Common Cardiac Diagnoses

The eight most common cardiac diagnoses in these patients were, in descending order, right-to-left shunt postoperative anastomosis (12%), left-to-right shunt with pulmonary hypertension (Eisenmenger's syndrome) (11%), postoperative tetralogy of Fallot (11%), unoperated tetralogy of Fallot (7%), cardiomyopathy (5%), postoperative atrioventricular canal (5%), postoperative Mustard operation for transposition of the great arteries (5%), and prolonged QT interval (5%). These eight diagnoses made up 61% of the patients. Each of the other diagnoses represented 4% or less of the patients. The characteristics of patients with these diagnoses are given in Tables 4-4 and 4-5.

Dysrhythmias

There were significant differences among the diagnoses with respect to the presence of dysrhythmias within 1 year before sudden death (Table 4-4). A low incidence of dysrhythmias (less than 25%) occurred in the patients with left-to-right shunt with pulmonary hypertension (Eisenmenger's syndrome) and those with unoperated or palliated tetralogy of Fallot. In all the other diagnoses, more than 50% of the patients had dysrhythmias in the year before death. The only diagnoses in which PVBs occurred in 25% or more of the patients were postoperative tetralogy of Fallot and a long QT interval. Atrial flutter was uncommon except in patients who had undergone the Mustard operation. Sinus bradycardia and junctional rhythm occurred in less than 25% of the patients, except those with a prolonged QT interval and those who had undergone the Mustard operation. Atrioventricular block was uncommon, except after repair of a complete atrioventricular canal or ventricular septal defect.

Table 4-4 *Dysrhythmias 1 week to 1 Year Before Death*

Diagnosis*	Number of patients	Any Dysrhythmia (%)	PVB (%)	AFL (%)	JR (%)	AVB (%)	Complex (%)
L-to-R shunt and PH	11	14	14				
TOF	7	17				17	
CM	5	60	20	20			20
LQTS	5	75	25		50		
R-to-L anas	12	10	10				
PO TOF	11	100	70		10	10	10
PO canal	5	75				75	
POM	5	100		50	25		25

* *AFL,* Atrial flutter; *AVB,* AV block; *CM,* cardiomyopathy; *Dys,* dysrhythmia; *JR,* junctional rhythm; *LQTS,* long QT syndrome; *L-to-R shunt,* left to right shunt; *PH,* pulmonary hypertension; *PO canal,* postoperative atrioventricular canal repair; *POM,* postoperative Mustard procedure; *PO TOF,* postoperative tetralogy of Fallot; *PVB,* premature ventricular beats, *R-to-L anas,* right to left shunt postoperative anastomosis, *TOF,* tetralogy of Fallot.

Table 4-5 *Circumstances of Death*

Diagnosis*	Number of patients	Deaths While Active (%)	Deaths During Sleep (%)	Dysrhythmis (%)	Age at Death and SEM	PO Interval and SEM
L-to-R shunt and PH	11	0	0	33	15.9 ± 2.0	—
TOF	7	0	67	25	10.6 ± 3.4	—
CM	5	50	50	100	10.6 ± 3.1	—
LQTS	5	67	0	100	11.4 ± 2.5	—
R-to L anas	12	0	0	30	10.4 ± 2.5	4.2 ± 1.5
PO TOF	11	28	14	100	16.2 ± 2.2	4.2 ± 1.3
PO canal	5	0	0	100	8.6 ± 2.9	1.7 ± .5
POM	5	50	50	100	11.5 ± 3.8	7.1 ± 2.6

* See Table 4-4 for abbreviations.

Circumstances of Death

The majority of patients died while at rest (Table 4-4). The only patients who died during sports had prolonged QT intervals, cardiomyopathy, Mustard repair, or repair of tetralogy of Fallot. The diagnoses of patients who died during sleep included unoperated tetralogy of Fallot, cardiomyopathy, postoperative Mustard repair, and postoperative tetralogy of Fallot. Either a probable or possible dysrhythmia was present in the majority of these diagnoses. A dysrhythmia did not appear to be involved in patients with a left-to-right shunt and pulmonary hypertension, unoperated tetralogy of Fallot, or patients with a right-to-left shunt postoperative anastomosis.

Two groups of patients were significantly older at the time of death: those who had postoperative tetralogy of Fallot and left-to-right shunt with pulmonary hypertension ($P < .01$). Patients who underwent repair of atrioventricular canal died at a significantly younger age than the rest of the group because they died relatively early postoperatively. The postoperative Mustard patients actually died significantly longer after surgery than the other patients, and the postoperative tetralogy of Fallot patients died at an older age, presumably because their reparative operations occurred at an older age than the Mustard operation.

Dysrhythmias in the Year Preceding Sudden Death

The specific dysrhythmias that were found differed among the diagnoses. PVBs were found in 50% or more of the following diagnoses: acquired cardiomyopathy, ostium primum atrial septal defect, transposition of the great arteries/

ventricular septal defect/postoperative Mustard repair, and postoperative tetralogy of Fallot. Atrial flutter was foung in 50% or more of the patients with aortic insufficiency, acquired cardiomyopathy, and postoperative Mustard repair. More than 50% of patients with transposition of the great arteries/ventricular septal defect/postoperative Mustard repair, of those with a prolonged QT interval had bradycardia or junctional rhythm. Complete atrioventricular block was found in more than 50% of patients with L-transposition of the great arteries, postoperative patent ductus arteriosus (congenital complete atrioventricular block), and postoperative tricuspid valve replacement.

The presence of dysrhythmias was related to poor hemodynamics at cardiac catheterization. A dysrhythmia was found in 11% of those with good hemodynamics compared with 50% of those with poor hemodynamics ($P < .01$). All of the specific dysrhythmias (e.g., PVBs), except junctional rhythm, were associated with poor hemodynamics. Junctional rhythm was significantly ($P < .01$) related to good hemodynamics: 56% of those with junctional rhythm had good hemodynamics whereas only 5% of the patients without junctional rhythm ($P < .01$) had good hemodynamics. This indicates that the postoperative patients with junctional rhythm (predominantly postoperative Mustard repair) who died suddenly had good hemodynamics.

The presumed direct cause of death was significantly related to the presence of dysrhythmias in the year before death. There were some exceptions, however. Among the 17 patients without previous dysrhythmia noted on routine ECGs within 1 year before death, 4 had a probable dysrhythmia at the time of death and 13 died of other causes. Of the 28 patients with a dysrhythmia in the year preceding death, only 4 of the 28 had another known cause of death, leaving 24 out of 28 with either a probable or possible dysrhythmia as the cause of death.

Historical Comparison

Between 1958 and 1983, 23,402 patients were seen in the Section of Pediatric Cardiology at Texas Children's Hospital; 981 (4.2%) of these patients are known to have died. Sudden death, by our criteria, occurred in 101, nonsudden death in 730, accidental death in 10, and there was insufficient information in 140 of the patients. A trend since 1958 is an increasing number of total patients in each 5-year period (Table 4-6). Within the last 5 years, there have been two major changes in dysrhythmia management: aggressive drug treatment of PVBs and

Table 4-6 *Historical Perspective from 1959 to 1983*

	1959–1963	1964–1968	1969–1973	1974–1978	1979–1983
Number of patients	2330	1716	4668	6562	8126
Number of sudden deaths (%)	3 (0.13)	27 (0.92)	21 (0.43)	37 (0.54)	22 (0.27)

aggressive pacemaker treatment of bradydysrhythmias. In the last 5 years, none of the 18 sudden deaths occurred in patients with a history of ventricular dysrhythmias; 16 of the 69 patients who died suddenly in the previous 20 years had ventricular dysrhythmias ($P < .05$). Since 1978 one patient died suddenly after surgery for tetralogy of Fallot, and this was due to a documented pacemaker failure and surgical complete atrioventricular block. Since 1977 there has been no sudden death in patients undergoing a Mustard procedure for transposition of the great arteries.

SUMMARY AND CONCLUSIONS

In this study of sudden death in patients previously seen in the Section of Pediatric Cardiology, we attempted to identify factors that might have been associated with later sudden death. The true denominator of these factors is unknown. For example, the number of patients with cardiac defects who have dysrhythmias and do not die is not known in all cases. Further studies are planned to document the incidence of the factors that might have been associated with sudden death in patients with similar cardiac lesions who did not die. The following conclusions can be drawn from the study:

1. Over three quarters of the patients who died suddenly had severe limitation of activity, cardiac enlargement on chest radiographic examination, and poor hemodynamics at cardiac catheterization.
2. The majority of patients who died suddenly had a dysrhythmia in the 12-month period preceding death. A significant number of these dysrhythmias developed for the first time in the year preceding death.
3. The presence of dysrhythmias was generally related to poor hemodynamics in patients who died suddenly.
4. Approximately one quarter of the patients with dysrhythmias received therapy that is currently believed to be appropriate.
5. Most sudden deaths occurred with the patient at rest, and approximately one quarter occurred during sports.
6. Specific dysrhythmias are associated with specific lesions and appear to be correlated with the risk of sudden death in that group.
7. Conspicuously absent from the list of diagnoses are children with a normal heart and children with mitral valve prolapse.
8. With improvement in treatment practices, that is, more aggressive drug treatment of ventricular dysrhythmias and more aggressive pacemaker treatment of bradydysrhythmias in the last 5 years, the incidence of sudden death at Texas Children's Hospital has been reduced significantly from previous years.

REFERENCES

1. Garson A, McNamara DG, Sudden Death in a Pediatric Cardiology population, 1958 to 1983: Relation to prior arrhythmias. J Am Coll Cardiol 1985; 5:1343–6.

Thomas A. Buckingham
Harold L. Kennedy

5

EXERCISE TESTING AND AMBULATORY ELECTROCARDIOGRAPHY IN NORMAL INDIVIDUALS AND IN PATIENTS AT RISK OF SUDDEN CARDIAC DEATH

COMPARISON OF EXERCISE TESTING AND AMBULATORY ELECTROCARDIOGRAPHY

Exercise testing and ambulatory electrocardiography are two noninvasive techniques used to diagnose cardiac disease and to assess therapeutic interventions. They also can be used to assess the risk of sudden cardiac death and to provide prognostic information. Both techniques employ the recording of ECG information. With exercise testing the person is physiologically stressed in a controlled manner while the physical and ECG responses are monitored. The stress is achieved by exercise using a step test, motorized treadmill, or bicycle ergometer. Ambulatory electrocardiography (Holter monitoring) records data on a magnetic tape for an extended period, usually 24 hours. The subject is thus examined during typical activities in a usual day-to-day environment. Since both these noninvasive ECG examinations are often used in the same patient, it is useful to point out their differences and similarities. In doing so, we will review the knowledge obtained from various populations studies with both techniques, in normal or asymptomatic individuals, and in those at risk of sudden cardiac death.

SUDDEN CARDIAC DEATH
0-8089-1725-0

Table 5-1 *Differences Between Exercise Testing and Ambulatory Electrocardiography*

	Exercise Testing	Ambulatory Electrocardiography
Personnel	Physician in attendance	No personnel required during recording
Environment	Controlled, limited external variables	Uncontrolled; exposed to natural stimuli
ECG leads	1, 3, or 12 leads for less than 30 minutes	2 leads for 24 hours
Interpretation	On-line monitoring, with immediate results	Usually some delay
Risks	Very low; emergency equipment necessary	Essentially none
Patient limitations	Must be able to exercise; certain cardiac medications interfere with results	No activity requirements
Variables with prognostic importance	Exercise-induced ventricular ectopy, exercise duration, and ST segment shift	Ventricular ectopic activity

Modified from Kennedy HL: Comparison of ambulatory electrocardiography and exercise testing. Am J Cardiol 47:1359, 1981. With permission.

Differences and Similarities

Ambulatory electrocardiography and exercise testing differ in several respects. Exercise testing, as noted in Table 5-1, provides on-line monitoring (i.e., immediate awareness) during a prescribed protocol of activity.[1] Ambulatory electrocardiography provides delayed awareness as data are obtained and later analyzed. With ambulatory electrocardiography, a rigid protocol is neither required nor desirable. The environment in ambulatory electrocardiography is variable, and there are multiple physical and emotional stimuli during usual daily activities. With exercise testing the environment is controlled and variables are minimized. The progressive development of hemodynamic stress is the objective in exercise testing, whereas in ambulatory monitoring the goal is the recording of ECG disturbances during usual activity. During ambulatory monitoring 2 leads are usually monitored, whereas 3 or 12 leads are monitored during exercise testing. Risks are minimal in exercise testing, with significant morbidity occurring in only 1 in 50,000 to 100,000 man-hours of exercise of cardiac patients.[2] During exercise testing, it is necessary to have a physician and supportive emergency equipment available. The only risk of ambulatory electrocardiography is epidermal irritation in areas of electrode contact in a small proportion of patients. Multiple variables are observed during both tests. During ambulatory monitoring, ventricular arrhythmias have been shown to correlate with prognosis, whereas in exercise testing multiple variables carry prognostic importance.

Ambulatory electrocardiography and exercise testing represent noninvasive cardiologic techniques frequently employed in many disease states to make a diagnosis or assess disease severity. Both techniques require instrumentation operated by experienced personnel for analysis, and both employ electrocardiography to monitor cardiac electrical changes. This includes observation of heart rate, arrhythmias, and ST segment changes. Information obtained by either test carries different diagnostic and prognostic values, depending on the population studied.

Electrocardiographic Parameters

Both exercise testing and ambulatory electrocardiography provide information on several ECG parameters, but ST segment changes and arrhythmias are particularly valuable. Other ECG parameters examined during exercise testing that may be of importance include R wave amplitude, Q wave amplitude and inverted U waves. In addition, several non-ECG variables monitored during exercise testing may be predictive of outcome.

Changes in ST segment are influenced by many factors, including medications, electrolyte imbalances, hyperventilation, conduction disturbances, and ventricular hypertrophy. Independent of these factors, ST segment changes demonstrated during exercise testing classically indicate ischemia. Exercise-induced ST segment depression has been shown to have both diagnostic and prognostic value. The degree of ST segment depression chosen as significant influences the sensitivity and specificity observed in the diagnosis of coronary artery disease (i.e., the deeper the ST segment depression, the less sensitive but more specific this diagnosis).

Although one early study[3] reported a high degree of correlation between the detection of ST segment depression during ambulatory monitoring and the presence of coronary artery disease at cardiac catheterization, others have shown a high prevalence of ''ischemic'' ST segment changes on ambulatory monitoring with other conditions, including mitral valve prolapse, neurocirculatory asthenia, orthostasis, or during high-temperature saunas.[4-6] Also, a recent report[5] describes the occurrence of diagnostic ST segment depression in as many as 30% of asymptomatic men, indicating a significant degree of inaccuracy when such changes are used to diagnose myocardial ischemia. ST segment changes detected by ambulatory electrocardiography thus have not been predictive of myocardial ischemia because of the variations in posture and autonomic tone encountered throughout the day. Although ST segment changes may indicate ''silent'' ischemia or spasm during ambulatory monitoring,[7] it may be misleading to base clinical decisions solely on such changes.[8] Exercise testing is superior to ambulatory monitoring in examining the ST segment for diagnostic and prognostic information, and a large body of data exists to support the relationship of exercise-induced ST segment shifts with outcome.[9]

Arrhythmias are fairly common in most cardiac disease states, but they are also common in normal persons. Although data exist that correlate arrhythmias detected by exercise testing with severity of coronary anatomy and subsequent mortality in certain subgroups of patients with cardiac disease, more data exists that correlate arrhythmias detected by the ambulatory ECG with prognosis. Ambulatory monitoring is a superior method for detecting arrhythmias.[10-12] The detection of arrhythmias is influenced by the total time of ECG examination,[10] which is longer with ambulatory electrocardiography. Prognostic information is thus primarily related to ST segment changes for exercise testing and arrhythmias for ambulatory monitoring. These two noninvasive studies provide complementary information because each correlates different ECG parameters to prognosis.

STUDIES IN NORMAL OR ASYMPTOMATIC POPULATIONS

Treadmill Exercise Testing

Ventricular Arrhythmias

Several studies have addressed the issue of exercise-induced arrhythmias in the asymptomatic, clinically normal individual. Early studies did not use coronary angiography and therefore probably inadvertently included patients with occult coronary artery disease. McHenry et al.[13] studied 561 men ages 25–54 with no apparent heart disease by means of maximal exercise testing. Single ventricular ectopic beats were seen in 35% and were noted to increase with age. Of those with one or more ventricular ectopic beats, 32% had frequent ventricular ectopy, but complex forms were rare. Blackburn, Taylor, and Keys[14] studied 12,000 employed men from seven countries using the Master 2-step test and found that exercise-induced ectopy was associated with a slight but nonsignificant increased incidence of subsequent cardiac events in a 5-year follow-up.[2] Froelicher et al.[15] studied 1390 asymptomatic U.S. Air Force crewmen and found exercise-induced ventricular ectopy to be a poor indicator of coronary events during a 6-year follow-up. All of the aforementioned studies were confined to men and did not include coronary angiography. A second study by McHenry et al.[16] examined 141 patients with chest pain and normal coronary angiograms (group IA), 144 asymptomatic persons in whom angiography was not performed (group IB), and 197 patients with coronary artery disease documented by angiography (group II). The incidence of exercise-induced ectopy at heart rates up to 130 beats/min was found to be 9% for groups 1A, 6% for group 1B, and 27% for group II. There was a slight increase in ventricular ectopy with exercise in patients who had coronary artery disease. The incidence of exercise-induced ectopy was similar in patients with normal angiograms and in those who were asymptomatic.

Studies of ventricular arrhythmias in clinically normal populations thus show an incidence of exercise-induced ventricular ectopy ranging from 16% to 50%, depending on the population studied. Exercise-induced ectopic activity tends to increase with age and with increasing workload but correlates poorly with the incidence of subsequent coronary events in this group of patients. Because these studies were conducted primarily in men, the incidence and significance of exercise-induced ventricular ectopy in asymptomatic or normal women remains unknown. Studies of ventricular ectopy induced by stress testing in patient populations with known or suspected coronary disease yield different conclusions and will be discussed later in this chapter.

ST Segment Changes

One study of an asymptomatic population using exercise testing was that of Allen et al.[17] As has been previously mentioned, treadmill exercise testing is a multifactorial test and requires the interpretation of several variables. In their study of an asymptomatic population of 577 men and 311 women, Allen et al. found that an exercise duration of less than 3 minutes correlated with subsequent coronary events only in women. In men over 40, however, ST depression, an increase or no change in the R wave, and an exercise duration of 5 minutes or less all correlated with subsequent cardiac events. These findings may be due, in part, to preexisting occult coronary artery disease in some subjects. Giagnoni et al.[18] studied 195 asymptomatic normotensive subjects with exercise-induced ST depression of 1 mm or more and compared them to 379 controls. During 6 years of follow-up, coronary events (angina pectoris, myocardial infarction, and sudden death) were more common and occurred earlier in the normotensive subjects than the controls. Using the same coronary events as endpoints, Froelicher et al.[15] followed up 1390 asymptomatic men for 6.3 years and showed that those with exercise-induced ST depression developed manifestations of coronary artery disease more often than those with a negative test results.

In summary, exercise testing can be used as a screening test for coronary artery disease in asymptomatic men at risk for the development of coronary artery disease, but it has a low predictive value. ST segment depression induced by exercise is a more specific marker for latent coronary artery disease than ventricular ectopy.

Ambulatory Monitoring Studies

Ventricular Arrhythmias

Ventricular ectopic beats are known to occur commonly in otherwise healthy individuals and can be detected by physical examination, electrocardiography, exercise testing, and ambulatory ECG recording.[19] Frequent and complex ventricular ectopic activity in normal populations has been regarded as an ominous sign in the past[20-22] and was believed to be associated with increased risk of sudden death. An early study was the 1969 Tecumseh epidemiologic study, reported by Chiang et al.,[22] which indicated that ventricular ectopic beats were a bad prognostic sign. Later studies of this and other populations, some using ambulatory monitoring, indicated that the predictive value of ventricular ectopic beats in identifying the patient at risk of sudden death largely depends on the presence of organic heart disease such as coronary artery disease, cardiomegaly, and hypertrophic cardiomyopathy or primary risk factors.[19-21, 23-29]

Several studies have addressed the issue of how much ventricular ectopy is normal.[30-40] These studies varied greatly in design and populations examined. Most studies have shown an increasing frequency, as well as complexity, of ectopy with older age. These studies are represented in Table 5-2, roughly arranged in order of increasing patient age. In the pediatric age group, Southall et al.[30] studied healthy newborn infants with 24-hour ambulatory electrocardiography and found no ventricular ectopy. A similar study included 104 school children ages 7–11, and only one child had a few, isolated ventricular ectopic beats.[31] Clarke, Hamer, and Shelton[40] studied 86 men and women, 16–65 years of age, who were free of cardiac disease and found ventricular ectopic beats in 63 subjects. More frequent ectopy was noted in the older patients. Verbaan, Pool, and VanWanrooy[36] studied 74 subjects ages 20–80 and found ventricular ectopy in 76%. Multiform beats were seen in 28, couplets in 7, R-on-T phenomena in 4, and ventricular tachycardia in 1. This study also noted more ventricular ectopy in older patients. In young adults, three studies by one group addressed the issue of ventricular ectopic beats in otherwise normal young men, women, and long-distance runners ages 19–28.[32-34] Patients with organic heart disease detected by history, physical examination, chest x-ray film, ECGs, and M-mode echocardiography were excluded from these three studies. Ventricular ectopic beats were found in approximately 50% of the young men and women but slightly more often (70%) in long-distance runners.

DeMaria et al.[41] studied 40 adults with chest pain and normal coronary arteriograms and found ventricular ectopic beats in 25%, with complex forms occurring in 8%. In a middle-aged group of adults, Kostis et al.[35] studied 101 patients who had organic heart disease ruled out by a rigorous protocol that included standard methods of examination plus exercise testing, cardiac catheterization, and coronary angiography. They found that 39% of the patients had some form of ventricular ectopy. Studies in elderly populations[37-39] have found ventricular ectopic beats in 80% of the subjects, with approximately one third having frequent and complex forms. These data indicate that the incidence of ventricular ectopic beats appears to increase with age even in the absence of organic heart disease.

An often cited study by Hinkle, Carver, and Stevens[27] showed a high prevalence of ventricular ectopic beats (62%) in a group of 296 employed middle-aged men. Complex forms were found in 19% of the subjects. Hinkle et al.[42] subsequently reported on a larger group of 811 employed American men between the ages of 35 and 65 studied with 6-hour or 24-hour ambulatory ECG recordings. An important conclusion of the studies of Hinkle is that the occurrence of frequent and complex ventricular arrhythmias was almost solely limited to those with significant cardiopulmonary disease or hypertension. Hinkle's study has been cited as evidence that frequent and complex ventricular ectopic activity on ambulatory ECG recordings is a benign finding in the absence of heart disease. The data of Kennedy and co-workers are in accord with these findings.[43] Horan and Kennedy[43] have followed up 72 asymptomatic individuals with frequent ventricular ectopic beats since 1973; after 7 years of observation, none of the individuals had experienced a fatal event. Others also have suggested that there is no increased risk of sudden cardiac death in this group of "normal" patients.[27,28] Califf et al.[44] performed 24-hour ambulatory monitoring on 260 patients without significant coronary artery disease documented by cardiac catheterization. Ventricular arrhythmias were found in 62% and complex forms (Lown grades 3, 4, and 5) in 28%. Follow-up over a period of 3 years revealed sudden death in only one subject. Frequent and complex ventricular ectopic beats in apparently healthy persons

Table 5-2 *Selected 24-Hour Ambulatory ECG Studies of "Normal" Population According to Increasing Age*

Reference	Year	Number of Patients	Patient group	Age Range (years)	Record Time (hr)	Ventricular ectopic beats†	More Than 30 beats/hr†	Multiform beats†	Couplets†	Ventricular tachycardia†	R-ON-T phenomenon†
30	1980	134	Neonates		24	0 (0)					
31	1981	104	Children	7–11	24	1 (1)					
32	1977	50	Medical students	23–27	24	25 (50)		6 (12)	1 (2)	1 (2)	3 (6)
33	1981	50	Students	22–28	24	27 (54)		5 (10)	0 (0)	1 (2)	2 (4)
34	1982	20	Runners	19–28	24	14 (70)		4 (20)			
35	1981	101	Adults free of heart disease*	16–68	24-48	39 (39)		4 (4)	0 (0)	0 (0)	2 (2)
36	1977	74	Adults	20–80				28 (38)	7 (9)	1 (1)	4 (5)
37	1979	15	Elderly	60–84	24	8 (53)	2 (13)	1 (7)	3 (20)	0 (0)	
38	1980	106	Elderly	75–95	24	73 (69)		23 (22)	4 (4)	4 (4)	
39	1982	98	Elderly	60–85	24	78 (88)	17 (17)	34 (35)	11 (11)	4 (4)	1 (1)

* Heart disease ruled out by complete physical examination, exercise testing, and cardiac catheterization.
† Numbers in parentheses refer to percentages (%).

thus may represent an idiopathic syndrome with a benign course and a good prognosis.

In summary, studies of ventricular ectopy in asymptomatic populations have shown that rare, isolated ventricular ectopic beats are common and are found more frequently in the elderly. Frequent and complex ventricular ectopy is usually associated with coronary risk factors, occult coronary artery disease, or subtle left ventricular dysfunction. Ventricular ectopy has not been shown to increase the risk of mortality or sudden cardiac death in the absence of organic heart disease.

ST Segment Changes

Technical factors can make recording and playback of the ST segment on ambulatory monitoring systems difficult, particularly in normal persons, and few studies therefore have been done. Changes in posture, high temperatures, orthostasis, and neurocirculatory asthenia may cause changes in the ST segment, suggesting that the autonomic nervous system plays an important role.[4-6, 8, 45]

Two studies examined ST segment changes in normal populations. Armstrong et al.[5] studied 50 asymptomatic middle-aged men with continuous ambulatory monitoring and found a 30% prevalance of "ischemic" ST segment changes. Crawford et al.[46] studied 31 patients without coronary artery disease on coronary angiography and found that 39% had a greater than 1 mm ST segment depression. Based on these limited data, it appears that intermittent ST segment shifts on 24-hour ambulatory monitoring are common in normal individuals and may be due to technical factors postural changes, or changes in autonomic tone.

PATIENT GROUPS AT RISK OF SUDDEN CARDIAC DEATH

The extensive data available on several cardiovascular diseases and conditions correlates the findings of exercise testing and ambulatory monitoring with subsequent mortality and sudden death. In particular, prognosis can be ascertained by these noninvasive tests in patients with chronic coronary artery disease, survivors of acute myocardiopathy, and survivors of sudden death. The available data regarding the rate of exercise testing and ambulatory monitoring will be discussed for each of these categories.

In this chapter, coronary artery disease is subdivided into chronic coronary artery disease and a history of myocardial infarction. The extensive data on exercise testing and ambulatory monitoring in survivors of myocardial infarction during the first 6 weeks after the acute event are included in the latter group.

Chronic Coronary Artery Disease

Coronary artery disease is a risk factor for sudden cardiac death, and severe coronary disease (e.g., left main artery or triple-vessel disease) carries a greater risk. The degree of damage to the myocardium is also a strong predictor of

Table 5-3 *Ventricular Arrhythmias in Coronary Artery Disease Detected with Exercise Testing and Ambulatory Electrocardiography*

	Exercise Testing	Ambulatory Electrocardiography
Chronic coronary artery disease		
Percentage of patients detected (%)	38–65	75–90
Percentage with frequent and complex arrhythmias (%)	30	50–60
Prognostic value	For identifying multivessel disease and increased mortality	For identifying multivessel disease and increased risk of sudden death
Early after myocardial infarction		
Percentage of patients detected (%)	38–43	77–84
Percentage with frequent and complex arrhythmias (%)	17–31	33–42
Prognostic value	For identifying increased risk of sudden death and multivessel disease	For identifying increased risk of sudden cardiac death

Modified from Kennedy HL: Comparison of ambulatory electrocardiography and exercise testing. Am J Cardiol 47:1359, 1981. With permission.

outcome. Findings on exercise tests and ambulatory monitoring can be correlated to the severity of coronary disease, as well as to left ventricular dysfunction.[47-48] It therefore seems logical that such findings would also correlate with long-term outcome and the incidence of sudden death. This has been shown in many studies.[46, 49-51] Table 5-3 summarizes the results of several studies on the role of exercise testing and ambulatory monitoring in these patients.

Exercise Testing

Although exercise testing can be used in the noninvasive diagnosis of coronary artery disease, this discussion will be confined to its use in predicting outcome and detecting severe coronary artery disease. Multiple variables observed during an exercise test include both non-ECG parameters, such as chest pain, exercise duration, peak exercise level attained, percentage of predicted maximal heart rate reached, blood pressure and pulse response, and ECG parameters, such as ST segment changes, arrhythmias, R wave amplitude, septal Q wave amplitude, and U waves. Variables that have been correlated with severe coronary artery disease include short exercise duration,[49, 52-53] ST segment depression greater than 0.2 or 0.3 mV,[53-55] hypotension during exercise,[54-57] and failure to achieve 85% of predicted heart rate.[58-59] As expected, a number of these same variables correlate with outcome. Treadmill exercise testing studies vary widely in terms of the populations included and the variables examined. Different exercise protocols are used by different centers, and those reporting follow-up varied in the duration of follow-up and the endpoints studied. The most common endpoint used was the "cardiac event" defined as death, myocardial infarction, or progression of angina. Some studies examined survival separately, but few specifically examined the incidence of sudden cardiac death. In exercise testing, the incidence of coronary artery disease in the population strongly affects the sensitivity, specificity, and predictive accuracy of the test in detecting coronary artery disease. It can likewise be expected that the incidence of coronary disease in the study population will strongly affect outcome during long-term follow-up. All of these factors make analysis and comparison of the many studies difficult.

VENTRICULAR ARRHYTHMIAS. Another variable examined during treadmill exercise testing is ventricular ectopy. This has been defined and quantified in several ways. An early study by Zaret and Conti[58] examined 32 patients with exercise-induced complex ventricular ectopy by cardiac catheterization compared to age-matched controls and found that exercise-induced ectopy indicated severe double or triple coronary artery disease. They failed to show an association between exercise-induced ectopy and ejection fraction or left ventricular and diastolic pressure. Goldschlager, Cake, and Cohn[59] examined ventricular ectopic beats before, during, or after exercise testing in 81 patients compared to 89 age-matched controls without ectopy and found that patients with exercise-induced arrhythmias had a significantly greater incidence of double- or triple-vessel disease and abnormal ventricular contractile patterns. Helfant et al.[60] also were able to correlate exercise-induced ventricular ectopic beats with double- and triple coronary artery disease and left ventricular contraction abnormalities in their study of 60 patients evaluated because of chest pain. McHenry et al.[16] examined 482 subjects with treadmill exercise testing and cardiac catheterization. They found it necessary to compare the incidence of exercise-induced ventricular ectopic beats at a heart rate of 130 beats/min to show a significant difference between those with and without coronary artery disease. In their study the incidence of exercise-induced ectopy up to a heart rate of 130 beats/min was 6%–9% in patients without and 27% in those with coronary disease. They also found that patients with three-vessel disease and abnormal left ventricular wall motion had a higher incidence of exercise-induced ventricular arrhythmias. In contrast to these results, a recent study by Nair et al.[61] of 280 patients evaluated because of chest pain failed to show a relationship between exercise-induced ventricular ectopy and multivessel coronary disease. These authors provide no explanation as to why their results differ from others.

In summary, most of these data indicate that in a population with chest pain or known coronary artery disease, exercise-induced ventricular ectopic beats reflect an increased likelihood of multivessel coronary artery disease and left ventricular wall motion abnormalities.

Additional studies have attempted to define whether exercise-induced ventricular ectopy can predict outcome in patients with chest pain or coronary artery disease. The previously cited study by Nair et al.[61] found that during a mean follow-up of 47 months, exercise-induced ventricular ectopy did not predict increased incidence of coronary events (cardiac death or myocardial infarction). In contrast, Udall and Ellestad,[62] in their 5-year follow-up of 6500 patients found that the annual incidence of coronary events was 1.7% among patients without ventricular ectopic beats or ST changes, 6.4% in patients with ventricular ectopic beats, and 11.4% in patients with both ventricular arrhythmias and ST segment change. They also showed an increased incidence of cardiac deaths in patients with ventricular ectopy before, during, or after exercise. The incidence of new coronary events was further increased if ventricular ectopy was "ominous" (multiform, bigeminal, or repetitive) or if ventricular ectopy increased during treadmill testing. In their study of 1852 men with coronary artery disease in the Seattle Heart Watch, Bruce et al.[51] used multivariate analysis to generate a logistic probability estimate of the risk of sudden cardiac death. This equation included an exertional arrhythmia score as one of its significant variables, although maximal systolic blood pressure and duration of exercise were more important predictors. The increasing frequency and complexity of ventricular ectopy determined an increasing risk of sudden cardiac death during 3 years of follow-up. In the Soviet Union, Ivanova et al.[63] followed-up 144 patients with known coronary artery disease for 2 years. They found that Lown class 2 or greater ventricular ectopic beats during exercise testing were associated with a fourfold increased risk of sudden cardiac death and a predictive accuracy of 20%. The risk of sudden death was further increased if ventricular ectopy was associated with other variables such as ST segment changes.

In conclusion, ventricular ectopy occuring during or after exercise testing in patients with coronary artery disease is associated with more severe coronary vessel involvement and left ventricular abnormalities, as well as coronary events and sudden cardiac death during follow-up. This association is strengthened as the frequency and complexity of ectopy increases or if ectopy is augmented during exercise. As might be expected, association of exercised-induced ventricular ectopy with other positive variables observed during treadmill testing increases the incidence of multivessel disease and sudden cardiac death still further.

ST SEGMENT. Several studies have examined the relationship between ST segment depression produced by exercise and findings at cardiac catheterization. Helfant et al.[60] studied 60 patients who underwent exercise testing because of chest pain. They noted that 20 of 22 patients who were found to have coronary disease developed ST depression greater than 0.2 mV with exercise. Sammarco, Pontims, and Selvester[55] examined 378 patients referred because of known ischemic heart disease or presumed angina pectoris by maximal treadmill exercise testing and coronary angiography. They found that ST depression greater than 0.3 mV measured 80 msec after the J point indicated patients with triple-vessel or left main coronary artery disease with a sensitivity of 38.6%, a specificity of 89.8%, and a predictive value of 74.1%. In their larger study of 1472 patients, McNeer et al.[49] found that a positive ST segment response greater than 0.1 mV and exercise duration both predicted the presence and extent of coronary artery disease. Of these two parameters, the ST segment response was superior in its predictive value. Weiner[56] also found that a combination of variables was useful in predicting left main coronary artery or triple-vessel disease. The combination of 0.2 mV ST depression, downsloping ST depression, depression beginning at less than 5 metabolic equivalents (METS), persistence of ST depression 6 minutes into recovery, and ST depression in at least 5 leads had a sensitivity of 49% and a predictive value of 74% for severe coronary artery disease. The differences in these various studies probably can be explained by differing populations and ST segment criteria. In addition, some studies examined diagnostic criteria for triple-vessel disease, whereas others only examined diagnostic criteria for left main coronary artery disease. Although the results of these studies are conflicting, it seems that in patients with known ischemic heart disease or chest pain typical of angina pectoris, severe ST segment depression (greater than 0.2 mV) or global ST segment depression (greater than 0.1 mV in inferior and anterior leads) suggest the presence of significant coronary artery disease.

Not surprisingly, several studies also have correlated severe ST segment depression with outcome during long-term follow-up. Dagenais et al.[64] examined 220 patients selected because they had ST segment depression greater than or equal to 0.2 mV during exercise. Patients who underwent coronary surgery were excluded. In this study they found that the duration of exercise required to achieve 0.2 mV ST segment depression was strongly correlated with survival. Most deaths occurring during this study were sudden cardiac deaths. In patients who underwent coronary angiography, mortality was associated with more severe coronary disease. McNeer et al.[49] found ST segment depression to be the most powerful predictor of outcome out of several exercise variables examined. Ellestad and Wan[65] obtained follow-up data on 2700 subjects referred for maximal treadmill exercise testing because of known or suspected coronary artery disease and found that ST segment depression of 0.15 mV occuring 0.08 sec from the J point predicted an annual incidence of some new coronary event of 9.5% compared to 1.7% in those with a negative test. Coronary events were again defined as death, myocardial infarction, or progression of angina. Over 4 years a mortality of 13.2% was observed in those with a positive test compared to 1.1% in those with a negative test. Sudden cardiac death was not examined specifically. In another study, Stuart and Ellestad[66] showed that 0.2 mV of both downsloping and upsloping ST segment depression indicated an increased incidence of coronary events during the 6-year follow-up. Bruce et al.[51] examined 1852 men with known coronary artery disease treated medically using a slightly different exercise protocol. Multivariate analysis did not show ST segment depression to be a significant predictor of outcome. In a separate analysis of a subset of 1808 men, Bruce found that ST segment depression of 0.15 mV after exercise predicted death within 3 years with a sensitivity of 41% and a specificity of 91%. In sharp contrast to these studies, Podrid, Graboy, and Lown[67] examined 212 men with known coronary artery disease and reproducible ST segment depression of more than 0.2 mV during exercise. During follow-up an annual mortality of 1.4% was observed, and survival was correlated with the duration of exercise but not the degree of ST segment depression. This finding is noteworthy, since several reports have found multivessel coronary artery disease in 85%–96% of patients with more than 0.2 mV ST segment depression. The results of Podrid, Graboy, and Lown may differ from other studies because they excluded patients with overt congestive heart failure, who are known to be at the highest risk of cardiac death.

In summary, the data indicate that patients with known or suspected coronary artery disease who develop severe ST segment depression (0.15–0.2 mV) during exercise testing are at increased risk for coronary events and death during follow-up. Although severe ST depression correlates with worse coronary disease, studies to date have not shown a relationship to sudden cardiac death.

OTHER VARIABLES. Several studies have stressed the importance of *exercise duration* in predicting severe coronary artery disease and prognosis. McNeer et al.[49] found a correlation with the stage of exercise achieved on the Bruce protocol and the presence of multivessel or left main coronary artery disease. The stage of exercise reached also predicted survival during 48 months of follow-up. Ellestad and Wan[65] also found that the early onset of ischemia predicted a worse outcome in their study of 2700 subjects. Bruce et al.[51] found that the duration of exercise could predict the incidence of sudden cardiac death during a 3-year follow-up period. In their analysis and follow-up of 220 patients with a strongly positive exercise test, Dagenais et al.[64] concluded that exercise duration was a powerful predictor of survival. The incidence of sudden cardiac deaths was not examined specifically in this study, but most deaths occurring during follow-up were sudden. Podrid, Graboy, and Lown[67] also found that exercise tolerance (exercise duration) correlated with survival during a 59-month follow-up.

These studies varied in their definitions of exercise duration and in endpoints used, but it is fair to say that exercise duration correlates with mortality in patients with chronic coronary artery disease. Other studies have confirmed that a short exercise duration is strongly correlated with survival rate[49,50,64] In summary, variables on exercise testing in patients with chronic coronary artery disease shown to be predictive of outcome include diminished exercise duration, severe ST segment depression, hypotension, exercise-induced ventricular ectopic beats, and failure to achieve 85% of predicted maximal heart rate. All of these same variables also have been correlated to an increased incidence of severe (left main or multivessel) coronary artery disease.

Ambulatory Monitoring

Ambulatory monitoring can be used to detect cardiac arrhythmias, but the incidence of ventricular arrhythmias varies depending on the population studied and the total time of monitoring. As mentioned earlier, 50% of normal adults will have ventricular arrhythmias on a 24-hour recording, with the incidence increasing to 75% on a 48-hour tracing.[1] Some normal people will have frequent (more than 30 each hour) and complex (Lown classes 3 to 5) ventricular arrhythmias (2%– 12%). Coronary artery disease patients have ventricular arrhythmias more often (75%–90%) and a greater prevalence of complex forms (50%–60%).[10,68] Even when patients with ventricular dysfunction are excluded, complex ventricular arrhythmias remain significantly more common in the presence of coronary artery disease. Unfortunately, the low yet definite prevalence of complex ventricular arrhythmias in the normal population, as well as the greater relative number of normal people, does not allow accurate identification of ischemic heart disease on the basis of complex arrhythmia detection alone. Ventricular arrhythmias are seen more often in patients with chronic coronary disease when they are examined by 24-hour ambulatory monitoring as compared to treadmill testing.[10,11] Ryan, Lown, and Horn[11] found ventricular ectopic beats in 88% of patients with coronary disease who were tested by ambulatory monitoring compared with 56% by exercise testing. Frequent and complex ventricular ectopy thus is seen more commonly in patients with ischemic heart disease than normal individuals and is more readily detected by means of 24-hour monitoring than by exercise testing. The incidence of ventricular ectopy in various studies of patients with chronic coronary disease is shown in Table 5-3.

Although the literature contains conflicting data, there appears to be a relationship between ventricular ectopic activity observed by ambulatory monitoring and the extent of coronary artery disease and left ventricular dysfunction. Calvert, Lown, and Giorlin[69] studied 124 patients by cardiac catheterization and ambulatory 24-hour monitoring and found an increased prevalence and grade of ventricular ectopic activity in patients with multivessel disease. Those with single-vessel disease did not differ from normal individuals. Elevated left ventricular end diastolic pressure and left ventricular asynergy were also associated with increased ventricular ectopy. In 115 patients undergoing cardiac catheterization and 10-hour ECG recording, Vismara et al.[70] confirmed that serious ventricular ectopic beats were more common in those with multivessel disease. Vismara did not find a relationship between ventricular ectopic activity and left ventricular dyssynergia or coronary collateral circulation. Sharma, Ballantyne, and Goldstein[71] studied 64 patients by means of 24-hour monitoring and cardiac catheterization and found that left ventricular asynergy correlated with the frequency of VPBs. They found no relationship between ventricular ectopy and the number of diseased vessels. In their study of 244 patients, Califf et al.[72] found that the presence of myocardial fibrosis as indicated by abnormal left ventricular contraction and abnormal initial QRS on ECG correlated with both frequent and complex ventricular arrhythmias on 24-hour monitoring. In their study, the number of significantly diseased coronary vessels depended on abnormal left ventricular contraction in its association with ventricular ectopy. Although these studies give somewhat conflicting results, it appears that there is some relationship between the frequency and complexity of ventricular ectopy recorded on 24-hour ambulatory ECGs and left ventricular dysfunction, the severity of coronary artery disease, or both.

Further studies have shown that there is a relationship between ventricular arrhythmias seen by ambulatory monitoring and the risk of subsequent sudden death.[44,73,74] In a second study of patients with coronary artery disease, Califf et al.[44] showed that ventricular arrhythmias were strongly related to abnormal left ventricular function in 395 patients. They also showed that a modification of the Lown grading system was useful in classifying ventricular ectopic activity according to prognostic importance. Although their data indicated that ventricular arrhythmias were useful in identifying patients at risk of sudden cardiac death, left ventricular ejection fraction was a more useful predictor. Furthermore, when invasive measurements of left ventricular function were considered, the ventricular arrhythmia score did not contribute independent prognostic information.

A combined study from the Soviet Union compared exercise testing to 24-hour ambulatory monitoring with respect to outcome during long-term follow-up by means of prognostic stratification.[63] These workers found that the variables most strongly associated with subsequent sudden death were reduced maximal exercise heart rate, exercise-induced frequent ventricular arrhythmias, complex ventricular arrhythmias revealed by 24-hour monitoring, and the onset of ST segment depression during exercise. Combinations of these variables were associated with an increase of up to twenty-fold in the incidence of sudden death.

Summary of Exercise Testing for Chronic Coronary Artery Disease

Several variables observed during exercise testing, including ventricular ectopy, can be correlated with more severe coronary artery disease and left ventricular dysfunction. Many of these same variables have been found to correlate with long-term survival and the risk of sudden cardiac death. Similarly, the occurrence and severity of ventricular ectopy on 24-hour ambulatory monitoring have been correlated with more severe coronary disease and left ventricular dysfunction in patients with chronic coronary artery disease. Follow-up of these patients has shown a relationship between ventricular ectopy and the incidence of sudden death in several studies. The studies suggest the complementary nature of these techniques in evaluating the prognosis and risk of sudden death in patients with ischemic heart disease. Several studies have shown a strong relationship between ventricular ectopic activity and left ventricular dysfunction. It is somewhat controversial whether these two variables are independent predictors of sudden death or not.

Post Myocardial Infarction

Treadmill Exercise Testing

VENTRICULAR ECTOPY. In recent years various types of modified exercise testing protocols have been carried out in patients convalescing from acute myocardial infarction.[75] Although initially believed to be a dangerous procedure in such patients, experience has shown that this is not the case. Most centers performing these tests have used either a heart rate–limited or symptom-limited procedure 2–3 weeks after the infarction. There is strong interest in using exercise testing in myocardial infarction patients to select those who are at high risk of sudden cardiac death during the initial months following the acute event. Although exercise testing will not detect frequent or complex ventricular ectopy as often as ambulatory monitoring,[76,77] much interest has been focused on exercise-induced ventricular ectopy in patients recovering from myocardial infarction. The prognostic significance of exercise-induced ventricular ectopy has been a controversial issue, however. Theroux et al.[77] found the risk of sudden death to be 2.5 times higher in patients with ventricular ectopic beats during predischarge treadmill exercise than in those without such ectopy. An increased mortality in patients with exercise-induced ventricular ectopy following infarction was confirmed by the study of Granath et al.[78] Ericsson et al.[79] found that the presence of exercise-induced ectopy was associated with a mortality risk ratio of 4.3 : 1 during a subsequent 3-month follow-up. In the study by Granath, exercise testing was carried out 3 weeks after infarction in 205 patients with follow-up over 2–5 years. Repeat exercise testing was carried out 9 weeks after infarction and also showed a predictive value with exercise-induced ventricular ectopy. Similarly, Weld et al.[80] performed low-level exercise testing in 236 patients just before hospital discharge and found ventricular arrhythmias in 43%. Using multiple logistic regression analysis to investigate exercise variables, they found that exercise-induced ventricular arrhythmias were a strong predictor of the subsequent 1-year mortality.

On the other hand, studies by DeBusk et al.[76, 81-83] have shown that ventricular ectopy during a single exercise test 3 weeks after infarction has no prognostic value independent of results of peak workload and ST segment changes. In these studies even complex ventricular arrhythmias (Lown classes 3 to 5) did not add prognostic information. DeBusk's study excluded patients with congestive heart failure who are known to be the highest risk group for subsequent mortality. A similar study by Smith et al.[84] of 62 patients followed up for a review of 21 months found no prediction value for exercise-induced ectopy in the early postinfarction period.

Other differences in these studies can be attributed to variations in study populations, exercise protocols, timing of exercise testing, cardiac drug use, and other uncontrolled factors. It is probably fair to say that exercise-induced ectopy is a risk factor for mortality and sudden death in postmyocardial infarction patients. Whether exercise-induced ectopy is a risk factor independent of left ventricular function is still controversial. One study[76] found that ventricular ectopic beats seen during serial exercise testing after infarction in 90 patients free of left ventricular dysfunction failed to predict mortality. This study suggests the possibility that left ventricular dysfunction may be the prime determinant of outcome, but further data on this question are needed.

ST SEGMENT CHANGES. In addition to ventricular ectopy, a number of studies show ST segment changes during low-level exercise testing before discharge to be predictive of subsequent mortality. Recent work has shown that the occurrence of ST segment changes in such a population correlates with the presence of multivessel coronary disease and with worse ejection fractions on ventriculography.[85,86] An important study in this area was reported by Theroux et al.[77] in 1979. They studied 210 patients an average of 11 days after infarction by submaximal treadmill testing. The 1-year sudden death and mortality were significantly increased in patients with exercise-induced ST segment depression. Sudden death occurred in 0.7% of patients without ST segment depression and in 16% of patients with ST segment depression. Much of the early work in this field has been done by the Stanford group and is reported in a series of publications.[76, 83, 87)] For example, Sami, Kraemer, and DeBusk[83] studied 200 patients who had had a myocardial infarction and did not have unstable angina or heart failure. The patients with subsequent cardiac arrest all had ST segment depression of more than 0.2 mV during exercise. Patients with ST segment depression of 0.1 mV or more had a 33% risk of sudden death or recurrent infarction compared to a risk of 5% in those without ST depression. DeBusk et al.[76] used stepwise multiple logistic regression analysis to determine that exercise-induced ST segment depression of 0.2 mV or more was the single most valuable indicator out of various clinical and exercise-related variables in predicting subsequent coronary events. Similar results were obtained by Smith et al.,[84] who studied 62 patients 18 days after infarction and noted a higher mortality and reinfarction rate during a 21-month follow-up in those with ST segment changes. Conflicting results were obtained by Weld et al.[80] who enrolled 250 patients recovering from myocardial infarction in a study of risk related to low-level exercise testing. In this study, multiple logistic regression analysis showed exercise duration and ventricular ectopic beats to be significant predictors of 1-year cardiac mortality, whereas exercise-induced ST depression was not predictive. Weld states that the differences in his results may be due to the fact that he included more patients with congestive heart failure in his study group than prior studies.

Although these authors examined slightly different populations of patients recovering from myocardial infarction, performed exercise testing at different intervals after infarction, and used slightly different exercise protocols, most studies agree that exercise-induced ischemia (ST segment depression) is a significant predictor of mortality and sudden death in this group of patients.

OTHER VARIABLES. Two additional exercise variables have been associated with mortality following myocardial infarction, but not specifically with the incidence of sudden cardiac death. Granath et al.[78] performed exercise testing at 3 and 9 weeks after myocardial infarction in 205 patients and found that although exercise-induced angina at 3 weeks did not predict increased mortality, exercise-induced angina at 9 weeks was. Koppes et al.[88] studied patients with maximal exercise tests at 8 weeks after infarction and found that those who could not achieve maximal predicted heart rate suffered more cardiac complications, including death, during follow-up. Another study stressing the importance of exercise duration is that of Weld et al.[80] Although exercise-induced angina and decreased exercise duration after myocardial infarction have been correlated with mortality during follow-up, a specific relationship to sudden cardiac death has not yet been clearly established for these variables.

Ambulatory Monitoring Studies

Few studies have assessed the prognostic importance of ST segment changes in ambulatory monitoring in the postinfarctional patient. This may be due, in part, to the difficulty in recording and analyzing the ST segment by this technique. On the other hand, a large amount of literature deals with the significance of ventricular ectopy predicting outcome in patients recovering from myocardial infarction. Work has shown that ambulatory monitoring is more effective at detecting frequent and complex ventricular ectopy than exercise testing in patients convalescing from infarction[12,76] These results are similar to those obtained in patients with chronic coronary artery disease and are not surprising. One study[89] has shown that complex ventricular ectopy on 24-hour ambulatory monitoring before discharge in patients who have had a myocardial infarction indicates a greater incidence of multivessel disease and lower ejection fraction. Many studies have shown a relationship between ventricular ectopic beats detected by ambulatory monitoring during the late hospitalization phase and subsequent mortality. Fewer studies have examined the specific endpoint of sudden cardiac death. Initial examination gives conflicting results, and the studies vary greatly in populations, duration of monitoring, definitions of frequent and complex arrhythmias and endpoints. Nevertheless, most of the data indicate that the presence of frequent or complex ventricular ectopic beats on predischarge 24-hour ambulatory monitoring after myocardial infarction predicts an increased incidence of sudden cardiac death during follow-up.

In one such study, Vismara, Amsterdam, and Mason[90] studied 68 survivors of acute myocardial infarction and found that although ventricular arrhythmias noted in the coronary care unit did not predict an increased incidence of sudden death, the presence of "complicated" ventricular ectopic beats before discharge did. Ruberman et al.[26] studied mortality and the incidence of sudden cardiac death in 1739 survivors of myocardial infarction examined by 1-hour recordings at variable times after the infarction. They found increased mortality and sudden death in those with complex ectopy (such as R-on-T phenomenon, runs of two or more, or multiform or bigeminal complexes). Schulze et al.[73,74] studied 81 patients who had had myocardial infarctions with 24-hour ambulatory monitoring and radionuclide gated blood pool scans. All eight patients who died suddenly during follow-up were in the subgroup of 26 patients with an ejection fraction of less than 40% and complicated arrhythmias (Lown classes 3 to 5).

The Multicenter Post Infarction Research Group[91] recently published data on 866 patients entered into a large prospective study in which most underwent 24-hour ambulatory monitoring and radionuclide ventriculography. Stepwise multivariate analysis identified four independent risk factors for death: ejection fractions less than 40%, ventricular ectopy of 10 or more depolarizations each hour, advanced New York Heart Association functional classes before infarction, and rales in the upper two thirds of the lung when the patient was in the coronary care unit.

Using somewhat different methods, the studies of Rehnqvist et al.[92-94] confirmed that complex ectopy before discharge predict an increased incidence of sudden cardiac death and reinfarction rate. In another study Kotler et al.[95] examined 160 patients and again found that complex ventricular ectopy predicted an increased risk of sudden death during follow-up. In their study, complex ectopy was defined as Lown class 2 or higher. Moss et al.[96-101] have performed a number of studies on survivors of myocardial infarction and found that Lown class 2 or higher identified a group of patients at risk of cardiac death or recurrent infarction. Ventricular tachycardia on 24-hour ambulatory monitoring identified a group at twofold risk,[100] and a separate analysis[101] showed that complex ectopy increased the risk of subsequent sudden cardiac death even when controlling for 10 other clinical variables. Bigger et al.[102-103] also found that ventricular tachycardia 2 weeks after infarction increased the risk of cardiac death.

Two studies found no correlation with ventricular ectopy and mortality after myocardial infarction. One study[104] suggested that complex ectopy did not indicate worse outcome; however, it did not include multiform or bigeminal beats or the R-on-T phenomenon in the complex category. The study of DeBusk et al.[76] also failed to show a relationship between ventricular ectopy and outcome. This study required patients to exercise on a treadmill at 3 weeks and thus excluded patients with poor left ventricular function, who are known to be at greatest risk. Also, this study did not examine arrhythmia complexity or frequency—only its presence or absence.

Although the data from most of the studies are in agreement that complex or frequent ventricular ectopy in the period immediately before or after hospital discharge predict increased risk of sudden death, there is some confusion as to which forms of arrhythmias are most dangerous. The relative importance of frequency of ventricular ectopic beats compared to complexity is difficult to determine. Each study used a slightly different classification of complex ectopy. Some studies included bigeminy and others did not. In one effort to solve this problem, Moss et al.[101] have developed a simple outcome-oriented system of classification. In this scheme, two categories of ventricular ectopy are recognized: "low-risk" ventricular ectopy (late cycle, with RR′/QT greater than 1, and uniform beats) and "high-risk" ventricular ectopy (early cycle, with RR′/QT less than or equal to 1, and multiform beats). During 2 years of follow-up, patients with high-risk ventricular ectopy had twice the mortality of those with low-risk ectopy. In the experience of Moss et al., increased frequency of ventricular ectopic beats did not improve this outcome-oriented classification. This scheme does not take into account the adverse effect of other complex forms of ectopy demonstrated in other studies and has not been universally adopted.

Controversy exists as to how long after myocardial infarction ambulatory monitoring is of prognostic value. Moss et al.[99] found that in contrast to the predictive value of ventricular ectopy on a 3- week postinfarction examination, a recording done at 5 months was of no value.

Summary of Exercise Testing for Myocardial Infarction

A number of excellent review have covered the use of various noninvasive tests following myocardial infarction.[1,70,96,105-109] In recent years low-level exercise testing has been used to predict outcome of patients before discharge following myocardial infarction. Review of the data published shows that there is general agreement that exercise-induced ischemia (ST depression), angina, ventricular arrhythmias, or poor exercise tolerance predict a poor outcome. Data from 24-hour ambulatory monitoring can be used to predict increased mortality and sudden death of complex forms of ventricular ectopy are seen, especially if there is coexisting evidence of poor left ventricular function. The data of Schulze and the Multicenter Post Infarction Research Group[73,74,91] seem to confirm that poor left ventricular function and frequent ventricular ectopy detected soon after myocardial infarction are independent risk factors for death.

Cardiomyopathy

Diffuse cardiomyopathy has been divided into three functional classes: obliterative, congestive, and restrictive and has many possible etiologies.[110] These conditions are generally characterized by a progressively deteriorating clinical course, a high prevalence of ventricular arrhythmias, and increased risk of sudden death.[111] Few population studies exist that report the frequency, type, and complexity of ventricular ectopy in these patients. No data exist relating exercise testing or ambulatory monitoring to prognosis of patients with restrictive cardiomyopathy.

Congestive Cardiomyopathy

Few studies have assessed the role of exercise testing in predicting outcome in patients with congestive cardiomyopathy. Two studies have examined ambulatory monitoring prognostic factors.[29,112] Follansbee, Michelson, and Morganroth[29] identified 37 patients with nonsustained ventricular tachycardia on 24-hour ambulatory monitoring. Of these patients, 19 had congestive cardiomyopathy, and 9 died suddenly during follow-up. These results would seem to indicate that ventricular tachycardia on 24-hour ambulatory monitoring predicts a poor outcome. A subsequent study by Huang, Messer, and Denes[112] identified 35 consecutive patients with idiopathic dilated cardiomyopathy who then underwent ambulatory monitoring. Although 60% of the patients had ventricular tachycardia, no difference in incidence of sudden death was observed between those with or without nonsustained ventricular tachycardia. Wilson et al.[113] studied 77 patients with class 3 or 4 congestive heart failure due to coronary artery disease, idiopathic cardiomyopathy, or valvular heart disease and found that five or more consecutive ventricular depolarizations predicted early and increased mortality. These apparently contradictory results probably can be explained by differences in study design and patient population.

In conclusion, not enough data are available to draw major conclusions regarding the role of exercise testing in determining prognosis in idiopathic congestive cardiomyopathy. Whether frequent or complex ventricular ectopy, including ventricular tachycardia, on ambulatory moitoring predicts a worsening of prognosis is still an area of controversy.

Hypertrophic Cardiomyopathy

Sudden cardiac death is commonly how death occurs in patients with hypertrophic cardiomyopathy.[114] In many of these patients the symptoms and natural history suggest that arrhythmias cause death. Ventricular arrhythmias are noted on exercise testing and ambulatory electrocardiography in the majority of such patients (61% and 83%, respectively).[115,116] Frequent and complex ventricular ectopic beats constitute more than 50% of such detected arrhythmias and are unrelated to symptoms or evidence of outflow tract obstructions.[116] Ventricular tachycardia is observed in 20%–28% of this population.[114,117] Again, ambulatory electrocardiography is superior to exercise testing in detecting complex ventricular arrhythmias (58% and 28%, respectively).[114,117] Although ventricular ectopy is often seen on exercise ECGs of patients with hypertrophic cardiomyopathy, the prognostic significance of this finding is unknown.

The prognostic value of these detected ventricular arrhythmias has recently been established in several studies.[28,114,117] McKenna et al.[17] noted that of 86 patients, 24 had ventricular tachycardia. In a mean follow-up of 2.6 years, 7 died suddenly, and 5 of the 7 had ventricular tachycardia compared with 2 of the 64 who did not have ventricular tachycardia. Supraventricular tachyarrhythmias were not associated with death. Maron et al.[114] examined 84 patients by ambulatory electrocardiography and observed ventricular tachycardia in 17 (20%). During follow-up sudden death occurred in 6 patients. Of these 4 had ventricular tachycardia, 1 had high-grade ventricular arrhythmias but without tachycardia, and 1 had low-grade arrhythmias. These two studies suggest that when 24-hour ambulatory electrocardiography detects ventricular tachycardia in a patient with hypertrophic cardiomyopathy, that patient is at increased risk of sudden death.

Survivors of Sudden Cardiac Death and Patients with Recurrent Sustained Ventricular Tachycardia

The widespread use of basic and advanced cardiac life support techniques such as those used in the Seattle Heart Watch[118] has demonstrated that a substantial proportion of patients suffering out-of-hospital ventricular fibrillation can be successfully resuscitated. Sudden cardiac death can be caused by the onset of ventricular tachycardia that degenerates into ventricular fibrillation or primary ventricular fibrillation alone.

Experience with such survivors of sudden death has shown that during the first year after hospitalization, there is 30% mortality, with three fourths of the deaths due to a recurrence of the sudden death syndrome.[119] Survivors of sudden death may have a variety of structural heart diseases including coronary artery disease (most common), cardiomyopathy, and valvular heart disease, or they may have no detectable structural heart disease. Although in recent years invasive electrophysiologic testing has achieved great popularity as a means to predict outcome and guide therapy in such patients, useful predictive data still can be obtained from noninvasive tests as well.

Weaver, Cobb, and Hallstrom[120] examined 90 ambulatory patients previously resusciated from out-of-hospital ventricular fibrillation by means of treadmill exercise testing an average of 11.5 months after the episode. During follow-up over a period of 2 years, 27 patients died, 19 with sudden unexpected cardiac arrest. Two findings on exercise evaluation were associated with subsequent fatalities: angina during treadmill testing and failure of systolic arterial pressure to rise 10 mm Hg or more during exercise. Weaver, Cobb, and Hallstrom[121] also examined the importance of 24-hour ambulatory monitoring in 124 similar patients who were resuscitated from out-of-hospital ventricular fibrillation. Ambulatory monitoring was performed 5 months (median) after cardiac arrest and showed that a high percentage of such patients had ventricular ectopy (90%). During a follow-up of 31.7 months (mean), 51 patients died, 32 from unexpected sudden cardiac arrest. Complex ectopy was present in 20% or more of the 30-minute recording intervals and occurred more often in patients who subsequently suffered cardiac arrest compared to those who survived ($P < .005$, specificity 72%, relative risk 2.3). Although complex arrhythmias were associated with a past history of congestive heart failure and remote myocardial infarction, they were predictive of outcome regardless of the clinical history.

Lown's group[122,123] has advocated the use of treadmill testing and ambulatory monitoring for the evaluation of patients with malignant ventricular arrhythmias. Patients in their study group included those with ventricular fibrillation, as well as those with recurrent, sustained ventricular tachycardia associated with either syncope or hemodynamic compromise. They have evolved a four-phase approach to the management of such patients involving baseline drug-free evaluation with exercise testing and 48 hours of ambulatory monitoring, acute drug testing, chronic drug testing, and posthospital management with individually selected drugs. In their experience, ambulatory monitoring or exercise testing expose frequent or complex arrhythmias that can be used as a target to assess drug efficacy in 85% of patients. The remaining 15% require electrophysiologic testing to guide therapy. With their individualized approach, a drug program that could eliminate certain complex forms of ventricular arrhythmias was achieved in 80% of patients, with an incidence of sudden death during follow-up of only 3% each year. Although these results are interesting and of clinical relevance, they do not bear directly on the question of which findings on ambulatory monitoring or exercise testing predict outcome and sudden death in such patients. They do point out the importance of complex arrhythmias on ambulatory monitoring in such patients and are consistent with the observations of Weaver, Cobb, and Hallstrom[121] in this regard. Weaver, Cobb, and Hallstrom[120] did not find exercise-associated arrhythmias to be predictive of outcome in their study, however. These differing results may be attributed to differences in study populations and other variables. The predictive value of exercise-associated arrhythmias in such patients remains unclear. Also, even though complex ectopy on 24-hour ambulatory monitoring can predict mortality and sudden cardiac death in patients with malignant ventricular arrhythmias, the relative importance of this technique compared to electrophysiologic testing is still very much in dispute.

CONCLUSION

Exercise testing and ambulatory electrocardiography are complimentary techniques that are useful for examining distinct forms of ECG data. Ambulatory monitoring is clearly superior to exercise testing in detecting ventricular ectopy and relating such ectopy to anatomy and outcome. Only one variable (ventricular ectopy) on ambulatory monitoring has proven prognostic value. Exercise testing can relate multiple variables to subsequent outcome. Exercise testing is clearly more useful at relating the ST segment to results during follow-up. Other variables observed during exercise testing, such as exercise duration, angina, ventricular ectopy, and blood pressure response, also can be related to coronary anatomy, left ventricular function, and subsequent mortality in different patient groups.

Studies of exercise testing and ambulatory monitoring in normal persons without signs or symptoms of heart disease generally agree that ventricular ectopy is a benign finding. The incidence, frequency, and complexity of ventricular ectopy recorded by ambulatory monitoring tend to increase with advancing age. Studies of individuals without detectable heart disease and frequent (greater than 60 ventricular ectopic beats each hour) or complex (Lown class 3 or greater) ventricular ectopy have been carried out. Approximately one fourth of these patients have occult coronary artery disease and another one fourth have signs of mild left ventricular dysfunction. The significance of these findings is unknown, but follow-up of this subset of patients reveals a good outcome.

Studies of these two noninvasive tests in various patient populations at risk of sudden cardiac death have been carried out and show that these tests can predict sudden death in many instances. The usefulness of these tests in predicting sud-

Table 5-4 *Summary of Relative Prognostic Value of Exercise Testing and Ambulatory Electrocardiography in Different Cardiac Diseases*

Disease	Exercise Testing	Ambulatory Electrocardiography
Coronary artery disease		
Venticular arrhythmias	Identify multivessel disease, impaired left ventricular function, and increased risk of death	Identify multivessel disease and sudden death risk
ST segment depression	Identify multivessel disease and increased mortality	Undefined
Postmyocardial infarction		
Ventricular arrhythmias	Identify increased sudden death risk	Indicate increased mortality and sudden death risk
ST segment	Identify multivessel disease; indicate risk of angina, coronary events, and sudden death	Undefined
Hypertrophic cardiomyopathy		
Ventricular arrhythmias	No diagnostic or prognostic value	Sudden death correlated with ventricular tachycardia
ST segment	Undefined	Undefined
Survivors of sudden death		
Ventricular arrhythmias	Undefined	Identify patients at increased risk of death
ST segment	Undefined	Undefined

den death using ventricular ectopy of ST segment criteria is summarized in Table 5-4. In patients with known coronary artery disease, exercise-induced frequent ventricular ectopy seems to be associated with an increased risk of sudden death. Similarly, several studies have shown a relationship between frequent and complex ventricular ectopy in patients with chronic coronary artery disease and subsequent sudden death. Similar results have been shown for exercise-induced ventricular ectopy and frequent or complex ectopy detected in patients shortly after myocardial infarction. ST segment depression on exercise testing of survivors of myocardial infarction also seems to correlate with sudden cardiac death during follow-up. Several studies using multivariate analysis have indicated that ventricular ectopy is a risk factor for sudden cardiac death in patients with ischemic heart disease independent of left ventricular dysfunction. Although most studies agree that complex forms of ectopy are aminous in this group of patients, the relative importance of complex ectopy to frequent ectopy is not clear.

Most studies have used the Lown classification or some variation thereof to grade ventricular ectopy. In patients with ischemic heart disease, few studies have directly compared the prognostic importance of exercise testing with ambulatory monitoring. Preliminary data seem to indicate that these two noninvasive, ECG tests can provide independent prognostic information. In patients with hypertrophic cardiomyopathy, independent studies indicate that nonsustained ventriuclar tachycardia demonstrated on 24-hour monitoring predicts an increased risk of sudden death. In survivors of out-of-hospital sudden death, factors associated with cardiac arrest during follow-up include complex ectopy on ambulatory monitoring, angina during exercise testing, or an abnormal blood pressure response during exercise.

It is hoped that further studies will determine if other exercise testing variables are related to sudden death in these populations. Although the role of ambulatory monitoring in examining the clinical and prognostic importance of the ST segment is limited because of technical factors, advances in this field may overcome this shortcoming in the near future. Additional studies that compare exercise testing to ambulatory monitoring and control for differences in age and left ventricular function are needed in all patient groups at risk of sudden death.

REFERENCES

1. Kennedy HL: Comparison of ambulatory electrocardiography and exercise testing. Am J Cardiol 47:1359, 1981
2. Haskell WL: Cardiovascular complications during exercise training of cardiac patients. Circulation 57:1920, 1978
3. Stern S, Tzivoni D, Stern Z: Diagnostic accuracy of ambulatory ECG monitoring in ischemic heart disease. Circulation 52:1045, 1975
4. Tzivoni D, Stern Z, Keren Z, et al: Electrocardiographic characteristics of neurocirculatory asthenia during everyday activities. Br Heart J 44:426, 1980
5. Armstrong WF, Jordan JW, Morris SN, et al: Prevalence and magnitude of S-T segment and T wave abnormalities in normal men during continuous ambulatory electrocardiography.
6. Taggart E, Parkinson P, Carruthers M: Cardiac responses to thermal, physical, and emotional stress. Br Med J 3:71, 1972
7. Biagini A, Mazzei MG, Carpeggiani C, et al: Vasospastic ischemic mechanism of frequent asymptomatic transient ST-T changes during continuous electrocardiographic monitoring in selected unstable angina patients. Am Heart J 103:13, 1982
8. Armstrong WF, Morris SN: The ST segment during ambulatory electrocardiographic monitoring. Ann Intern Med 98:249, 1983
9. Ellestad MH: Stress Testing: Principles and practice. FA Davis, Philadelphia, 1980, pp 77–96.
10. Poblete PF, Kennedy HL, Caralis DG: Detection of ventricular ectopy in patients with coronary heart disease and normal subjects by exercise testing and ambulatory

electrocardiography. Chest 74:402, 1978

11. Ryan M, Lown B, Horn H: Comparison of ventricular ectopic activity during 24-hour monitoring and exercise testing in patients with coronary heart disease. N Engl J Med 292:224, 1975
12. DeSoyza N, Murphy ML, Bissett JK, et al: Detecting ventricular arrhythmia after myocardial infarction: Comparison of Holter monitoring and treadmill exercise. South Med J 70:403, 1977
13. McHenry PL, Fisch C, Jordan SW, et al: Cardiac arrhythmias observed during maximal treadmill exercise testing in clinically normal men. Am J Cardiol 29:331, 1972
14. Blackburn H, Taylor H, Keys A: The electrocardiogram in prediction of five-year coronary heart disease incidence among men aged forty through fifty-nine. Circulation 41:154, 1970
15. Froelicher V, Thomas M, Pillow C, et al: Epidemiologic study of asymptomatic men screened by maximal treadmill testing for latent coronary artery disease. Am J Cardiol 34:770, 1974
16. McHenry PL, Morris SN, Kavalier M, et al: Comparative study of exercise-induced ventricular arrhythmias in normal subjects and patients with documented coronary artery disease. Am J Cardiol 37:609, 1976
17. Allen WH, Aranow WS, Goodman P, et al: Five-year follow-up of maximal stress test in asymptomatic men and women (abstract). Am J Cardiol 45:419, 1980
18. Giagnoni E, Secchi MB, Wu SC, et al: Prognostic value of exercise EKG testing in asymptomatic normotensive subjects: A prospective matched study. New Engl J Med 309:1085, 1983.
19. Kennedy HL, Underhill SJ: Frequent or complex ventricular ectopy in apparently healthy subjects. Am J Cardiol 38:141, 1976
20. Rabkin SW, Mathewson FA, Tate RB: Relationship of ventricular ectopy in men without apparent heart disease to occurrence of ischemic heart disease and sudden death. Am Heart J 101:135, 1981
21. Chiang BN, Perlman, Fulton M, et al: Predisposing factors in sudden cardiac death in Tecumseh, Michigan: A prospective study. Circulation 41:31, 1970
22. Chiang B, Perlman L, Ostrander L Jr, et al: Relationship of premature systoles to coronary heart disease and sudden death in the Tecumseh epidemiologic study. Ann Intern Med 79:1159, 1969
23. Crow RS, Prineas RJ, Dias V, et al: Ventricular premature beats in a population sample: Frequency and associations with coronary risk characteristics. Circulation 51-52 (suppl 3):211, 1975
24. Crow RC, Prineas R, Blackburn H: The prognostic significance of ventricular ectopic beats among the apparently healthy. Am Heart J 101:244, 1981
25. Ruberman W, Weinblatt E, Goldberg JD, et al: Ventricular premature beats and mortality after myocardial infarction. N Engl J Med 297:750, 1977
26. Ruberman W, Weinblatt E, Goldberg JD, et al: Ventricular premature complexes and sudden death after myocardial infarction. Circulation 64:297, 1981
27. Hinkle LE, Carver ST, Stevens M: The frequency of asymptomatic disturbances of cardiac rhythm and conduction in middle-aged men. Am J Cardiol 24:626, 1969
28. Maron BJ, Savage DD, Wolfson JK, et al: Prognostic significance of 24-hour ambulatory electrocardiographic monitoring in patients with hypertrophic cardiographic monitoring in patients with hypertrophic cardiomyopathy: A prospective study. Am J Cardiol 48:252, 1981
29. Follansbee WP, Michelson EL, Morganroth J: Non-sustained ventricular tachycardia in ambulatory patients: Characteristics and associa-

tion with sudden cardiac death. Ann Intern Med 92:741, 1980

30. Southall DP, Richards J, Mitchell P, et al: Study of cardiac rhythm in healthy newborn infants. Br Heart J 43:14, 1980
31. Southall DP, Johnston F, Shinebourne EA, et al: Twenty-four hour electrocardiographic study of heart rate and rhythm patterns in population of heatlhy children. Br Heart J 45:281, 1981
32. Brodsky M, Wu D, Denes P, et al: Arrhythmias documented by 24-hour continuous electrocardiographic monitoring in 50 male medical students without apparent heart disease. Am J Cardiol 39:390, 1977
33. Sobotka PA, Mayer JH, Bauernfeind RA, et al: Arrhythmias documented by 24-hour continuous ambulatory electrocardiographic monitoring in young women without apparent heart disease. Am Heart J 101:753, 1981
34. Talan DA, Bauernfeind RA, Ashley WW, et al: Twenty-four hour continuous ECG recordings in long-distance runners. Chest 82:19, 1982
35. Kostis JB, McCrone K, Moreyra AE, et al: Premature ventricular complexes in the absence of identifiable heart disease. Circulation 63:1351, 1981
36. Verbaan CJ, Pool J, VanWanrooy J: Incidence of cardiac arrhythmias in a presumed healthy population, in Stott FD, Raftery EB, Sleight P, et al (Eds): Proceedings of the International Symposium on Ambulatory Monitoring, New York, Academic Press Inc, 1977, p 1
37. Glasser SP, Clark PI, Applebaum HJ: Occurrence of frequent complex arrhythmias detected by ambulatory monitoring. Chest 75:565, 1979
38. Camm AJ, Evans KE, Ward DE, et al: The rhythm of the heart in active elderly subjects. Am Heart J 99:598, 1980
39. Fleg JL, Kennedy HL: Cardiac arrhythmias in a healthy elderly population: Detection by 24-hour ambulatory electrocardiography. Chest 81:302, 1982
40. Clarke JM, Hamer J, Shelton JR: The rhythm of the normal human heart. Lancet 2:508, 1976
41. DeMaria AN, Amsterdam EA, Vismara LA, et al: Arrhythmias in the mitral valve prolapse syndrome. Ann Intern Med 84:656, 1976
42. Hinkle LE, Carver ST, Argyros DC, et al: The prognostic significance of ventricular premature contractions in healthy people and in people with coronary heart disease. Acta Cardiol (suppl) 18:5, 1974
43. Horan MJ, Kennedy HL: Characteristics and prognosis of apparently healthy patients with frequent and complex ventricular ectopy: Evidence for a relatively benign new syndrome with occult myocardial and/or coronary disease. Am Heart J 102:809, 1981
44. Califf RM, McKinnis RA, Burks J, et al: Prognostic implications of ventricular arrhythmias during 24-hour ambulatory monitoring in patients undergoing cardiac catheterization for coronary artery disease. Am J Cardiol 50:23, 1982
45. Lachman AB, Semler HJ, Gustafson RH: Postural ST-T wave changes in the radioelectrocardiogram simulating myocardial ischemia. Circulation 31:557, 1965
46. Crawford MH, Mendoza CA, O'Rourke RA, et al: Limitations of continuous ambulatory monitoring for detecting coronary disease. Ann Intern Med 89:1, 1978
47. Patterson RE, Horowitz SF, Eng C, et al: Can noninvasive exercise test criteria identify patients with left main or 3-vessel coronary disease after a first myocardial infarction? Am J Cardiol 51:361, 1983
48. Calvert A, Lown B, Gorlin R: Ventricular premature beats and anatomically defined coronary heart disease. Am J Cardiol 39:627, 1977
49. McNeer JF, Margolis JR, Lee KL, et al: The role of the exercise test in the

evaluation of patients for ischemic heart disease. Circulation 57:64, 1978
50. Bruce RA, DeRouen TA, Hammermeister KE: Noninvasive screening criteria for enhanced 4-year survival postaortocoronary bypass surgery. Circulation 60:638, 1979
51. Bruce RA, DeRouen TA, Peterson DL, et al: Noninvasive predictors of sudden cardiac death in men with coronary heart disease: Predictive value of maximal exercise stress testing. Am J Cardiol 39:833, 1977
52. Nixon JV, Lipscomb K, Blomquist CG, et al: Exercise testing in men with significant left main coronary disease. Br Heart J 42:410, 1979
53. Levites R, Anderson GJ: Detection of critical coronary lesions with treadmill exercise testing: Fact or fiction? Am J Cardiol 42:533, 1978
54. Blumenthal DS, Weiss JL, Mellits ED, et al: The predictive value of a strongly positive stress test in patients with minimal symptoms. Am J Med 70: 1005, 1981
55. Samarco ME, Pontims S, Selvester RH: Abnormal blood pressure response and marked ischemic ST segment depression as predictors of severe coronary artery disease. Circulation 61:572, 1980
56. Weiner DA: Exercise testing for the diagnosis and severity of coronary artery disease. J Cardiac Rehab 1:438, 1981
57. Morris SN, Phillips JF, Jordan JW, et al: Incidence and significance of decreases in systolic blood pressure during graded treadmill exercise testing. Am J Cardiol 41:221, 1978
58. Zaret B, Conti CR: Exercise-induced ventricular irritability: Hemodynamic and angiographic correlations (abstract). Am J Cardiol 29:298, 1972
59. Goldschlager H, Cake D, Cohn K: Exercise-induced ventricular arrhythmias in patients with coronary artery disease: Their relation to angiographic findings. Am J Cardiol 31:434, 1973
60. Helfant RH, Pine R, Kabde V, et al: Exercise-related ventricular premature complexes in coronary heart disease: Correlations with ischemia and angiographic severity. Ann Intern Med 80:589, 1974
61. Nair CK, Aronow WS, Sketch MH, et al: Diagnostic and prognostic significance of exercise-induced premature ventricular complexes in men and women: A 4-year follow-up. J Am Coll Cardiol 1:1201, 1983
62. Udall JA, Ellestad MH: Predictive implications of ventricular premature contractions with treadmill stress testing. Circulation 56:985, 1977
63. Ivanova LA, Mazur NA, Smirnova TM, et al: Electrocardiographic exercise testing and ambulatory monitoring to identify patients with ischemic heart disease. Am J Cardiol 45:1132, 1980
64. Dagenais GR, Rouleau JR, Christen A, et al: Survival of patients with a strongly positive exercise electrocardiogram. Circulation 65:452, 1982
65. Ellestad MH, Wan MKC: Predictive implications of stress testing: Follow-up of 2700 subjects after maximum treadmill stress testing. Circulation 51:363, 1975
66. Stuart RJ, Ellestad MH: Upsloping ST segments in exercise stress testing. Am J Cardiol 37:19, 1976
67. Podrid PJ, Graboys TB, Lown B: Prognosis of medically treated patients with coronary artery disease with profound ST segment depression during exercise testing. N Engl J Med 305:1111, 1981
68. Uretz EF, Vasilomanolakis EC, Ruggie N, et al: Relationship between ventricular arrhythmias and heart disease. (abstracts). Am J Cardiol 49:1006, 1982
69. Calvert A, Lown B, Gorlin R: Ventricular premature beats and anatomically defined coronary heart disease. Am J Cardiol 39:627, 1977
70. Vismara, LA, Vera Z, Foerster JM, et al: Identification of sudden death risk factors in acute and chronic cor-

onary artery disease. Am J Cardiol 39:821, 1977
71. Sharma SD, Ballantyne F, Goldstein S: The relationship of ventricular asynergy in coronary artery disease to ventricular premature beats. Chest 66:358, 1974
72. Califf RM, Burks JM, Behar VS, et al: Relationships among ventricular arrhythmias, coronary artery disease, and angiographic and electrocardiographic indicators of myocardial fibrosis. Circulation 57:725, 1978
73. Schulze RA, Strauss HW, Pitt B: Sudden death in the year following myocardial infarction. Am J Med 62: 192, 1977
74. Schulze RA, Rouleau J, Rigo P, et al: Ventricular arrhythmias in the late hospital phase of acute myocardial infarction: Relation of left ventricular function detected by gated blood pool scanning. Circulation 52:1006, 1975
75. Miller DH, Borer JS: Exercise testing early after myocardial infarction: Risks and benefits. Am J Med 72:427, 1982
76. DeBusk RF, Davidson DM, Houston N, et al: Serial ambulatory electrocardiography and treadmill exercise testing soon after uncomplicated myocardial infarction. Am J Cardiol 45:547, 1980
77. Theroux P, Waters DD, Halpern C, et al: Prognostic value of exercise testing soon after myocardial infarction. N Engl J Med 301:341, 1979
78. Granath A, Sodermark T, Winge T, et al: Early workload tests for evaluation of long-term prognosis of acute myocardial infarction. Br Heart J 39:758, 1977
79. Ericsson M, Granath A, Ohlsen P, et al: Arrhythmias and symptoms during treadmill testing three weeks after myocardial infarction in 100 patients. Br Heart J 35:787, 1973
80. Weld FM, Chu K, Bigger JT, et al: Risk stratification with low-level exercise testing two weeks after acute myocardial infarction. Circulation 64: 306, 1981
81. Markiewicz W, Houston N, DeBusk RF: Exercise testing soon after myocardial infarction. Circulation 56:26, 1977
82. Davidson DM, DeBusk RF: Prognostic value of a single exercise test three weeks after uncomplicated myocardial infarction. Circulation 61:236, 1980
83. Sami M, Kraemer H, DeBusk RF: The prognostic significance of serial exercise testing after myocardial infarction. Circulation 60:1238, 1979
84. Smith JW, Dennis A, Gassmann A, et al: Exercise testing three weeks after myocardial infarction. Chest 75:12, 1979
85. Schwartz KM, Turner JD, Sheffield LT, et al: Limited exercise testing soon after myocardial infarction: Correlation with early coronary and left ventricular angiography. Ann Intern Med 94:727, 1981
86. Fuller CM, Raizner AE, Verani MS, et al: Early post-myocardial infarction stress testing: An accurate predictor of multivessel coronary disease and subsequent cardiac events. Ann Intern Med 94:734, 1981
87. Haskell WL, DeBusk RF: Cardiovascular responses to repeated treadmill exercise testing soon after myocardial infarction. Circulation 60: 1247, 1979
88. Koppes GM, Kruyer WB, Beckmann CH, et al: Response to exercise early after uncomplicated acute myocardial infarction in patients receiving no medication: Long-term follow-up. Am J Cardiol 46:764, 1980
89. Schulze RA, Strauss HW, Pitt B: Sudden death in the year following myocardial infarction: Relation to ventricular premature contractions in the late hospital phase and left ventricular ejection fraction. Am J Med 62:192, 1977.
90. Vismara LA, Amsterdam EA, Mason DT: Relation of ventricular arrhythmias in the late hospital phase of acute myocardial infarction to sud-

den death after hospital discharge. Am J Med 59:6, 1975
91. Multicenter Post Infarction Research Group: Risk stratification and survival after myocardial infarction. N Engl J Med 309: 331, 1983
92. Rehnqvist N: Ventricular arrhythmias after an acute myocardial infarction. Eur J Cardiol 7:169, 1978
93. Rehnqvist N: Ventricular arrhythmias prior to discharge after acute myocardial infarction. Eur J Cardiol 4:63, 1976
94. Rehnqvist N, Sjorgren A: Ventricular arrhythmias prior to discharge and one year after acute myocardial infarction. Eur J Cardiol 5:425, 1977
95. Kotler MN, Tabatznik B, Mower MB, et al: Prognostic significance of ventricular ectopic beats with respect to sudden death in the late postinfarction period. Circulation 47:959, 1973
96. Moss AJ: Clinical significance of ventricular arrhythmias in patients with and without coronary artery disease. Prog Cardiovasc Dis 23:33, 1980
97. Moss AJ, Schnitzler R, Green R, et al: Ventricular arrhythmias three weeks after myocardial infarction. Ann Intern Med 75:837, 1971
98. Moss AJ, DeCamilla J, Mietlowski W, et al: Prognostic grading and significance of ventricular premature beats after recovery from myocardial infarction. Circulation 52(suppl 3):204, 1975
99. Moss AJ, DeCamilla J, Davis HP, et al: Clinical significance of ventricular ectopic beats in the early posthospital phase of myocardial infarction. Am J Cardiol 39:635, 1977
100. Anderson KP, DeCamilla J, Moss AJ: Clinical significance of ventricular tachycardia (three beats or longer) detected during ambulatory monitoring after myocardial infarction. Circulation 57:890, 1978
101. Moss AJ, Davis HT, DeCamilla J, et al: Ventricular ectopic beats and their relation to sudden and nonsudden cardiac death after myocardial infarction. Circulation 60:998, 1979
102. Bigger JT, Heller CA, Wenger TL, et al: Risk stratification after acute myocardial infarction. Am J Cardiol 42:202, 1978
103. Bigger JT, Weld FM, Rolnitzky LM: Prevalence, characteristics and significance of ventricular tachycardia (three or more complexes) detected with ambulatory electrocardiographic recording in the late hospital phase of acute myocardial infarction. Am J Cardiol 48:815, 1981
104. De Soyza H, Bennett FA, Murphy ML, et al: The relationship of paroxysmal ventricular tachycardia complicating the acute phase and ventricular arrhythmia during the late hospital phase of myocardial infarction to long-term survival. Am J Med 64:377, 1978
105. Cohn P: The role of noninvasive cardiac testing after an uncomplicated myocardial infarction. Engl J Med 309:90, 1983
106. Spann JF: Changing concepts of pathophysiology, prognosis, and therapy in acute myocardial infarction. Am J Med 74:877, 1983
107. Vlay SC, Reid PR: Ventricular ectopy: Etiology, evaluation, and therapy. Am J Med 73:899, 1982
108. Winkle RA: Current status of ambulatory electrocardiography. Am Heart J 102:757, 1981
109. Winkle RA: Ambulatory electrocardiography and the diagnosis, evaluation, and treatment of chronic ventricular arrhythmias. Prog Cardiovasc Dis 23:99, 1980
110. Goodwin JR, Oakley CM: The cardiomyopathies. Br Heart J 34:545, 1972
111. Fowler NO: Differential diagnosis of cardiomyopathies. Prog Cardiovasc Dis 14:113, 1971
112. Huang SK, Messer JV, Denes P: Significance of ventricular tachycardia in idiopathic dilated cardiomyopathy: Observations in 35 patients. Am J Cardiol 51:507, 1983
113. Wilson JR, Schwartz JS, Sutton MS, et al: Prognosis in severe heart fail-

ure: Relation to hemodynamic measurements and ventricular ectopic activity. J Am Coll Cardiol 2:403, 1983

114. Maron BJ, Roberts WC, Edwards JE, et al: Sudden death in patients with hypertrophic cardiomyopathy: Characterization of 26 patients without functional limitation. Am J Cardiol 41:803, 1978

115. Savage DD, Serdes SF, Maron BJ, et al: Prevalence of arrhythmias during 24-hour electrocardiographic monitoring and exercise testing in patients with obstructive and nonobstructive hypertrophic cardiomyopathy. Circulation 59:866, 1979

116. McKenna WJ, Chetty S, Oakley CM, et al: Arrhythmia in hypertrophic cardiomyopathy: Exercise and 48-hour electrocardiographic assessment with and without beta-adrenergic blocking therapy. Am J Cardiol 45:1, 1980

117. McKenna WJ, England D, Doi YL, et al: Arrhythmia in hypertrophic cardiomyopathy. I. Influence on prognosis. Br Heart J 46:168, 1981

118. Eisenberg MS, Copass MK, Hallstrom AP, et al: Treatment of out-of-hospital cardiac arrests with rapid defibrillation by emergency medical technicians. N Engl J Med 382:1379, 1980

119. Cobb LA, Baum RS, Alvarez H, et al: Resusciation from out-of-hospital ventricular fibrillation: 4-year follow-up. Circulation 51-52(suppl 3):223, 1975

120. Weaver WD, Cobb LA, Hallstrom AP: Characteristics of survivors of exertion and nonexertion-related cardiac arrest: Value of subsequent exercise testing. Am J Cardiol 50:671, 1982

121. Weaver WD, Cobb LA, Hallstrom AP: Ambulatory arrhythmias in resuscitated victims of cardiac arrest. Circulation 66:212, 1982

122. Lown B: Management of patients at high risk of sudden death. Am Heart J 103:689, 1982

123. Lown B, Graboys TB: Management of patients with malignant ventricular arrhythmias. Am J Cardiol 39:910, 1977

Allan M. Greenspan

6

ELECTROPHYSIOLOGIC TECHNIQUES FOR EVALUATING PATIENTS AT RISK FOR SUDDEN DEATH

Sudden cardiac death accounts for some 300,000[1,2] deaths each year in the United States. Frequently, it occurs in patients with no previous symptoms or signs of organic heart disease and is wholly unexpected. Since the two major electrophysiologic derangements responsible for sudden cardiac death, asystole from any cause and ventricular tachyarrhythmias,[3] are frequently treatable, the development of reliable markers for patients at risk for these derangements would help reduce the incidence of sudden cardiac death.

In the last 10 years, the development of intracardiac recording and stimulation techniques have enabled cardiologists to more systematically evaluate and treat bradyarrhythmias (sinus node dysfunction and atrioventricular block) and ventricular tachyarrhythmias. These techniques have been applied to the following patients at a high risk of sudden cardiac death with encouraging results of therapy guided by electrophysiologic evaluation[4,5]:

1. Cardiac arrest survivors
2. Complex ventricular ectopic activity after myocardial infarction
3. Nonsustained ventricular tachycardia and poor left ventricular function

The purpose of this chapter is to analyze the electrophysiologic technqiues used to evaluate patients at high risk for sudden death and to discuss therapeutic modalities for its prevention.

SUDDEN CARDIAC DEATH
0-8089-1725-0

GENERAL CONSIDERATIONS

Three to five multipolar electrode catheters are inserted percutaneously (or via cutdown) in the femoral, brachial, or subclavian veins and, if necessary, in the femoral artery. These are placed under fluoroscopic guidance at specific intracardiac sites. Typically, the catheters are positioned at the high right atrium near the sinus node, at the atrioventricular junction to record bundle of His activity, in the coronary sinus, at the right ventricular apex, in the right ventricular outflow tract, and occasionally in the left ventricle. Baseline recordings are made, and then programmed atrial and ventricular stimulation are performed. If ventricular tachyarrhythmias are induced, programmed ventricular stimulation is performed during the tachycardia to effect termination. Antiarrhythmic drugs are then administered, and baseline recordings as well as programmed stimulation are repeated. Follow-up electrophysiologic studies may be performed with one or two catheters on subsequent days using additional oral or parenteral antiarrhythmic drugs.

The specific electrophysiologic techniques used in any evaluation of high-risk patients is based on the clinically documented arrhythmia that indexes the patient as high risk. Specifically, the finding of bifascicular block on Holter monitoring or marked bradycardia or asystole during the resuscitation procedure would focus the electrophysiologic evaluation on infranodal conduction characteristics. Alternatively, complex ventricular ectopic activity or nonsustained ventricular tachycardia associated with syncope, myocardial infarction, or ventricular tachycardia or fibrillation during resuscitation would focus the electrophysiologic evaluation on induction and suppression of ventricular tachyarrhythmias.

EVALUATION OF INFRANODAL CONDUCTION CHARACTERISTICS

Although most cases of sudden cardiac death are attributed to ventricular tachyarrhythmias, approximately 30% of the patients have asystole, frequently due to infranodal block.[3,6] Evaluation of infranodal conduction characteristics thus is essential in studying patients at high risk.

Technically, the critical factor in the evaluation is accurate and consistent measurement of the HV interval, or the conduction time from the bundle of His to the earliest site of ventricular activation. Care must be taken to position the tripolar catheter precisely to avoid an artifactually normal or shortened HV interval measurement.[7] This can be ensured by positioning the atrioventricular junctional catheter to record atrial and ventricular spikes of relatively equal amplitude. The normal HV interval is 35–55 msec. A moderate prolongation to 60–75 msec rarely indicates significant infranodal conduction disturbances; however, HV intervals greater than 90 msec are associated with frequent and rapid progression to complete atrioventricular block.[8] Other observations that suggest significant infranodal disease include widening of the His potential to greater than 25 msec[9];

split His potentials, indicating intra-His conduction disease (which is almost always associated with progression to infranodal block)[10] and the development of infranodal block with incremental atrial pacing.[11] An example of significant infranodal disease manifest by a widening of the His potential, a prolonged HV interval, and block below the bundle of His during sinus rhythm is shown in Figure 6-1. If the HV interval is only moderately prolonged and there is no other obvious abnormality, the infranodal conduction system can be stressed with a type IA antiarrhythmic agent (e.g., procainamide, 500–1000 mg, IV). Prolongation of the HV interval by more than 25% of baseline and beyond 90 msec indicates a severe underlying infranodal conduction disturbance.[12] The significance of infranodal block developing with programmed atrial stimulation is less clearcut. It may well be a normal phenomenon, depending on the atrial cycle length and refractory periods of the His-Purkinje system and atrioventricular nodes.

EVALUATION OF VENTRICULAR TACHYARRHYTHMIAS

The rationale for using programmed ventricular stimulation to evaluate patients at high risk for sudden death is based on the large percentage of patients who have clinically documented ventricular tachycardia (7%–26%) and ventricular fibrillation (62%–74%) after resuscitation.[3,5] Furthermore, recent studies of such patients have shown high rates of inducibility of ventricular tachyarrhythmias during electrophysiologic evaluation and excellent success in preventing recurrent arrhythmias or sudden death with antiarrhythmic therapy directed by serial electrophysiologic drug testing.[13] Assuming that ventricular tachyarrhythmias are frequently the cause of sudden death, a systematic approach to therapy would be advisable, such as that provided by programmed ventricular stimulation.

The use of programmed ventricular stimulation in designing therapy for ventricular tachyarrhythmias offers significant advantages over other, more empiric, approaches.[14] Since most ventricular tachyarrhythmias, particularly in patients with organic heart disease who are at risk for sudden death, are reentrant in mechanism, programmed ventricular stimulation allows reproducible induction of the arrhythmia.[15,16] This obviates the unpredictable interval between recurrences of the ventricular tachyarrhythmias that interfere with the evaluation of therapeutic modalities. Since most reentrant ventricular tachyarrhythmias can be terminated by programmed ventricular stimulation,[17] repeated cardioversions that are often required with failure of empiric drug trials may be avoided. Furthermore, programmed ventricular stimulation allows testing of multiple antiarrhythmic agents, thus facilitating rapid determination of effective drugs and their appropriate doses. Programmed ventricular stimulation also helps determine the effectiveness of pacer modalities[18] and can considerably shorten the hospitalization time for patients with often life-threatening tachyarrhythmias. Finally, programmed ventricular stimulation can rapidly and reliably predict failure of standard antiarrhythmic drug treatment[19] or pacer effectiveness and thereby allow planning for surgical or experimental electrical treatment.

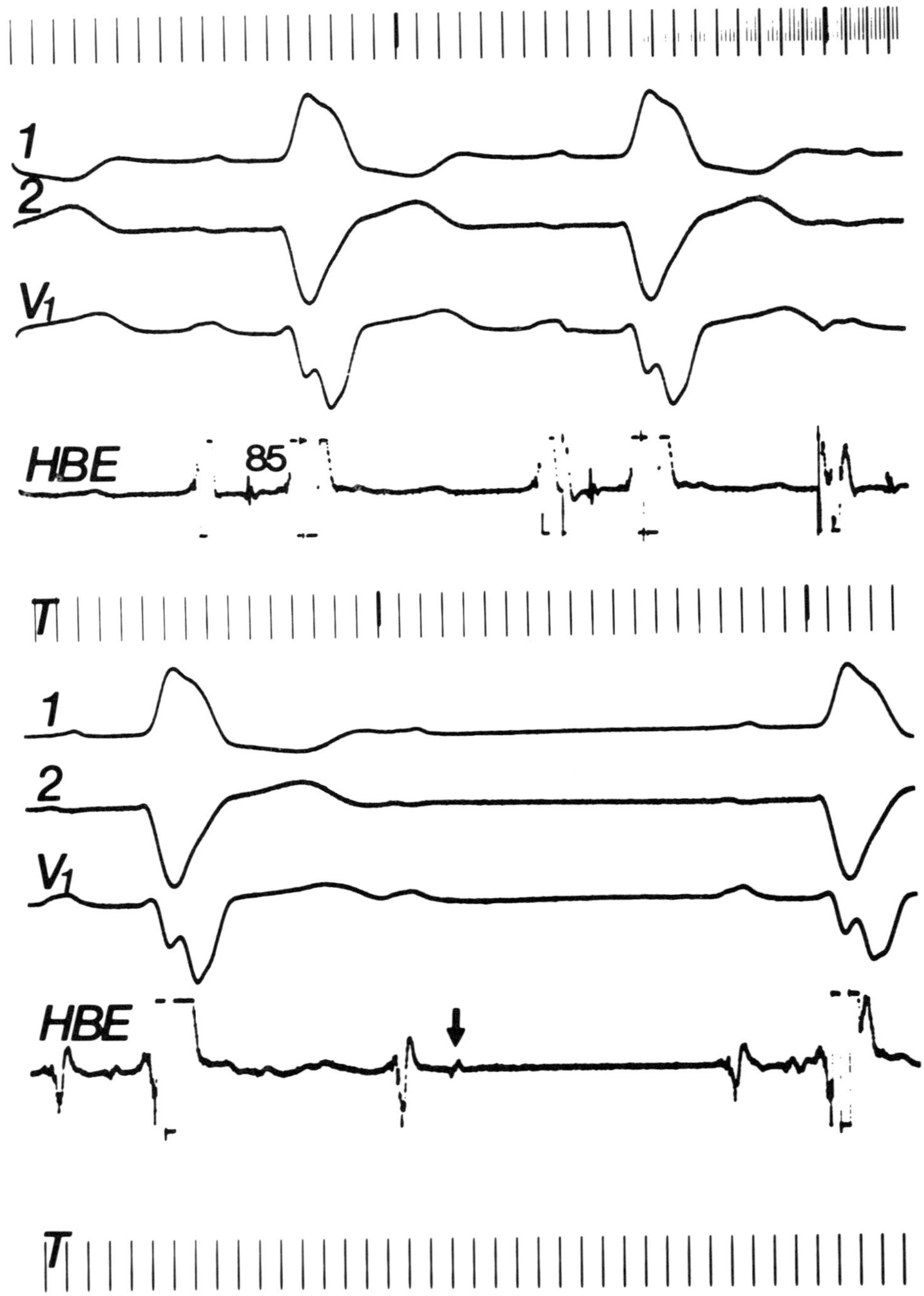

Fig. 6-1. Surface of ECG leads 1, 2, and V_1 and an intracardiac electrogram from the bundle of His area (*HBE*) in a patient with infranodal conduction disturbance. The upper panel demonstrates a prolonged HV interval (85 msec), and the lower panel shows widening of the His spike and infranodal block or block below the bundle of His (*arrow*). *T*, Time lines.

TECHNIQUE OF PROGRAMMED VENTRICULAR STIMULATION

The stimulation protocol employed in electrophysiology laboratories varies with respect to the pulse width, amplitude, standard paced cycle lengths, and number of extrastimuli introduced. The standard techniques used in our laboratory will be presented as a model; and the effects of variations in protocol on sensitivity and specificity of arrhythmia induction and the predictive accuracy of drug testing will also be discussed.

Bipolar stimulation is employed, using a constant current source that generates a rectangular pulse wave of 1 msec duration and twice the late diastolic threshold in amplitude. Pacing modalities include ventricular drive pacing at cycle lengths of 800–300 msec for 15–30 seconds and the introduction of single, double, and triple ventricular extrastimuli during sinus rhythm and two paced cycle lengths (600 and 450 msec). After every eight sinus or paced ventricular complexes (S_1), a single extrastimulus (S_2) is introduced at progressively shorter coupling intervals from late diastole to the ventricular refractory period. This is repeated at each cycle length, and then double (S_2, S_3) and triple (S_2, S_3, S_4) ventricular extrastimuli are introduced in a similar fashion. For multiple extrastimuli the S_1, S_2 interval is set at 50–100 msec greater than the refractory period at a given cycle length. The S_2, S_3 and S_3, S_4 extrastimulus coupling intervals are initially set equal to the S_1, S_2 coupling interval. The coupling interval of the last extrastimulus (e.g., S_2, S_3) is then progressively reduced until it fails to capture, at which point the preceding extrastimulus coupling interval (S_1, S_2) is shortened until S_3 once again captures. This process is repeated until the first extrastimulus (S_2) reaches its refractory period, and the whole procedure is repeated at another cycle length.[18] Not only are multiple cycle lengths used, but the protocol is applied at two right ventricular sites (the apex and outflow tract) and if necessary at one left ventricular site. The responses to programmed ventricular stimulation are as follows:

1. *Intraventricular reentrant responses:* Ventricular complexes induced by extrastimuli not involving reentry within the bundle branches.
2. *Nonsustained ventricular tachycardia:* Ventricular tachycardia lasting longer than 5 intraventricular reentrant responses and less than 30 seconds.
3. *Sustained ventricular tachycardia:* Ventricular tachycardia lasting longer than 30 seconds or requiring cardioversion due to hemodynamic compromise before 30 seconds.

If intraventricular reentrant responses or nonsustained or sustained ventricular tachycardia is induced, the protocol is repeated to demonstrate reproducibility, unless the patient requires cardioversion. Induction reproducibility is a critical requirement to ensure that the induced arrhythmia is not artifactual and that the lack of any intraventricular reentrant responses or ventricular tachycardia after drug intervention represents a drug effect.

When a ventricular tachyarrhythmia is induced, the patient's blood pressure response and clinical condition are intensively monitored, and the tachycardia is observed for 30 seconds to establish whether or not it is sustained. If there are signs of hemodynamic compromise (angina, hypotension, or syncope) the tachycardia is immediately terminated by programmed ventricular stimulation or cardioversion. Since most sustained ventricular tachycardia has a reentrant mechanism, programmed ventricular stimulation is frequently successful in terminating the tachycardia (65%–80% of cases.)[17] The most effective mode of termination is rapid ventricular pacing, although single, double, and sometimes triple ventricular extrastimuli can terminate the tachycardia.[20] Cardioversion always must be readily available as a backup modality because in up to 10% of the patients undergoing programmed stimulation, particularly with double extrastimuli or rapid pacing, the tachycardia may accelerate or degenerate to ventricular fibrillation.[16,17]

The use of both multiple cycle lengths and multiple sites of stimulation increases the sensitivity of the stimulation protocol for inducing a ventricular tachyarrhythmia.[14,21] The ability to induce a reentrant arrhythmia depends on the delivery of a critically timed extrastimulus, usually closely coupled to the previous stimulus, that dissociates conduction and refractoriness in the reentrant pathways. This in turn depends on the refractoriness and conduction characteristics of the intervening tissue between the site of stimulation and reentrant circuit and the tissue immediately surrounding the circuit. Factors that shorten the conduction time (proximity of the stimulation site to the circuit) or the refractoriness (shorter paced cycle lengths) of the intervening tissue will increase the likelihood of delivering an appropriately timed extrastimulus. The effects of cycle length on the abnormal tissue near the reentrant circuit is less predictable, so that multiple cycle lengths ensure a better chance of preventing entrance or exit block into or out of the reentrant circuit. Clearly, straight pacing allows uniformity of cycle lengths and obviates "long-short" cycle phenomena that occur in patients with frequent spontaneous ventricular premature depolarizations (VPDs) and that can artifactually induce repetitive responses.

Another method for altering conduction and refractoriness to facilitate induction of ventricular tachyarrhythmias is the use of isoproterenol infusions. The infusion is administered until the heart rate increases by 50% of the control or to a range of 130–150 beats/min. If the infusion alone does not induce ventricular tachyarrhythmias, programmed ventricular stimulation is repeated at one right ventricular site. Using this technique, ventricular tachyarrhythmias (sustained and nonsustained) were inducible in 75%–85% of patients in whom no arrhythmias were inducible by programmed ventricular stimulation alone.[22]

Programmed ventricular stimulation is highly effective in inducing ventricular tachyarrhythmias in patients with clinically documented sustained and nonsustained ventricular tachycardia and ventricular fibrillation. The arrhythmias can be reproducibly initiated in 80%–95% of patients.[23] Of the stimulation modes, single (20%–35%) and double (45%–60%) ventricular extrastimuli are the most commonly effective.[14] In addition, almost 90% of patients will have arrhythmias induced with right ventricular stimulation, and less than 10% require left ventricular stimulation.[14]

RELATION OF THE INDUCED VENTRICULAR TACHYARRHYTHMIA TO THE CLINICAL ARRHYTHMIA

For selection of antiarrhythmic therapy based on the response of the induced ventricular tachyarrhythmia to drugs to rational, it must be closely related to the clinically occurring arrhythmia. It has been well documented for patients with recurrent sustained ventricular tachycardia that the tachycardia induced by programmed stimulation is almost identical in cycle length and morphology to that observed clinically.[24]

Although other tachycardias are also inducible in the electrophysiology laboratory, they usually occur after antiarrhythmic drug administration or when programmed ventricular stimulation is performed during the induced arrhythmia in an effort to terminate it.[15,16] An example of this is shown in Figure 6-2 where burst pacing applied during ventricular tachycardia alters the tachycardia morphology. Many of these so-called nonclinical forms that are induced by programmed ventricular stimulation appear clinically if patients are monitored by telemetry or Holter monitoring for long durations.[14] Perhaps the clinical form is only the most stable configuration of the ventricular tachycardia so that on random sampling with a 12-lead ECG or single Holter monitor the clinical form is the most likely to be recorded. An inducible tachycardia, especially if it polymorphic, that differs completely from the clinically observed one and requires extraordinary measures for induction (3–4 extrastimuli at short paced cycle lengths) may be artifactual.[25]

SENSITIVITY AND SPECIFICITY OF PROGRAMMED VENTRICULAR STIMULATION

The applicability of programmed ventricular stimulation as a screening procedure in patients at high risk for sudden death depends on its sensitivity and specificity for identifying patients with clinical ventricular tachyarrhythmias. For the technique outlined above, excluding triple ventricular extrastimuli (i.e., single and double ventricular extrastimuli during three cycle lengths and at two sites in the right ventricle and one site in the left ventricle) in patients with documented or suspected sustained ventricular tachycardia, the sensitivity and specificity are 95% or greater.[24] As a number of recent studies have suggested, however, sensitivity and specificity of programmed ventricular stimulation for identifying patients with sustained ventricular tachyarrhythmias depends on a number of factors, including variation in the stimulation technique, clinical setting, type of underlying organic heart disease, and characteristics of the clinically observed arrhythmia.

The addition of a third extrastimulus at 1.5–2 times the diastolic threshold increases the sensitivity for right ventricular stimulation alone, but does not significantly alter sensitivity for double extrastimuli from both the right and left ventricle.[26] There is also no decrease in specificity with the third extrastimulus. The addition of a fourth extrastimulus has no effect on the sensitivity of the programmed ventricular stimulation but significantly reduces its specificity by causing induction of nonclinically observed ventricular tachyarrhythmias, specifically

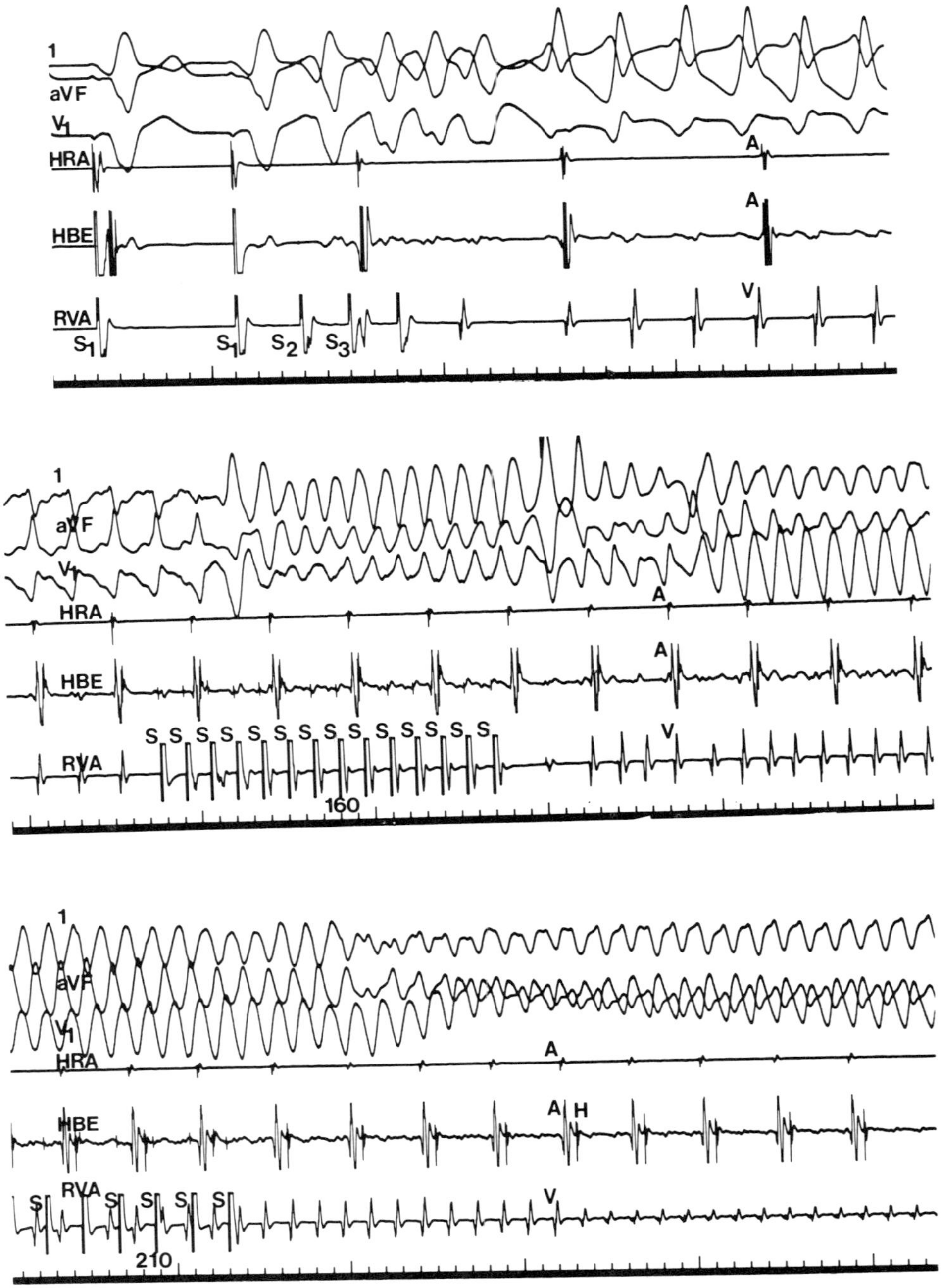

Fig. 6-2. Analog records from a patient with inducible sustained ventricular tachycardia. Surface ECG leads 1, aVF, and V_1 and intracardiac electrograms from the high right atrium (*HRA*), bundle of His region (*HBE*), and right ventricular apex (*RVA*) are recorded. Sustained ventricular tachycardia is induced with double ventricular extrastimuli, showing a nonspecific intraventricular conduction defect, right axis configuration (*upper panel*). Overdrive pacing (cycle length equals 160 msec) at the RVA during the tachycardia accelerates the tachycardia and alter its morphology to a right bundle, right axis configuration (*middle panel*). Repeat overdrive pacing (cycle length equals 210 msec) does not alter the morphology but does accelerate the tachycardia (*lower panel*).

polymorphic nonsustained ventricular tachycardia and ventricular fibrillation.[27] Increasing the stimulus strength by altering either the current amplitude or duration again adds nothing to sensitivity of programmed ventricular stimulation but significantly reduces the specificity. At 20 mA, with double extrastimuli polymorphic nonsustained ventricular tachycardia and ventricular fibrillation were induced in patients with documented sustained, uniform morphology ventricular tachycardia.[27]

The patient's clinical setting clearly influences the sensitivity and specificity of programmed ventricular stimulation. The specificity of programmed ventricular stimulation is low in patients with chronic coronary artery disease and no clinically documented or suspected ventricular tachyarrhythmias,[25,28,29] and it is even lower in the early postinfarction period.[28] The sensitivity of programmed ventricular stimulation is much reduced in patients with the long QT syndrome and ventricular tachyarrhythmias (usually polymorphic nonsustained ventricular tachycardia) whether they are idiopathic, drug related, or caused by transient metabolic disturbances.[14] Also, exercise-induced ventricular tachycardia is almost never inducible by programmed ventricular stimulation.[30]

The sensitivity of programmed ventricular stimulation in patients with clinically documented ventricular tachyarrhythmias also depends on the patient's underlying organic heart disease. In patients with coronary artery disease and left ventricular aneurysms, the sensitivity of programmed ventricular stimulation is approximately 95%.[24] It is somewhat lower in patients without organic heart disease (79%)[31] and is much lower in patients with cardiomyopathies and valvular heart disease (50%–65%).[32] Furthermore, in young patients with normal hearts, ventricular tachycardia is commonly not inducible.[33]

Finally, the electrophysiologic characteristics of the clinically observed arrhythmia influence the sensitivity of programmed ventricular stimulation. Patients with observed uniform morphology, sustained ventricular tachycardia have a 90%–95% inducibility rate, particularly if there is underlying heart disease.[24,31] The primary induced arrhythmia in this category is sustained ventricular tachycardia (91%). For patients with clinically documented, nonsustained ventricular tachycardia (monomorphic) the inducibility rate is 62%–80%[24,34] with about equal percentages of sustained and nonsustained ventricular tachycardia being induced. For patients with ventricular fibrillation observed during resuscitation, the sensitivity of programmed ventricular stimulation for induction of any ventricular tachyarrhythmia is 43%–83%, and the sensitivity for induction of ventricular fibrillation is quite low (0%–13%).[13,35] Many patients have no inducible ventricular tachyarrhythmia, and the overwhelming majority of those with inducible arrhythmias have rapid, monomorphic, sustained ventricular tachycardia that causes hemodynamic compromise.

ELECTROPHYSIOLOGIC DRUG TESTING

Once reproducible induction of a ventricular tachyarrhythmia is established, the impact of antiarrhythmic drugs on the reentrant circuit can be tested by programmed ventricular stimulation. If ventricular tachycardia that was previously inducible can no longer be induced after drug administration, the drug has rendered the reentrant circuit incapable of sustaining the arrhythmia and the drug should be clinically effective.[18] Most of the standard antiarrhythmic agents will be effective only if they interfere with the reentrant circuit. These drugs cannot totally eradicate the ambient ventricular ectopic activity that triggers the ventricular tachyarrhythmias. The efficacy of these agents therefore can be thoroughly evaluated with programmed ventricular stimulation and serial drug testing. In this way drug failure, as well as success, can be rapidly identified.[18] Newer, experimental agents (e.g., amiodarone and sotalol) are such effective suppressants of ambient ventricular ectopic activity that they also may be effective by eliminating the triggering phenomenon; this can only be tested by serial ambulatory monitoring and long-term clinical observation. Electrophysiologic drug testing may have a lower predictive accuracy for such agents.[36,37]

The technique of electrophysiologic drug testing is standardized. After discontinuing all antiarrhythmic agents for 5 half-lives, the patient undergoes baseline electrophysiologic evaluation, including the standard ventricular stimulation protocol. Reproducible induction of the ventricular arrhythmia is established by repeated initiation with the same or similar stimulation modes (although extrastimulus coupling intervals may vary), and a drug is given parenterally. Programmed ventricular stimulation is then repeated until the arrhythmia is induced or the standard stimulation protocol is completed. A plasma sample for drug-level determination is obtained at the time of the demonstrated electrophysiologic effect. An oral drug regimen is devised to achieve plasma levels greater than or equal to that shown to be effective actutely, and programmed ventricular stimulation is repeated after 5 half-lives, at the time of a trough plasma level, to confirm the efficacy of the oral regimen.[18,37]

Analog records from a serial drug study in a patient with inducible sustained ventricular tachycardia is shown in Figure 6-3. Although procainamide, mexiletine, and quinidine fail to prevent induction of ventricular tachycardia, amiodarone or a combination of quinidine and mexiletine are effective.

Drug efficacy using programmed ventricular stimulation is defined as prevention of induction of sustained and nonsustained ventricular tachycardia and fibrillation by the complete standard stimulation protocol (up to three extrastimuli during three cycle lengths at two right ventricular sites). No more than five repetitive responses can be reproducibly induced for a drug to be considered successful. Altering the mode of induction to a less physiologic one (e.g., double to triple

---

Fig. 6-3. Analog records from serial drug testing in a patient with inducible sustained ventricular tachycardia. In each panel surface ECG leads V_1, aVF, and 1 and an intracardiac electrogram from either the right ventricular apex (*RVA*) or right ventricular outflow tract (*RVOT*) are recorded. In the control state (*upper panel*) triple ventricular extrastimuli (S_2, S_3, S_4) introduced during pacing at a cycle length of 450 msec induced sustained ventricular tachycardia. Procainamide (*second panel*), mexiletine (*third panel*), and quinidine (*fourth panel*) all failed to prevent induction of sustained ventricular tachycardia, although quinidine substantially slowed the rate. The combination of mexiletine and quinidine (*fifth panel*), as well as amiodarone (*sixth panel*), did prevent induction of ventricular tachycardia with the complete stimulation protocol, including triple ventricular extrastimuli, during pacing at a cycle length of 450 msec.

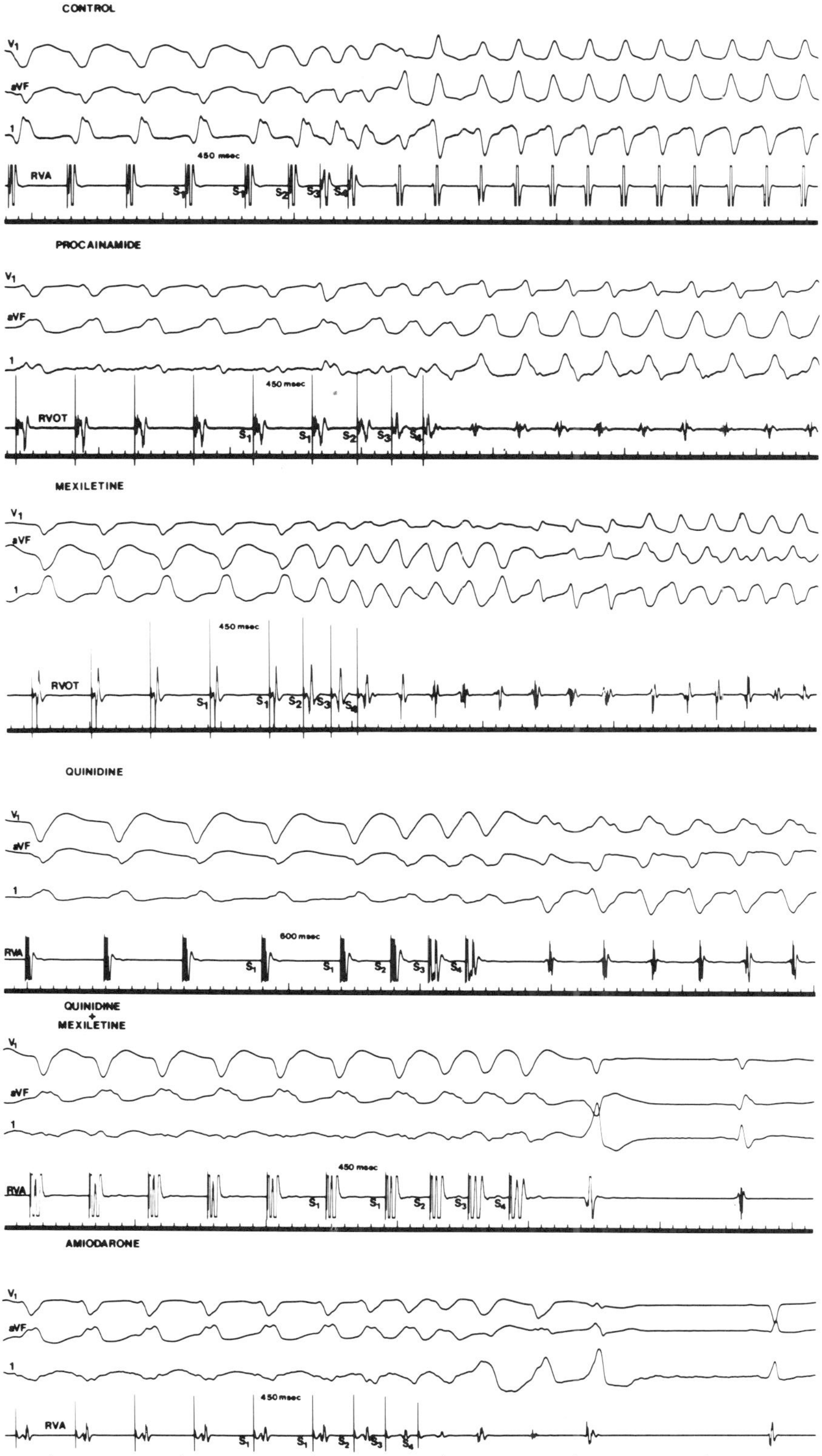

CONTROL
V1
aVF
1
450 msec
RVA
PROCAINAMIDE
450 msec
RVOT
MEXILETINE
450 msec
RVOT
QUINIDINE
600 msec
RVA
QUINIDINE
+
MEXILETINE
450 msec
RVA
AMIODARONE
450 msec
RVA

extrastimulii), narrowing the tachycardia zone, or changing the duration of the induced arrhythmia (e.g., from sustained to nonsustained ventricular tachycardia) has not correlated with drug efficacy.[14]

Ultimately, the most important index of drug efficacy is the ability to successfully prevent future clinical recurrences of the ventricular arrhythmia. Programmed ventricular stimulation is an excellent predictor of drug efficacy. With only standard antiarrhythmic agents, the predictive value for successful prevention of clinical sustained ventricular tachycardia is 93%, the predictive value for clinical recurrence is 90%, and the overall predictive accuracy is 92%.[38] The positive predictive value of programmed ventricular stimulation in resuscitated patients for prevention of recurrent cardiac arrest is equally high (90%–100%), but the negative predictive value is much lower (40%–50%).[13,35]

The experimental antiarrhythmic drugs are changing the predictive value of programmed ventricular stimulation, however. For amiodarone, which may suppress ventricular tachyarrhythmias by either interfering with the reentrant circuit or by eradicating the ambient ventricular ectopic activity, programmed ventricular stimulation still has a very high positive predictive value (approaching 100%) but a low negative predictive value (33.3%) for recurrence of ventricular arrhythmias.[36] A little over half of the patients receiving amiodarone who have arrhythmias reinduced with programmed ventricular stimulation have no subsequent clinical recurrence, perhaps because all the triggering phenomena are wiped out and the consequence of this cannot be tested by programmed ventricular stimulation.

PACING MODALITIES FOR TERMINATION OF VENTRICULAR TACHYARRHYTHMIAS

Besides severe infranodal conduction disturbances, the rationale for using pacemakers in the treatment of patients at high risk for sudden death is based on the inducibility of a reentrant ventricular tachyarrhythmia. Reentrant arrhythmias can be terminated by a critically timed extrastimulus that prematurely captures a portion of the circuit and renders it refractory to the oncoming reentrant wave front. By performing programmed ventricular stimulation during the induced ventricular tachyarrhythmia, the specific site and modality of pacing that most reliably and safely terminates the arrhythmia can be determined, and thus the characteristics of successful pacer therapy can be defined.

In addition to identifying a safe and effective pacing modality, programmed ventricular stimulation allows one to test three other prerequisites that must be met for the application of pacer therapy. First, the patient must tolerate the ventricular tachyarrhythmia hemodynamically so that the pacing modality can be activated. Second, the patient must readily recognize when the ventricular tachyarrhythmia is present and when it is terminated in order to appropriately inactivate the pacer. Finally, the effective pacing modality must be applicable at a technically feasible site of pacing (e.g., the right ventricular apex).

The modes of ventricular stimulation that terminate reentrant arrhythmias include the introduction of single and double extrastimuli and rapid overdrive pacing.[20,39,40] Sustained ventricular tachycardia can be terminated in 80% of the cases by programmed stimulation; only 20% require cardioversion.[14] Overdrive pacing is the most frequently successful modality for terminating ventricular tachyarrhythmias,[41] although single and double extrastimuli are also effective. If single VPDs can terminate the arrhythmia, then underdrive pacing (pacing at rates substantially slower than the ventricular tachyarrhythmia) will be effective. If two or more extrastimuli are required to terminate the ventricular tachyarrhythmia, then overdrive pacing (pacing at rates faster than the ventricular tachyarrhythmia) will be required for termination.[15] The importance of this distinction lies in the potentially life-threatening side effect that sometimes occurs with overdrive pacing: acceleration of the ventricular tachyarrhythmia culminating in hemodynamic compromise and syncope or degeneration to ventricular fibrillation.[43] Thus overdrive pacing thus can only be used when physicians and defibrillation equipment are immediately available and cannot be used as an outpatient therapeutic modality. On the other hand, underdrive pacing can be readily applied on an outpatient basis, using a patient-activated radiofrequency pacemaker.

In general, the applicable pacing modality can be predicted from certain electrophysiologic characteristics of the arrhythmia. If the rate of the ventricular tachyarrhythmia is less than 150 beats/min or the site of origin is close to the stimulation site (e.g., septal infarct and right ventricular apex stimulation), it can be terminated by a single VPD, or underdrive, pacing. If, however, the rate of the ventricular tachyarrhythmia is greater than 170/beats/min or its site of origin is remote from the stimulation site, termination will require double VPDs, or overdrive, pacing.[15] Occasionally, a drug can significantly slow a ventricular tachyarrhythmia to less than 170 beats/min (e.g., type IA antiarrhythmic agents, mexiletine, and amiodarone), rendering it susceptible to termination by a single ventricular extrastimulus. Combined drug and pacing therapy can be very effective and convenient, obviating the need for more experimental therapeutic modalities.[41]

Newer pacing modalities have been examined to determine their ability to terminate ventricular tachyarrhythmias. Introduction of extrastimuli during ventricular tachycardia at higher current strengths (5 and 10 mA) has increased the effectiveness of pacing, particularly for faster tachycardias that require VPDs introduced at shorter coupling intervals to interfere with the reentrant wave front.[42] Increasing the current strength shortens the ventricular effective refractory period, allowing extrastimuli to get to the reentrant circuit early enough to terminate the arrhythmia. Another modality which has improved the efficacy of pacing therapy in selected cases is the introduction of ventricular extrastimuli during overdrive pacing that captures the ventricle by pacing at cycle lengths 30–50 msec shorter than that of the ventricular arrhythmia.[43]

Two new modalities are being perfected that may radically alter the application of electrical/pacing therapy for ventricular tachyarrhythmias. The internal cardioverter, which is just starting clinical trials, terminates ventricular tachycardia by applying a 0.05–5 joule shock between leads on a specially designed catheter with large surface area poles.[44] The pulse generator circuitry allows recognition of the ventricular tachyarrhythmia and will spontaneously trigger the caridoverter output. The internal cardioverter also has the advantage of rarely accelerating the ventricular tachyarrhythmia, but will have a backup defibrillation mode for such an eventuality. Figure 6-4 demonstrates the comparative efficacy of

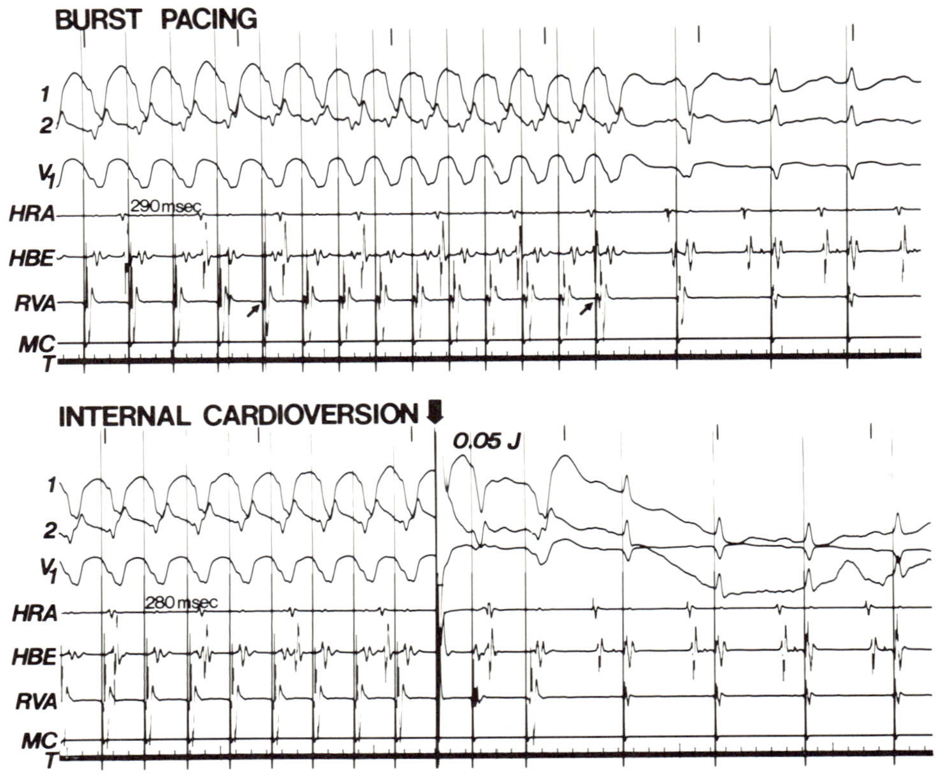

Fig. 6-4. Termination of sustained ventricular tachycardia by two electrical modalities. Surface ECG leads 1, 2, and V_1 and intracardiac electrograms from the high right atrium (*HRA*), bundle of His region (*HBE*), and right ventricular apex (*RVA*) are recorded along with the marker channel (*MC*) from the internal cardioverter and time lines (*T*). Sustained, uniform morphology ventricular tachycardia was induced and recorded in both panels. In the upper panel overdrive pacing was initiated at the arrow and terminates the tachycardia after 10 complexes (*second arrow*). In the lower panel internal cardioversion was successfully performed with a 0.05-joule shock delivered at the arrow and terminates the tachycardia.

burst pacing and internal cardioversion for termination of sustained ventricular tachycardia. The tachycardia is easily terminated by a relatively low-energy shock, 0–0.05 joule, without untoward effects.

The other development, which is farther along in clinical trials, is the automatic implantable cardioverter defibrillator. It consists of an electrode net applied epicardially, transvenous electrodes in the ventricle and atrium, and a generator that senses ventricular fibrillation and delivers a 25-joule output for defibrillation after a 30-second delay to allow for loss of consciousness. This device is particularly useful in patients with drug-resistant ventricular flutter that causes syncope or ventricular fibrillation.[45] These two new devices, which do not depend on the patient remaining conscious during the arrhythmia, will have wider application than standard pacing modalities in the future.

ELECTROPHYSIOLOGICALLY DIRECTED SURGICAL THERAPY FOR VENTRICULAR TACHYARRHYTHMIAS

Except for emergent infarctectomy in the setting of recurrent ventricular fibrillation complicating an acute myocardial infarction, surgical therapy for ventricular tachyarrhythmias before the application of electrophysiologic techniques has had a poor outcome. The surgical mortality associated with aneurysectomy or coronary artery bypass grafting performed for ventricular tachycardia has been high both in perioperative and late postoperative phases, and the cure rate for ventricular tachyarrhythmias has been low (40%–58%).[46] The low cure rate for such unguided surgical therapy may be related to its failure to excise or interrupt the reentrant circuit. Recently, endocardial mapping techniques have demonstrated that the site of origin of reentrant ventricular tachycardia in patients with coronary artery disease and left ventricular aneurysms is not in the aneurysm itself, but is located within a rim of viable tissue 1–2 cm of the border of the aneurysm,[47] a region not excised during clinical aneurysectomy. Based on this information, a new surgical technique was developed that uses preoperative catheter and intraoperative endocardial mapping to localize the site of origin of the ventricular tachycardia and direct endocardial resection of the specified region. The results with the endocardial resection technique are strikingly improved.[48]

Localization of the site of origin by endocardial mapping is based on the hypothesis that during ventricular tachycardia the electrical wave front emanates from the reentrant circuit and spreads over the endocardium, eventually invades the Purkinje system, and spreads from the endocardium to the epicardium. The earliest site of activation on the endocardium should be closest to the site of origin.[49] By recording the electrical wave front as it passes specific locations, indicated by the intrinsic deflections of the local electrograms, and then time aligning all the electrograms relative to a fixed reference, the earliest region of electrical activation can be determined and the site of origin localized.[47,49] An example of such an endocardial map is shown in Figure 6-5, where analog records of the left ventricular activation patterns are recorded during ventricular tachycardia.

Catheter endocardial mapping is performed with a multipolar electrode catheter inserted retrogradely into the left ventricle, and at least on additional catheter usually is inserted at the right ventricular apex for a stable reference recording. During ventricular tachycardia, the left ventricular mapping catheter is moved to each of 12 predetermined sites, and the local electrograms are recorded. Ventricular tachycardia may have to be repeatedly induced, since it frequently terminates with catheter manipulation. The localization of each catheter position must be verified by biplane fluoroscopic visualization. The endocardial map is generated by time aligning the recordings from each site and determining the site with the earliest activation time.[49]

During ventricular tachycardia, the earliest endocardial site of activation generally precedes the onset of ventricular activation as indicated by the surface QRS activity. Recordings from the site of origin of the ventricular tachycardia near the border of an aneurysm typically show such presystolic activity with wide (> 60 msec) low-amplitude (<1 mV) fragmented electrograms. Depending on

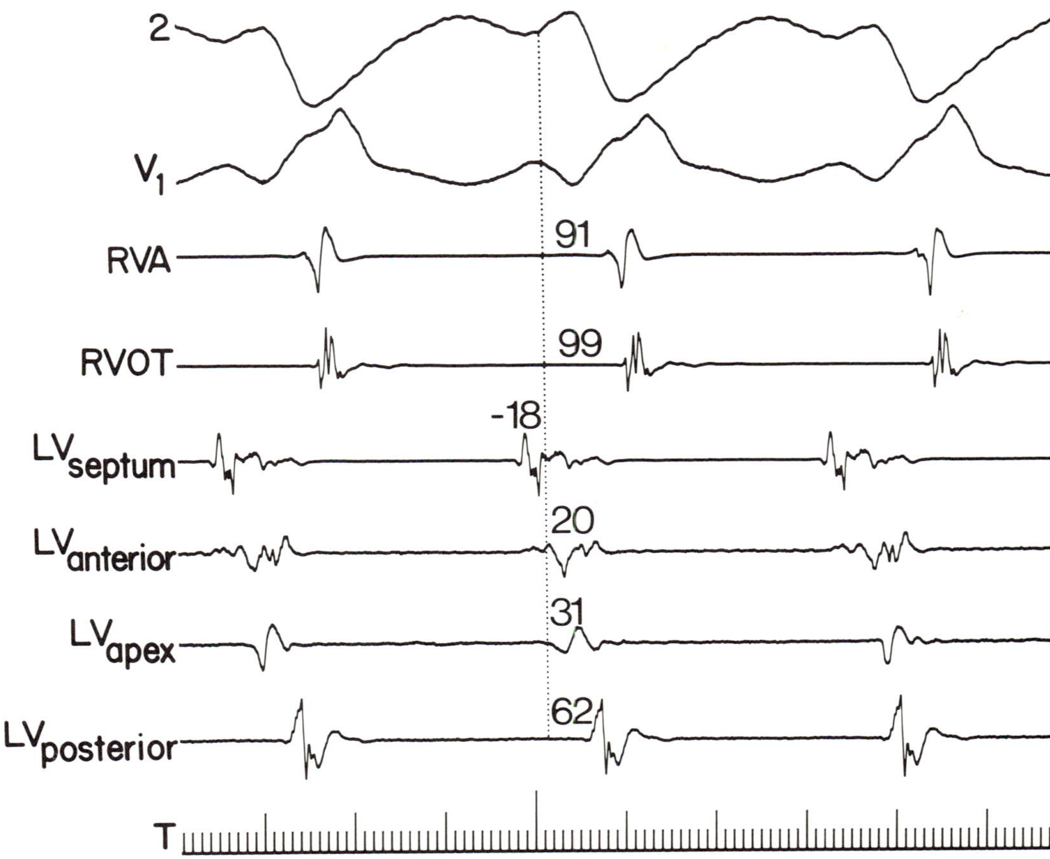

Fig. 6-5. An endocardial catheter map of the left ventricle during sustained ventricular tachycardia. Surface leads 2 and V_1 and intracardiac electrograms from the right ventricular apex (*RVA*), right ventricular outflow tract (*RVOT*), left ventricular septum (*LV septum*), left ventricular anterior wall (*LV anterior*), left ventricular apex (*LV apex*), and left ventricular posterior wall (*LV posterior*) were recorded sequentially and then time aligned on the same time axis. The activation times at each intracardiac site relative to the onset of surface QRS activity (*dotted perpendicular line*) are measured and recorded just above each electrogram. Earliest arrival of the electrical wave front during ventricular tachycardia occurs at the left ventricular septum 18 msec before the onset of surface QRS activity, which is 38 msec earlier than any other recorded site. This indicates that the left ventricular septal recording site is nearest the site of origin of the ventricular tachycardia. Note the increased width and fragmentation of the left ventricular septal electrogram that is frequently seen near the site of origin. *T,* Time lines.

catheter position, continuous electrical activity may be recorded throughout the cardiac cycle, which is believed to represent direct recording of the reentrant electrical wave front.[50]

Catheter endocardial mapping can localize the site of origin to a 4–8 cm^2 region in the ventricle.[47] Endocardial mapping with a hand-held probe has a higher resolution, however. During an aneurysectomy, similar multiple site recordings of endocardial electrical activity are made in concentric circles of increasing diameter from the edge of the clinical aneurysectomy. The recordings are time aligned in the operating room, and the earliest site of electrical activation during ventricular tachycardia is determined.[51] In this way, under direct visualization in the operating room, the site of origin can be localized to a 3–5 cm^2 region of the endocardium. Correlation between the two types of mapping is excellent.[47]

Data generated from both catheter and intraoperative endocardial mapping in conjunction with intraoperative epicardial mapping have demonstrated several interesting facts. First, in patients with coronary artery disease, previous myocardial infarctions, and left ventricular aneurysms, the site of origin of ventricular tachycardia is in the normal tissue within 1–2 cm from the border of the aneurysm,[48,52] whereas in patients with right ventricular dysplasia or ventricular tachycardia after repair of tetralogy of Fallot, the site of origin is in the right ventricle.[53] Second, surface ECG morphology of the ventricular tachycardia does not always correlate directly with the ventricular site of origin. In patients with coronary artery disease, left ventricular aneurysms, and ventricular tachycardia, almost all left bundle-branch block configuration tachycardias arise in the left ventricle.[47,54] This is understandable because the surface ECG morphology depends only on the epicardial activation pattern. A left ventricular site of origin, close to the septum, can generate a wave front that more rapidly penetrates the right ventricle, perhaps because of exit block to the left ventricle, resulting in a left bundle-branch block type of pattern. Third, multiple surface ECG morphologies of ventricular tachycardia do not necessarily imply multiple sites of origin.[54] Again, surface ECG morphology depends on an epicardial and in turn endocardial activation pattern. But a single site of origin can give rise to multiple endocardial and epicardial activation patterns due to differing exit points from a single reentrant circuit.

All these findings have practical implications for surgical therapy of ventricular tachycardia. The site of origin being in normal tissue near the border of the left ventricular aneurysm implies that the surgical approach must be more extensive than the clinical aneurysectomy, which leaves a rim of the aneurysm, in order to excise the site of origin. The fact that a left bundle-branch block configuration does not necessarily indicate a right ventricular site of origin means that an aneurysectomy in the left ventricle will be effective in treating patients with left bundle-branch block tachycardias and left ventricular aneurysms. Finally, surgical therapy can be applied in patients with multiple morphologies of ventricular tachycardia, as long as mapping identifies a single site of origin, and the left ventricle, after an aneurysectomy, is large enough to maintain normal left ventricular function.

The endocardial resection technique for therapy of ventricular tachycardia involves performance of a clinical aneurysectomy, followed by intraoperative endocardial mapping. When the site of origin of the ventricular tachycardia is adequately localized, the endocardium in that region is stripped from the myocardium and epicardium and excised.[55] The ventriculotomy is closed and coronary bypass grafting performed if indicated. Ten days postoperatively the patient undergoes repeat cardiac catheterization to evaluate left ventricular function and repeat programmed ventricular stimulation from the right and left ventricles to evalute the suppressant effect of surgery on the ventricular tachycardia.[48]

SUMMARY

The techniques of electorphysiologic evaluation of patients after resuscitation or at high risk for sudden death are aimed at identifying causative rhythm disturbances and then evaluating the three modalities of therapy for such rhythm disturbances. In addition to baseline recordings of the atrioventricular conduction system electrophysiologic characteristics, programmed ventricular stimulation is a key technique in both diagnosis and evaluation of antiarrhythmic drug and pacemaker therapy. The techniques are not yet standardized, and the sensitivity and specificity of programmed ventricular stimulation as a screening procedure for ventricular tachyarrhythmias will vary with differences in stimulation protocol, underlying heart disease, and clinically observed arrhythmias in the patients being studied. Programmed ventricular stimulation can be applied as well to arrhythmias other than recurrent sustained ventricular tachycardia and can be equally helpful in designing antiarrhythmic drug therapy for polymorphic nonsustained ventricular tachycardia and ventricular fibrillation. Failure to induce an arrhythmia in patients who have been resuscitated may indicate an acute intercurrent problem (drug-induced or metabolic derangement) that caused the spontaneous ventricular tachyarrhythmia. Despite this, a lack of inducibility of a ventricular tachyarrhythmia may not predict a lower recurrence risk for a sudden cardiac event. Finally, if drugs and pacer therapy are unsuccessful, endocardial mapping may be used to investigate the feasibility of surgical therapy. In the future, programmed stimulation also will be useful in evaluating patients for therapy with the internal cardioverter.

REFERENCES

1. Kuller L: Sudden death in arteriosclerotic heart disease: The case for preventive medicine. Am. J. Cardiol. 24:617–628, 1969.
2. Goldstein S: Sudden Death and Coronary Heart Disease. Mt Kisco, New York, Futura Publishing Co Inc, 1974, p 5
3. Myerberg RJ, Conde CA, Sung RJ, et al: Clinical electrophysiologic and hemodynamic profile of patients resuscitated from pre-hospital cardiac arrest. Am J Med 68:568, 1980.
4. Josephson ME, Horowitz LN, Greenspan AM, et al: Electrophysiologic findings in patients suffering cardiac arrest. Am J Cardiol 45:406, 1980
5. Ruskin JN, DiMarco JP, Garan H: Out-of-hospital cardiac arrest: Electrophysiologic observations and selection of long-term anti-arrhythmic therapy. N Engl J Med 303:607, 1980
6. Cobb LA, Werner JA, Trobangh GB: Sudden cardiac death: A decade's experience with out-of-hospital resuscitation. Mod Concepts Cardiovasc Dis 49:31, 1980
7. Josephson ME, Seides SF: Clinical Cardiac Electrophysiology: Techniques and Interpretations. Philadelpha, Lea & Febiger, 1979, p 24
8. Scheinman MM, Peters RW, Moding, et al: Prognostic value of infranodal conduction time in patients with chronic bundle branch block. Circulation 56:240, 1977
9. Gupta PK, Lichstein E, Chadda KD: Chronic His bundle block: Clinical, electrocardiographic, electrophysiolo-

gical and follow-up studies on 16 patients. Br Heart J 38:1343, 1976

10. Guimond C, Puech P: Intra-His bundle blocks (102 cases). Eur J Cardiol 4:481, 1976
11. Dhingra RC, Wyndham C, Bauernfeind R, et al: Significance of block distal to the His bundle induced by atrial pacing in patients with chronic bifascicular block. Circulation 60: 1455, 1979
12. Tonkin AM, Heddle WF, Tornos P: Intermittent AV block: Procainamide administration as a provocative test. Aust NZ J Med 8:594, 1978
13. Bendett DG, Benson DW Jr, Klein GJ, et al: Prevention of recurrent sudden cardiac arrest: Role of provocative electropharmacologic testing. JACC 2:418, 1983
14. Horowitz LN, Josephson ME, Kastor JA: Intracardiac electrophysiologic studies as a method for the optimization of drug therapy in chronic ventricular arrhythmia. Prog Cardiovasc Dis 23:81, 1980
15. Josephson ME, Horowitz LN, Farshidi A, et al: Recurrent sustained ventricular tachycardia. I. Mechanisms. Circulation 57:431, 1978
16. Mason JW, Winkle RA: Electrode-catheter arrhythmia induction in the selection and assessment of antiarrhythmic drug therapy for recurrent ventricular tachycardia. Circulation 58:971, 1978
17. Fisher JD, Mehra R, Furman S: Termination of ventricular tachycardia with bursts of rapid ventricular pacing. Am J Cardiol 41:94, 1978
18. Horowitz LN, Josephson ME, Farshidi A, et al: Recurrent sustained ventricular tachycardia. III. Role of the electrophysiologic study in selection of antiarrhythmia regimens. Circulation 58: 986, 1978
19. Ruskin JN, Garan H: Chronic electrophysiologic testing in patients with recurrent sustained ventricular tachycardia. Am J Cardiol 43:400, 1979
20. Josephson ME, Horowitz LN: Electrophysiologic approach to therapy of recurrent sustained ventricular tachycardia. Am J Cardiol 43:631, 1979
21. Doherty JU, Kienzle MG, Waxman HL, et al: Programmed ventricular stimulation at a second right ventricular site: Sensitivity, specificity, and characteristics of patients with induced ventricular tachycardia. Am J Cardiol 52:1184, 1983
22. Reddy CP, Gettes LS: Use of isoproterenol as an aid to electric induction of chronic recurrent ventricular tachycardia. Am J Cardiol 44:705, 1979
23. Wellen HJJ, Durrer DR, Lie KI: Observations on mechanisms of ventricular tachycardia in man. Circulation 54:237, 1976
24. Vandepol CJ, Farshidi A, Spielman SR, et al: Incidence and clinical significance of induced ventricular tachycardia. Am J Cardiol 45:725, 1980
25. Scheinman MM, Morady F, Shen EN, et al: Relevance of site of stimulation and number of extrastimuli. International Workshop— New Progress in the Identification of Patients at Risk of Ventricular Tachyarrhythmias, Altenburg, Germany, 1983, p 7a
26. Buxton AE, Waxman HL, Marchlinski FE, et al: Role of triple extrastimuli during electrophysiologic study of patients with documented sustained ventricular tachyarrhythmias. Circulation 69:532, 1984
27. Brugada P, Green M, Abdollah H, et al: Significance of ventricular arrhythmias initiated by programmed ventricular stimulation: The importance of the type of ventricular arrhythmia induced and the number of premature stimuli required. Circulation 69:87, 1984
28. Borgreffe M, Haerton K, Breithardt G: Prognostic significance of programmed ventricular stimulation in patients with coronary artery disease. International Workshop—New Progress in the Identification of Patients at Risk of Ventricular Tachyarrhythmias, Altenburg, Germany, 1983, p 16
29. Rosanowski C, Borgreffe M, Brei-

thardt G: Preliminary results with the use of three and four premature stimuli during basic drive. International Workshop—New Progress in the Identification of Patients at Risk of Ventricular Tachyarrhythmias, Altenburg, Germany, 1983, p 8
30. Wu D, Kou H-C, Hung J-S: Exercise-triggered paroxysmal ventricular tachycardia. Ann Intern Med 95:410, 1981
31. Prystowski EN, Miles WM, Evans JJ, et al: Induction of ventricular tachycardia: relationship to clinical arrhythmia and type of heart disease. International Workshop—New Progress in the Identification of Patients at Risk of Ventricular Tachyarrhythmias, Altenburg, Germany, 1983, p 14
32. Naccarelli GV, Prystowsky EN, Jackman WM, et al: Role of electrophysiologic testing in managing patients who have ventricular tachycardia unrelated to coronary artery disease. Am J Cardiol 50:165, 1982
33. Pedersen DH, Zipes DP, Foster PR, et al: Ventricular tachycardia and ventricular fibrillation in a young population. Circulation 60:988, 1979
34. Spielman SR, Yacone LA, Greenspan AM, et al: Electrophysiologic testing in high risk patients with nonsustained ventricular tachycardia and abnormal ventricular function. Circulation 68 (suppl 3):56, 1983
35. Josephson ME, Horowitz LN, Spielman SR, et al: Electrophysiologic and hemodynamic studies in patients resusciated from cardiac arrest. Am J Cardiol 46:948, 1980
36. Horowitz LN, Spielman SR, Greenspan AM, et al: Utility of elecrophysiologic testing of amiodarone for ventricular tachyarrhythmias. Circulation 68 (suppl 3): 382, 1983
37. Mason JW, Winkle RA: Electrode-catheter arrhythmia induction in the selection and assessment of antiarrhythmic drug therapy for recurrent ventricular tachycardia. Circulation 58:971, 1978
38. Horowitz LN, Spielman SR, Greenspan AM, et al: Role of programmed stimulation in assessing vulnerability to ventricular arrhythmias. Am Heart J 103:604, 1982
39. Fisher JD, Cohen HL, Mehra R, et al: Cardiac pacing and pacemakers. II. Serial electrophysiologic-pharmacologic testing for control of recurrent tachyarrhythmias. Am Heart J 93:658, 1977
40. Fisher JD, Mehra R, Furman S: Termination of ventricular tachycardia with bursts of rapid ventricular pacing. Am J Cardiol 41:94, 1978
41. Wellens HJJ, Bar FWHM, Lie KI, et al: Effect of procainamide, propranolol, and verapamil on mechanism of tachycardia in patients with chronic recurrent ventricular tachycardia. Am J Cardiol 40:579, 1977
42. Waxman HL, Cain ME, Greenspan AM, et al: Termination of ventricular tachycardia with ventricular stimulation: Salutary effect of increased current strength. Circulation 65:800, 1982
43. Greenspan AM, Horowitz LN, Josephson ME, et al: Unpublished observation, 1980.
44. Yee R, Zipes DP, Gulamhusein S, et al: Low energy countershock using an intravascular catheter in an acute cardiac care setting. Am J Cardiol 50:1124, 1982
45. Mirowski M, Reid PR, Watkins, L, et al: Clinical treatment of life-threatening ventricular tachyarrhythmias with automatic implantable defibrillation. Am Heart J 102:265, 1981
46. Horowitz LN, Harken AH, Kastor JA, et al: Surgical treatment of ventricular arrhythmias in coronary artery disease. Ann Intern Med 95:88, 1981
47. Josephson ME, Horowitz LN, Spielman SR, et al: Comparison of endocardial catheter mapping with intraoperative mapping of ventricular tachycardia. Circulation 61:395, 1980
48. Horowitz LN, Harken AH, Kastor JA, et al: Ventricular resection guided by epicardial and endocardial mapping

for treatment of recurrent ventricular tachycardia. N Engl J Med 302:589, 1980

49. Josephson ME, Horowitz LN, Farshidi A: Recurrent sustained ventricular tachycardia. II. Endocardial mapping. Circulation 57: 440, 1978
50. Josephson ME, Horowitz LN, Farshidi A, et al: Continuous local electrical activity: A mechanism of ventricular tachycardia. Circulation 57:659, 1978
51. Horowitz LN, Josephson ME, Kastor JA, et al: Intraoperative epicardial and endocardial mapping of ventricular tachycardia in man. Am J Cardiol 43:401, 1979
52. Josephson ME, Hanken AH, Horowitz LN: Endocardial excision: A new surgical technique for the treatment of recurrent ventricular tachycardia. Circulation 60:1430, 1979
53. Horowitz LN, Vetter VL, Harken AH, et al: Electrophysiologic characteristics of sustained ventricular tachycardia occurring after repair of tetralogy of Fallot. Am J Cardiol 446:62, 1980
54. Josephson ME, Horowitz LN, Farshidi A, et al: Recurrent sustained ventricular tachycardia. IV. Pleomorphism. Circulation 59:459, 1979
55. Harken AH, Josephson ME, Horowitz LN: Surgical endocardial resection for the treatment of malignant ventricular tachycardia. Ann Surg 190:456, 1979

J. Thomas Bigger, Jr.
James Coromilas
Francis M. Weld
James A Reiffel
Linda M. Rolnitzky

7

IDENTIFICATION OF HIGH-RISK PATIENTS AFTER MYOCARDIAL INFARCTION: POINTERS FOR MANAGEMENT

Supported in part by NIH Grants HL-22982, HL-12738, and HL-70204 from the National Heart, Lung, and Blood Institute, Bethesda, Md.; by a Grant-in-Aid from the American Heart Association, Dallas; and by grants from the Winthrop and Chernow Foundations, New York.

In this chapter, we will deal with the identification of high- and low-risk patients after myocardial infarction. This discussion is focused on the period just before hospital discharge for several reasons. Hospital discharge is a time when the patient and the physician are concerned with the uncertainties of the first postinfarction year. All physicians and most patients know that the death rate is high in the year after myocardial infarction. The physician finds a predischarge evaluation of the patient useful for assessing risk and the functional capacity of patients. These findings can be translated into management decisions about level of activity, rehabilitation plans, further diagnostic tests, and medical or surgical treatment.

SUDDEN CARDIAC DEATH
0-8089-1725-0

FUNCTIONAL EVALUATION

Early efforts at risk stratification used a variety of risk indicators to relate to total or cause-specific mortality. In 1978 a new approach, functional evaluation, emerged.[1] With functional evaluation, risk is classified as an arrhythmia, ischemia or left ventricular dysfunction, and each category is assessed by special tests. The worth of this concept is only now being evaluated in detail, since studies that incorporate functional evaluation are just being completed and have not involved intervention trials to any great extent. The concept of risk stratification judged by clinical status at baseline and randomization in risk strata has been used. Studies now under way are using physiologic tests to stratify risks. For example, only very recent studies of antiarrhythmic drugs have selected patients who have arrhythmias for treatment. Earlier trials enrolled all postinfarction patients who lacked exclusion criteria for the trial drug.

COMPETING RISKS

Before discussing specific physiologic risk variables, we should discuss briefly the concept of competing risks as it applies to the coronary heart disease patient who has just suffered a myocardial infarction. Such patients are catego-

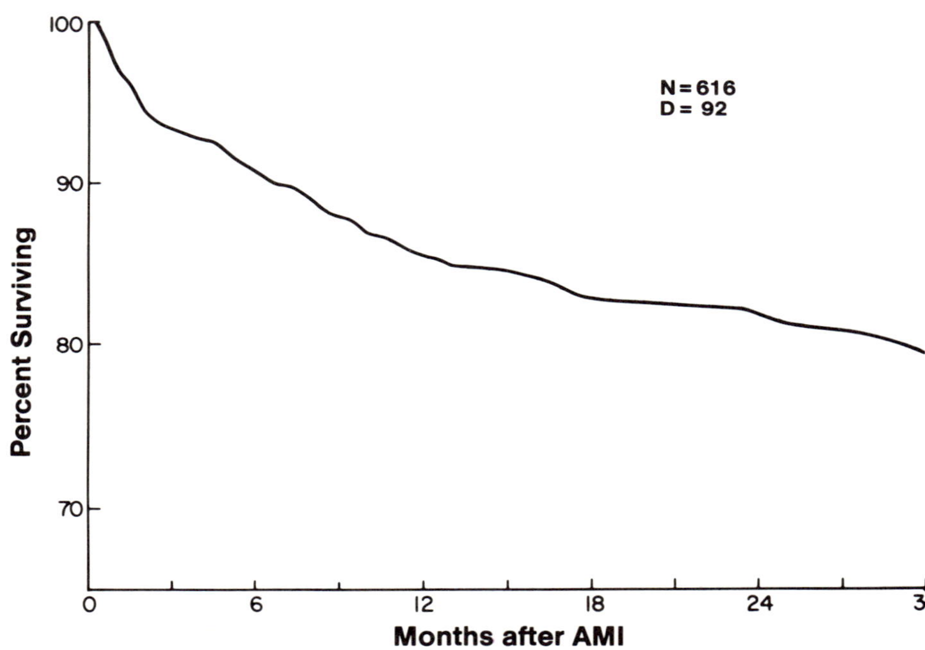

Fig. 7-1. Survivorship curve for 616 patients with definite acute myocardial infarction (*AMI*) followed up at The Presbyterian Hospital in the City of New York. In 30 months of follow-up, 92 deaths occurred; 55 deaths (60%) occurred within the first 6 months.

rized as being at low, intermediate, or high risk because of the presence and magnitude of arrhythmias, ischemia, or left ventricular dysfunction. Often one of these risk variables predominates, but all will be present to some extent and more than one may be clinically apparent. Left ventricular dysfunction and ischemia or left ventricular dysfunction and ventricular arrhythmias are two common combinations. It is reasonable to expect that patients in whom the arrhythmic risk predominates are most likely to die arrhythmia-related or sudden deaths. However, patients in whom arrhythmic risk predominates may die of ischemia-related causes. There is a severe problem in trying to link physiologic risk factors to functional mortality categories because the quality of the mortality information that is available even under the best of circumstances is usually inadequate. It is often difficult to ascribe the pathophysiologic sequences that lead to death even when the final episode occurs in the hospital under the view of skilled observers. To reconstruct the pathophysiologic sequence leading to death outside of the hospital is rarely possible. Even instantaneous death, which is equated with ventricular fibrillation, a paradigm of arrhythmic death, can be triggered by many different mechanisms: ischemia from coronary spasm, ischemia from tachycardia with fixed luminal obstruction, or scar-related ventricular tachycardia.

Despite these problems, functional categorization of risk factors and deaths has the best chance of accurately guiding our thinking and therapy.

TIME DISTRIBUTION OF DEATH AND REINFARCTION AFTER MYOCARDIAL INFARCTION

Mortality

The overall mortality between hospital discharge and the 1-year anniversary of infarction currently averages about 10%. The time distribution of the cumulative mortality is shown in Figure 7-1. About half of the deaths in the first year occur during the first 3 months, and about one third occur during the first 6 weeks.[2–6] The concentration of death and reinfarction in the first few weeks after discharge provides a strong rationale for predischarge evaluation of patients after infarction. The timing of common practices such as symptom-limited maximum exercise testing 3 or 4 months after infarction are questionable considering the number of postdischarge deaths and reinfarction events that occur in the first 3 months after infarction.

Moss et al.[7] categorized deaths as sudden or nonsudden as a function of time after myocardial infarction. There was an excess of nonsudden heart failure deaths in the 3 months after discharge. Thereafter, no factors measured before discharge could be identified that predicted the mode of death to be sudden or nonsudden. Even in the first few months, there were many sudden deaths.

Reinfarction

Figure 7-2 shows the time of nonfatal reinfarctions after the index myocardial infarction. It can be seen that reinfarction concentrates in the early postdischarge months even more than death. Again, the time distribution of reinfarction speaks

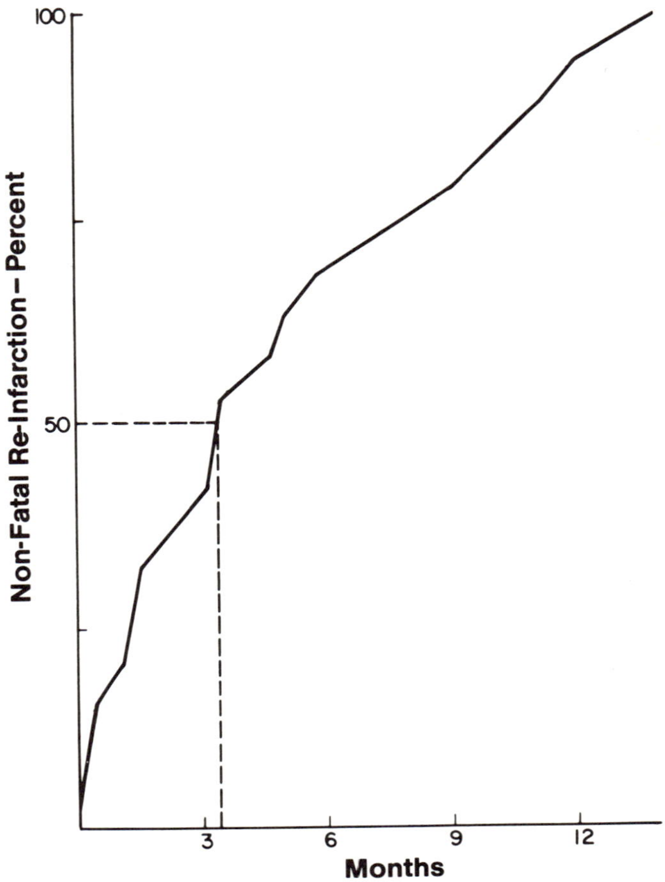

Fig. 7-2. Cumulative recurrence of nonfatal myocardial infarction in 866 patients followed up in the eight hospitals of the Multicenter Postinfarction Program. During 2 years of follow-up, almost half of the nonfatal reinfarctions occurred within the first 6 months.

for early detection of risk factors with predischarge diagnostic studies and early attempts to remove or neutralize the risks.

LEFT VENTRICULAR DYSFUNCTION

Clinical Measures

The degree of left ventricular dysfunction after myocardial infarction is closely related to the amount of myocardium rendered necrotic or severely ischemic.[8] Using radionuclide ventriculograms as a measure of left ventricular function, some abnormality can be detected in over 75% of patients with acute myocardial infarction, and patients with anterior wall infarctions have significantly lower left ventricular ejection fractions (EFs) than those with inferior infarctions.[9–11] About 50% of patients develop congestive heart failure as a manifestation of left ventricular dysfunction after infarction.[12] The Killip classification is the most widely used clinical scheme for the assessment of left ventricular function after acute myocardial infarction. In this system, shortly after admission to the cardiac care unit (CCU), patients are assigned to one of four arbitrary classes as follows: class I, no signs of heart failure; class II, mild or moderate heart failure with rales, an S_3 gallop, and pulmonary venous hypertension; class III, frank pulmonary edema; class IV, cardiogenic shock as defined by hypotension (systolic blood pressure < 90 mm Hg), peripheral vasoconstriction, and evidence of low blood flow (oliguria and impaired mental status). Using this classification in a series of 250 patients, Killip and Kimball[13] found that the incidence of life-threatening arrhythmias and in-hospital mortality increased markedly from classes I to IV. Other studies have confirmed that the presence of left ventricular dysfunction in the CCU assessed by clinical examination and chest x-ray findings is predictive of both in-hospital and late postdischarge mortality.[6,14,15] There is a relationship between the clinical findings and hemodynamic measurements of left ventricular dysfunction, but marked individual discrepancies are also noted.[12,16] Shell et al.[16] prospectively compared clinical signs of left ventricular dysfunction and hemodynamic measurements in 90 patients with evolving transmural myocardial infarction. All patients were studied within 12 hours of the onset of symptoms and before any therapy (other than morphine, oxygen, and lidocaine) was initiated. The clinical class was related to the pulmonary capillary wedge (PCW) pressure, with the mean PCW pressure increasing from 17 mm Hg in Killip class I patients to 22 in class II and 24 in classes III and IV patients. Despite this correlation, 13 of 43 Killip class I patients had a PCW pressure greater than 18, and 16 of 47 Killip classes II to IV patients had a PCW pressure less than or equal to 18 mm Hg. Individually the clinical classification did not reliably predict the PCW pressure. Also in this study, the PCW pressure was a much better predictor of early (30-day) mortality than was the clinical classification. The clinical evidence of the early left ventricular dysfunction disappears in over 60% of the patients by the time they are discharged from the CCU, although there is still considerable left ventricular dysfunction as measured by EF.[9,10,12,17] The presence of an enlarged heart on standard posteroanterior and lateral chest x-ray films at the time of discharge from the hospital is associated with a fivefold increased risk of dying in the following year.[14]

Left Ventricular Ejection Fraction

Utility of Ejection Fraction

The left ventricular ejection fraction (LVEF) is the best and most sensitive indicator of left ventricular dysfunction after myocardial infarction.[9–11] It has been shown with contrast ventriculography and radionuclide ventriculography that global LVEF is a good measure of infarct size.[18–20] The depression of LVEF reflects the cumulative loss of myocardium due to the index infarction, previous infarction, or other preexisting heart disease. In a subset of patients, some of the LVEF depression may be due to persistent yet reversible ischemic dysfunction[17] or to "stunned myocardium" that has been spontaneously reperfused but has not yet recovered mechanical function.[21] A low LVEF is the best single predictor of both early and late cardiac death after myocardial infarction.[9,11,22–25] An LVEF of 30% within 24 hours of acute myocardial infarction is associated with a 30%–55% in-hospital mortality.[11] For patients who survive to be discharged, LVEF of less than 30% is associated with a fivefold increased risk of dying in the year after discharge and a 1-year mortality of 35%.[23,24] Of the deaths in the year after infarction, 50% occur in this subset of patients with an LVEF less than 30%, and 70% of all the deaths are accounted for by an EF less than 40%.[23–25]

Variation with Time

Wackers et al.[26] have performed serial measurements of LVEF during the first 24 hours after myocardial infarction. They found that 56% of the patients had spontaneous changes in LVEF during the first 24 hours, with improvement occurring in 32% and deterioration occurring in 24% of the patients. The changes in LVEF ranged from a 32% absolute increase to a 14% absolute decrease. These spontaneous changes occurred most often in patients who had a low LVEF to begin with but could not be predicted by clinical variables. After the first 24 hours, the mean LVEF stabilizes and does not change during the hospital course or during the year after infarction.[9,10,27,28] Constancy of LVEF from 3 days to discharge has been shown by careful serial measurements of LVEF during hospitalization after acute myocardial infarction[10,27] (Figure 7-3). Similarly, the constancy of LVEF from time of discharge to 6–14 months after discharge has been demonstrated.[28] Although the group means do not change (Table 7-1), about 50% of the patients have a significant change in EF during hospitalization. Of the patients who have a change in EF, about one half will show significant improvement and the other half will show deterioration. The changes in EF tend to occur within the first few days after infarction, with any subsequent changes being less common and usually in the same direction as the initial changes.[27] Even in patients who demonstrate these changes in global LVEF, the regional wall motion did not change in the sequential studies, suggesting that sequential changes in LVEF are due largely to changes in loading conditions of the ventricle rather than to changes in intrinsic ventricular function.[27] Only the initial LVEF and not any sequential changes in LVEF was predictive of early (30-day) mortality and morbidity (due to congestive heart failure and conduction disturbances).[27]

Early Measurement of Ejection Fraction

Because the LVEF does not vary significantly after the first 24 hours of myocardial infarction, we recommend obtaining radionuclide ventriculograms at about the time of discharge from the CCU, at 3–5 days after admission. Although many patients with a low EF die of progressive left ventricular failure, many of the deaths in the low EF group have arrhythmic or ischemic causes.[22–25] Since a low EF (< 30%) is also of prognostic value in predicting in-hospital morbidity and mortality, the determination of LVEF at 3–5 days becomes useful in identifying patients at high risk of developing congestive heart failure, hypotension, shock, or an extension of myocardial infarction.[11] It may be possible to prevent some of the morbidity and mortality in this group of patients when they are identified as having

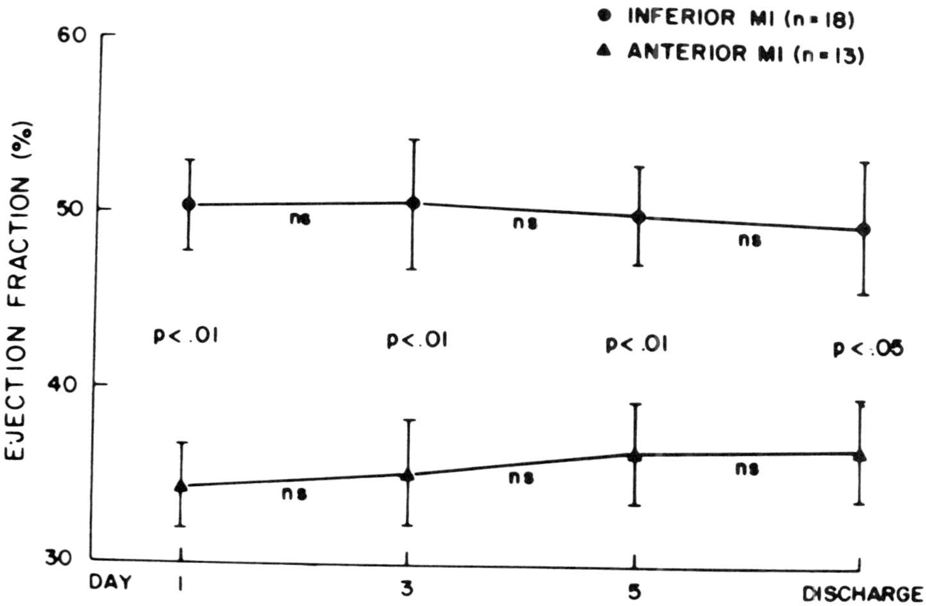

Fig. 7-3. Sequential measurement of left ventricular ejection fractions (*LVEF*) in patients with inferior and anterior wall myocardial infarction (*MI*). No significant sequential change occurs in LVEF from day 1 until discharge. From Reduto LA, Berger HJ, Cohen LS, et al: Sequential radionuclide assessment of left and right ventricular performance after acute transmural myocardial infarction. Ann Intern Med 89:441, 1978. With permission.

Table 7-1 *EF as a Function of Time after Myocardial Infarction*

Study	Number of Patients	Day 1	5–21 days before discharge	6 wk–20 mo after discharge
Schelbert et al.[9]	50	42 ± 2*	45 ± 2*	49 ± 1
Ramanathan et al.[17]	16	35 ± 11	38 ± 11	40 ± 9
Borer et al.[28]	45	—	39 ± 5	42 ± 4

* Forty-three patients had an EF measured both on day 1 and on day 5 after infarction.

a low EF early by instituting therapy promptly (digitalis and afterload reduction) or by performing specialized studies early to search for potentially revisable problems (electrophysiologic studies to identify arrhythmic risk, early catheterization looking for potentially reversible ischemic jeopardy, and ischemic dysfunction). The use of the radionuclide ventriculogram to identify these patients is most compelling, because up to 50% of the cases of a severely depressed EF are not detected by clinical evaluation.[11]

Comparison of Clinical Evaluation and Radionuclide Ventriculography to Detect Left Ventricular Dysfunction

Clinical classification of cardiac function using the Killip classification correlates poorly with LVEF.[29] Although a higher Killip class is associated with a lower group mean LVEF, there are frequent discrepancies between Killip classification and LVEF. The range of LVEF found in Killip classes I and II patients is extremely wide, with up to 25% of class I patients and 50% of class II patients having an LVEF below 40%[9,29] (Table 7-2). More than 80% of patients with acute infarction are in Killip classes I or II; within this large group of patients, many have severe left ventricular dysfunction that is not detected by clinical evaluation.

In a recent study by Sanford et al.[29] stepwise linear regression analysis was used to evaluate the ability of clinical variables to predict LVEF within 24 hours of infarction. They found that the best combination of clinical variables to predict LVEF included (1) location of the infarction, (2) an abnormal chest x-ray film, (3) rales to two thirds of the posterior thorax, (4) previous myocardial infarction, (5) transmural myocardial infarction, and (6) sinus tachycardia. However, the *r* value between a predicted and observed LVEF was only 0.418.

The discrepancy between clinical evidence of left ventricular dysfunction and depression of LVEF is more marked in the phase of infarction after the CCU when many of the patients who were initially in class II have no evidence of left

Table 7-2 *The Relationship between Killip Class and LVEF*

Study	Killip Class	Number of Patients	LVEF	Percentage with EF < 40 (%)
	I	27	52 ± 5	11
Schelbert et al.[9]	II	24	40 ± 5	50
	III	12	33 ± 7	83
	I	41	50 ± 14	22
Sanford	II	52	42 ± 17	46
et al.	III	7	27 ± 7	86

ventricular dysfunction on clinical examination, yet may have a severely depressed LVEF.[10–12,17]

Cardiac size determined from a standard chest x-ray examination correlates poorly with LVEF.[30] Although cardiomegaly (a cardiothoracic ratio > 0.50 or a cardiac volume > 540 ml/m²) is usually associated with a severely depressed LVEF (< 30%), patients with normal heart size often have a depressed LVEF. Cardiomegaly on chest x-ray examination thus is a relatively specific, but less sensitive, measure of left ventricular dysfunction than EF.[29,30]

Exercise Testing to Detect Left Ventricular Dysfunction

When we instituted routine postmyocardial infarction exercise testing in 1974, we postulated that decreased exercise time would correlate with clinical left ventricular failure and that exercise time would be important not only in posthospital exercise prescription but also in prognostic stratification.[31] The standardized low-level exercise protocol used at the Columbia–Presbyterian Medical Center consists of three stages as shown in Table 7-3. The exercise period is preceded by a supine observation period of 9 minutes and followed by a recovery period of 9 minutes. The final 3 minutes of exercise are identical to stage I of the standard Bruce exercise protocol, equivalent to 4–5 multiples of resting oxygen consumption (METS). We do not exercise patients who have rest angina, congestive heart failure that is symptomatic at rest, tachycarrhythmias that compromise hemodynamic function, or a standing systolic blood pressure less than 90 mm Hg. Patients who have these contraindications to low-level exercise testing at the time of hospital discharge have a 50% 1-year cardiac mortality.[31]

During the exercise test, shortness of breath or fatigue are nonspecific symptoms but raise the question of left ventricular failure. Physical examination immediately after cessation of treadmill exercise may disclose pulmonary rales, S_3 gallop, or a transient murmur of mitral regurgitation to indicate left ventricular failure. All of these exercise test variables are subject to interobserver variation, and, to obtain a more objective exercise test variable, we investigated the usefulness of decreased exercise time as a measure of left ventricular failure (Table 7-4).

Table 7-3 *Protocol for Low-Level Treadmill Exercise Test*

Stage	Incline (%)	Speed (mph)	Duration (min)	METs
Pretest Supine	—	—	9	1.0
0	0	1.7	3	2.3
½	5	1.7	3	3.5
1	10	1.7	3	4.6
Recovery	—	—	9	—

Table 7-4 *Relationship of Exercise Time under 6 Minutes to Clinical Measures of Left Ventricular Failure*

Measure of Left Ventricular Failure	Exercise Time under 6 Minutes: Yes	No	Chi Totals	Odds Square	Ratio
Rales ($\leq \frac{1}{3}$) or S_3 gallop in CCU					
Yes	90	91	181	13.1	2.1
No	89	186	275		
TOTAL	179	277	456		
Digoxin therapy in CCU					
Yes	82	73	155	17.2	2.3
No	100	208	308		
TOTAL	182	281	463		
Rales or S_3 gallop at exercise*					
Yes	33	31	64	6.4	2.1
No	126	243	369	6.4	2.1
TOTAL	159	274	433		
Digoxin therapy at exercise					
Yes	97	73	170	33.7	3.2
No	86	208	294		
TOTAL	183	281	464		
Cardiomegaly on x-ray examination					
Yes	103	128	231	4.8	1.6
No	80	154	234		
TOTAL	183	282	465		
Pulmonary congestion on x-ray examination					
Yes	57	38	95	11.7	2.3
No	104	163	267		
TOTAL	161	201	362		

* Present either before or after exercise.

There is a strong association of exercise time under 6 minutes with radiographic cardiomegaly, radiographic pulmonary vascular congestion, rales, or S_3 gallop in the CCU or at the time of exercise testing, and digoxin therapy either in the CCU or at the time of exercise testing.

Decreased exercise time compared to a decreased EF as a measure of left ventricular failure is shown in Table 7-5. Left ventricular failure is associated with

Table 7-5 *Relationship between LVEF and Exercise Time to Clinical Left Ventricular (LV) Failure*

Variable	Number of patients	Percentage with Variable* (%)	Percentage with LV Failure (%)	Odds Ratio	*P* Value
LVEF					
< 30%	170	36	55	5.7	< .01
Exercise					
Time < 6 min	425	42	35	2.6	< .01

* Conditional probability of having left ventricular failure if the variable is present.

both variables, but the association with LVEF is much stronger. We found that the odds of having clinical left ventricular failure were about three times greater if a patient had an EF less than 30% compared to an exercise time of less than 6 minutes.

Both low LVEF and decreased exercise time are strongly associated with 1-year cardiac mortality. We thought that most of the relationship between exercise time and subsequent mortality was due to the relationship between exercise duration and left ventricular dysfunction. To test this hypothesis, we examined the realtionship between exercise duration and LVEF in the 145 patients in Table 7-5. We were surprised to find no significant association between these two variables. This finding probably indicates that exercise duration and LVEF reflect left ventricular failure in qualitatively different ways. Analysis of the three-way association among exercise duration, LVEF, and mortality indicates that exercise duration and LVEF are independent predictors of mortality as well. There is not much redundancy between a low LVEF and short exercise time in terms of predictive value for cardiac death after hospital discharge. Patients who have both an LVEF less than 30% and decreased exercise time have a very high 1-year mortality (> 30%).

VENTRICULAR ARRHYTHMIAS AFTER MYOCARDIAL INFARCTION

Holter ECG Studies to Determine the Prevalence and Significance of Ventricular Arrhythmias

Stemming from observations made in the early days of the CCU, studies have been done using Holter technology to determine the prevalence and significance of ventricular arrhythmias in the various phases of coronary artery disease. Despite these studies, considerable controversy still exists about the prognostic significance of ventricular arrhythmias in coronary artery disease.

Frequency of Ventricular Premature Depolarizations

A number of studies have given estimates for the prevalence of ventricular arrhythmias just before discharge after the myocardial infarction.[14,33–41] Only recently have reports of 24-hour ECG analysis in large groups of patients become available.[7,42] Figure 7-3 shows the cumulative frequency distribution of VPD frequency 10–20 days after acute myocardial infarction in 616 patients studied at the Columbia–Presbyterian Medical Center. A predischarge 24-hour Holter ECG recording for each patient was analyzed by a digital computer program, and the patients were followed up for at least 1 year.[42–44] The average frequency, that is, the total VPD count in the 24-hour recording divided by the number of analyzable hours in the recording, is plotted on the *X*-axis. Because the VPD frequency distribution is so markedly skewed, a log scale is used. The cumulative frequency is plotted on the *Y*-axis. Slightly less than 50% of the patients have more than 1 VPD/hr, 20%–25% have more than 10 VPDs per hour, and less than 10% have more than 100 VPDs per hour. On the basis of conventional criteria (e.g., 30, 60,

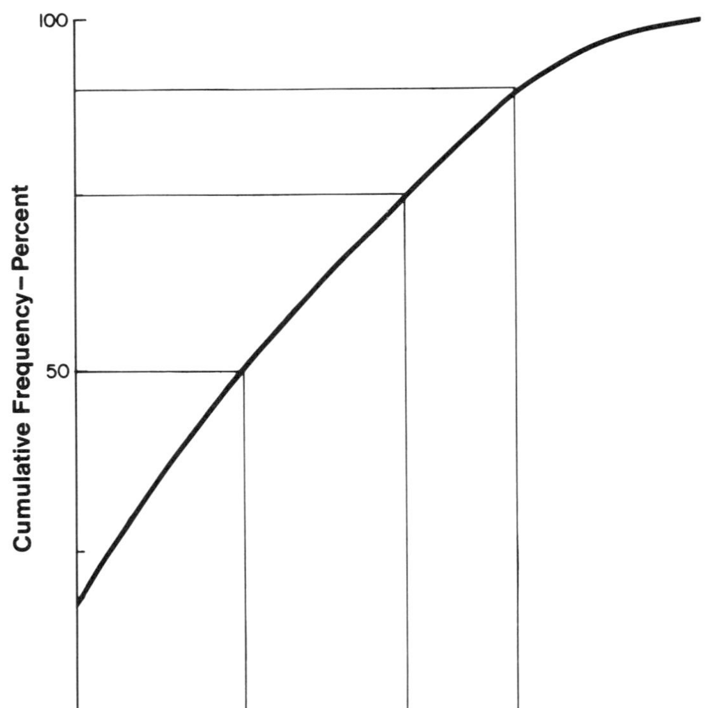

Fig. 7-4. Cumulative frequency distribution of VPD frequency expressed as the hourly average over a 24-hour period. The fiftieth percentile is just below 1 VPD/hr, the seventy-fifth percentile is 10 VPD/hr, and the ninetieth percentile is 60 VPD/hr.

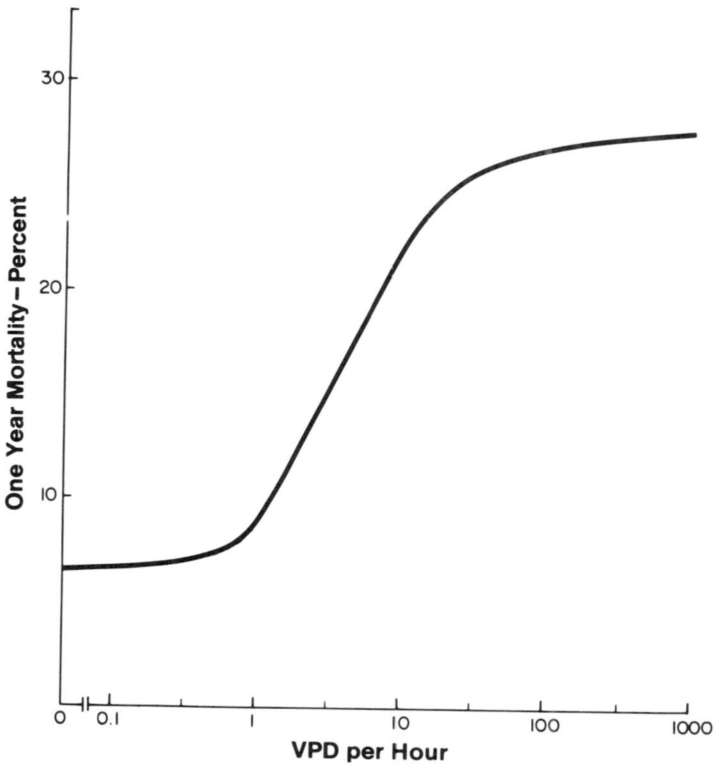

Fig. 7-5. Mortality as a function of average hourly VPD frequency. Patients with less than 1 VPD/hr have a low mortality. The mortality rises sharply as a function of VPD frequency and reaches a plateau between 10 and 30 VPD/hr.

or 100 VPDs per hour, less than 15% of the patients are candidates for treatment of ventricular arrhythmias at the time of discharge after myocardial infarction. The mortality force of VPD, unadjusted for any other factor, is shown in Figure 7-4. In a population with an overall 1-year mortality of 13%, the mortality for patients who have less than 1 VPD/hr is 7% (22/332). Mortality is an S-shaped function of VPD frequency on a log scale (see Fig. 7-5). Mortality increases sharply as a function of VPD frequency, beginning at 1 VPD/hr and essentially plateaus at frequencies between 10 and 30 VPDs/hr. The risk of dying steeply increases as VPD frequency increases from 1–10 VPDs/hr. These data suggest that current criteria for antiarrhythmic treatment should be decreased to 10 or even 3 VPDs per hour.

Complex Features

Studies in biased samples of chronic ischemic heart disease and postinfarction groups have suggested that complex features have greater significance than VPD frequency in terms of predicting mortality.[45,46] Table 7-6 shows the prevalence of complex features assessed by 24-hour Holter ECG recordings made 10–

Table 7-6 *Relationship between VPD Characteristics and 1-Year Cardiac Death*

	Patients		Deaths		
Characteristic	Number	Percentage (%)	Number	Percentage (%)	Odds Ratio
Bigeminy	192	31	32	17	1.6
Multiform	325	53	54	16	1.9
R on T	152	25	32	21	2.4
Pairs	187	30	42	22	3.2
Ventricular tachycardia	75	12	21	28	3.3

20 days after myocardial infarction. Almost half of the patients had multiform VPD; of the patients with more than 1 VPD/24 hr, that is, potentially having multiform VPD, two-thirds had multiple VPD configurations. This high prevalence occurred even though a stringent definition for multiform VPD was used: only four VPD configurations were permitted in either of the two ECG leads. About 30% of the patients had paired VPD and 25% had R-on-T VPD. Only 12% of the patients had ventricular tachycardia defined as 3 or more VPD at any rate. The strength of association of these complex features with 1-year death was estimated using the corrected odds ratio (o′): the odds of dying with the complex feature

Table 7-7 *Relationship between VPD Frequency and Complexity in the Late-Hospital Phase of Myocardial Infarction*

		Complexity (%)				
Frequency	Number of Patients	Bigeminy	Multiform	R on T	Pairs	VT
< 0.1	164	0	9	4	1	1
0.1–0.9	168	11	51	18	15	4
1–9.9	136	42	74	33	35	14
10–99	102	72	83	47	73	21
≥ 100	44	96	87	50	80	63
TOTAL	616	31	53	25	30	13

versus the odds of dying without the complex feature.[47] The odds of dying were increased most by repetitive forms: pairs, o′ equals 3:2; and VT, o′ equals 3:3. The 1-year mortality for pairs and ventricular tachycardia were 22% and 28%, respectively. Despite the brief and asymptomatic form of unsustained ventricular tachycardia after infarction, ventricular tachycardia detected by 24-hour ECG recordings just before discharge is a lethal condition.[48–50]

Frequency of Ventricular Premature Depolarizations and Complex Forms

We examined the relationships between VPD frequency and complex forms. Table 7-7 shows that as VPD frequency increases, the proportion of patients with each complex feature increases. The weakest relationship is between frequency and multiform VPD; the proportion having multiform VPD increases only slightly as a function of frequency at VPD frequencies above 0.1 VPD/hr (2.4/day). Table 7-8 shows the correlations among the complex features and VPD frequency dichotomized at its optimum value of 10 VPD/hr. The phi coefficient is used to express the strength of association among the VPD characteristics. Phi is interpreted as the correlation coefficient, although the values of phi are somewhat smaller than conventional r values.[47] Bigeminy and paired VPDs have strong relationships with VPD frequency. Also, pairs and runs of three or more in a row are strongly associated (phi = 0.42; o′ = 14:1). A multiple logistic regression was used to relate VPD frequency (log transform) and the complex features listed in Table 7-6 to 1-year cardiac mortality. A step-down procedure selected VPD frequency, pairs, and runs as having statistically significant independent associations with mortality. One purpose in this evaluation was to determine if there is independent prognosis significance for frequency and some or all of the complex features. Table 7-9 illustrates the relationships among VPD frequency of 10 or greater, repetitive VPD (either pairs or runs), and 1-year mortality. These data show that repetitive VPD increase the odds of dying to about the same degree either in patients with low or high VPD frequency.

Table 7-8 *Strength of Association among VPD Characteristics*

	F-10*	Bigeminy	Multiform	R on T	Pairs	VT
F-10	1.00	0.59	0.23	0.32	0.55	0.34
Bigeminy		1.00	0.28	0.33	0.53	0.35
Multiform			1.00	0.24	0.28	0.24
R on T				1.00	0.24	0.24
Pairs					1.00	0.42
VT						1.00

* Numbers represent phi coefficients.

Table 7-9 *Relationship between Repetitive VPDs and Mortality Adjusted for the Effects of VPD Frequency*

Frequency (per hr)	Repetitive VPDs	Patient Status		Number of Patients	Mortality (%)	Odds Ratio
		Dead	Alive			
<10	Absent	31	349	380	8	
	Present	16	68	84	19	2.7
≥10	Absent	6	36	42	14	
	Present	31	79	110	28	2.2
Total	84	532	616	14		

Time Dependence of VPD Frequency and Complexity

After 20 years of intense interest in the ventricular arrhythmias that accompany myocardial infarction, the time course of VPD frequency and complexity is still poorly defined. The best information is available for VPD frequency, runs (3 or more consecutive VPD), and ventricular fibrillation. In the prehospital phase of myocardial infarction, that is, the first 4–6 hours, VPD frequency is not great. Although 90% of the patients have some VPDs,[51] only about 10% have 10 or more VPD/hr. During the period between 6 and 72 hours after the onset of the ischemic symptoms in myocardial infarction, about 70% of patients will have 10 or more VPD/hr. There is very little information on VPD frequency between the fourth and tenth days of myocardial infarction. Preliminary data suggest that VPD frequency reaches a nadir on the fourth to sixth days of myocardial infarction. By the time of discharge, 20%–25% of the patients have 10 or more VPD/hr. The prevalence of frequent VPD continues to increase until it reaches a second peak 6–12 weeks after infarction and remains relatively constant for at least a year. The time course of ventricular tachycardia prevalence parallels that of VPD frequency. In the first 4–6 hours of myocardial infarction, the incidence of ventricular tachycardia is only about 4%.[51] During the 6–72 hour period, almost 40% of the patients with myocardial infarction will experience ventricular tachycardia. During the 4–6 day period the prevalence of ventricular tachycardia drops to about 5%. At about the time of discharge, 10–16 days after the infarction, the incidence of ventricular tachycardia is about 10%. This rises to a peak of 15%–20% at 6–12 weeks after infarction. The prevalence of ventricular fibrillation as a function of time after onset of infarction is completely different. About 15% of patients with myocardial infarction will experience ventricular fibrillation in the first 4–6 hours.[51] The incidence falls rapidly and is only 3%–4% in the 6–72 hour period. The incidence of primary ventricular fibrillation is about 5% between 3 and 16 days after infarction and perhaps 6%–7% between hospital discharge and the 1-year anniversary of infarction.

Interestingly, the ventricular arrhythmias recorded near the time of discharge after myocardial infarction are more predictive of subsequent mortality than those recorded in the CCU. Table 7-10 shows the relationships among ventricular tachycardia in the CCU and in a 24-hour ECG recording made at the time of hospital discharge. About 40% of the patients with myocardial infarction had at least one episode of ventricular tachycardia during their stay in the CCU, whereas only 12% of the patients had ventricular tachycardia in a 24-hour ECG recording at the time of discharge in 554 patients. Patients who had ventricular tachycardia in the CCU were were twice as likely to have ventricular tachycardia in a predischarge ECG recording than those who did not; however, their likelihood of dying was not significantly increased. The overall 1-year mortality in patients who experienced ventricular tachycardia in the CCU was 17%, not significantly different from those who did not have ventricular tachycardia. Patients with ventricular tachycardia detected in a predischarge 24-hour ECG recording had a 1-year mortality of 28%, or a 3.9 fold increase in the likelihood of dying.

Ventricular Arrhythmias and Left Ventricular Dysfunction

For many years it was believed that there was a relationship between ventricular arrhythmias and left ventricular dysfunction in ischemic heart disease. Several clinical and experimental studies show that ventricular arrhythmias were more frequent and complex when left ventricular scarring was present or global left ventricular dysfunction was apparent by EF measurements.[41,52–55] Califf, Wagner, and Rosati[56] analyzed a heterogeneous group of 611 patients with coronary artery disease who were studied in the cardiac catheterization laboratory. Ventricular arrhythmias, LVEF, and coronary anatomy as univariates each were strongly associated with mortality during follow-up. When the independent significance of these three variables was assessed using a step-up procedure in a multiple logistic regression model, ventricular arrhythmias were found not to be significantly associated with mortality independent of left ventricular dysfunction and

Table 7-10 *Relationships between Ventricular Tachycardia (VT) in the CCU, and at Time of Discharge and 1-Year Death*

VT in CCU	VT at 2 Weeks	Patient Status		Number of Patients	Mortality (%)	Odds Ratio
		Dead	Alive			
Absent	Absent	29	271	300	10	
	Present	8	22	30	27	3.4
Present	Absent	25	164	189	13	
	Present	13	22	35	37	3.8
Total	75	479	554	14		

severity of coronary atherosclerosis. Ruberman et al.[45] examined the relationships among clinical heart failure, ventricular arrhythmias in a 1-hour ECG analysis, and subsequent sudden cardiac death in 1739 men who had had myocardial infarction within 3 months. These workers found that complex ventricular arrhythmias (defined as bigeminal, multiform, paired, R on T, or runs) and congestive heart failure were independently associated with sudden cardiac death. Moss et al.[7] set out to confirm the findings of Ruberman in a group of 940 men who had had recent myocardial infarction. Clinical heart failure was used as the index of left ventricular dysfunction, and ventricular arrhythmias were detected by manual analysis of a 6-hour predischarge (about 3 weeks) ECG recording and classified by Ruberman's criteria. Moss et al. also found complex ventricular arrhythmias to have an independent association with cardiac mortality. These two studies have been criticized for their crude measures of left ventricular dysfunction and for their brief ECG recordings. In 1975, Schulz et al.[41] published a preliminary study that used, for the first time, a quantitative and continuous measure of left ventricular dysfunction, LVEF, to evaluate the relationships among left ventricular dysfunction, ventricular arrhythmias, and sudden cardiac death in 81 patients recovering from myocardial infarction. Poor left ventricular function was defined as an EF less than 40% and complex ventricular arrhythmias as Lown grades 3 to 5 in 24-hour ECG recordings. There were only 8 deaths, but these all occurred in the 26 patients who had *both* left ventricular dysfunction and complex ventricular arrhythmias, making it impossible to separate the risk of left ventricular dysfunction from arrhythmic risk. In May of 1982, the Multicenter Investigation of the Limitation of Infarct Size (MILIS) gave a preliminary report of their findings in 388 postinfarction patients.[26] Each patient had LVEF measured by radionuclide ventriculography and a 24-hour ECG recording analyzed by digital computer (Table 7-11). Poor left ventricular function was defined as an EF less than or equal to 40%, and repetitive (two or more consecutive VPD) were used as the index of ventricular arrhythmias. During the first year of follow-up, 25 deaths occurred. The MILIS data suggest that the associations of left ventricular dysfunction and repetitive

Table 7-11 *Mortality 1 Year after Infarction as a Function of LVEF and Repetitive VPD*[25]

EF	Repetitive VPDs	Patient Status: Dead	Patient Status: Alive	Number of Patients	Mortality (%)	Odds Ratio
>40%	Absent	3	196	199	2	
	Present	4	51	55	7	4.9
≤40%	Absent	6	81	87	7	
	Present	12	35	47	25	4.4
TOTAL	25	363	388	6		

VPD are additive. The lowest mortality occurred in the group with an EF greater than 40% and no repetitive VPD; 65% of the patients were in this group and their 1-year mortality was only 2%. The highest mortality rate was found in the group with a low EF and repetitive VPD present; only 12% of the patients were in this group and their mortality was 25%. The risk of dying within a year was increased more than fourfold if repetitive VPD were found; this step-up in mortality was identical in both the high and low EF groups, indicating that the arrhythmic variable predicted mortality after adjusting for left ventricular dysfunction. The Multicenter Post Infarction Program (MPIP) recently issued a preliminary report of very similar data in 765 patients.[32] Men and women, ages 70 and under, were enrolled within 2 weeks of myocardial infarction. Each had a radionuclide ventriculogram and a 24-hour ECG recording before discharge; the ECG recordings were analyzed by digital computer. The a priori variables used in their primary analysis were angina pectoris during ambulation before discharge (ischemic variable), an LVEF dichotomized at 40%, and a VPD frequency dichotomized at 10 VPD/hr. The total 2-year mortality was used as the endpoint for the analysis; 101 patients died during follow-up. A Laird-Olivier regression model was used (similar to Cox regression analysis). The LVEF and ventricular arrhythmias were found to be significantly and independently related to mortality; angina pectoris did not improve the prediction of mortality. The MILIS and MPIP studies both indicate that ventricular arrhythmias are more likely to occur in patients with a low EF, but, after adjusting for LVEF there is still a significant association between ventricular arrhythmias and mortality. These data suggest that it is rational to treat frequent or repetitive VPD in the hope of reducing the arrhythmic mortality during the first year or two after myocardial infarction. Large-scale trials to evaluate the validity of this practice have not been done, however.

Exercise Testing to Evaluate Postinfarction Ventricular Arrhythmias

Ventricular arrhythmias can be detected by predischarge exercise testing, as well as by Holter ECG recording. In the exercise test protocol outlined in Table 7-3, three ECG leads were continuously recorded during the 9-minute preexercise period, during exercise (a maximum of 9 minutes), and during the 9-minute recovery period. Continuous hard-copy recording is important for detection of ventricular arrhythmias. For comparison, we define exercise VPD as those occurring during exercise and the first 3 minutes of recovery. Rest VPD are defined as those occurring during the 9-minute preexercise period and the final 3 minutes of recovery. There is no association whatsoever between exercise ST segment displacement (either elevation or depression) or angina pectoris and exercise arrhythmias,[31] indicating that ischemia is rarely a mechanism of exercise arrhythmias during low-level exercise. VPD occurring both at rest and during exercise probably result from the same pathophysiologic mechanisms that produce resting VPD. VPD that occur only during exercise are probably related to the increased sympathetic activity produced by exercise.

Table 7-12 shows the strong association between exercise VPD and 1-year cardiac mortality in postinfarction patients.[31] The prevalence of any exercise VPD

Table 7-12 *Exercise Test VPDs and 1-Year Cardiac Mortality*

Exercise Test VPD	Cardiac Death Within 1 Year		Number of Patients	Mortality (%)
	Yes	No		
None	6	154	160	4
Either exercise or rest	7	70	77	9
Rest only	1	27		4
Exercise only	6	43		12
Both exercise and rest	14	74	88	16
TOTAL	27	298	325	8

is 43% in our sample, whereas the prevalence of pairs or runs of VPD is less than 10%. Considering the brevity of the exercise and recovery period, 4–12 minutes, the occurrence of VPD during an exercise test is a remarkable predictor of death in the subsequent year. The odds of dying are increased fourfold by the occurrence of VPD during the exercise test. Several other groups also have found an association between exercise VPD and subsequent mortality.[57–61] Some investigators have failed to find this association, however.[62,63] There could be many reasons for the differences in significance of exercise VPD among these studies. Perhaps the most important factor is whether or not continuous recording was done to detect arrhythmias during the test; less sensitive methods will fail to detect many VPD. Other factors such as patient selection, concomitant drug therapy, or time between infarction and exercise testing may also contibute to the differences among the studies.

Postinfarction Electrophysiologic Tests

Electrophysiologic testing is a new approach for evaluating postinfarction risk. This approach is an outgrowth of the now well-established observation that electrophysiologic studies are valuable in evaluating patients with known ventricular tachyarrhythmias and in guiding their therapy.[64–83] In such patients, programmed ventricular stimulation can usually induce the arrhythmia the patient has suffered spontaneously (e.g., ventricular tachycardia or ventricular fibrillation). Therapy that results in loss of arrhythmia inducibility usually is effective in long-term follow-up.* Although not all patients with known sustained ventricular tachycardia are inducible in the electrophysiology laboratory, the majority are, especially those who have coronary heart disease. Similarly, the large majority of patients who have suffered sudden cardiac death, which is most often secondary to ventricular fibrillation, also have inducible ventricular tachycardia in the electrophysiology laboratory.[75]

* See references 64, 67, 72, 73, 75, 77, and 83.

Programmed Ventricular Stimulation

Programmed ventricular stimulation for sustained ventricular tachycardia uses two or three electrode catheters placed in the right side of the heart chambers. Single, double, and occasionally triple ventricular premature stimuli of 1–2 msec in duration and usually twice the diastolic threshold in intensity are delivered to the right ventricular apex during ventricular pacing. Basic paced complexes are denoted as A1 if atrial and V1 if ventricular; ventricular premature stimuli are denoted as V2 (single), V2V3 (double), and V2V3V4 (triple). Pacing protocols often include (1) the use of several drive rates; (2) stimulation of several right ventricular sites, (3) stimulation of the left ventricle, (4) stimulation with several current intensities, and (5) the use of rapid burst pacing.

Repetitive Ventricular Responses

Few electrophysiologic studies have been done in patients with recent myocardial infarction. In 1978, Greene, Reid, and Schaeffer[84] published the first postinfarction electrophysiologic study. Using A1V2 stimulation, they found that the presence of repetitive ventricular responses (RVR) was associated with an increased risk for ventricular tachycardia or cardiac death in the first year after infarction (Table 7-13). Of the 19 patients who suffered cardiac death or ventricular tachycardia, 15 (79%) had RVR, whereas 4 of 29 patients (14%) without ventricular tachycardia or cardiac death had RVR. These results await confirmation in other centers.

In a comparison group of patients with known ventricular tachycardia, Greene, Reid, and Schaeffer[84] found an 88% prevalence of RVR, which is much higher than the 10% found by other investigators. The disproportionately high prevalence of RVRs reported by Greene, Reid, and Schaeffer could be a problem of definition since this group included bundle of His reentry in their RVR definition, and other authors do not.

The difference between the observations of Greene, Reid, and Schaeffer in patients recovering from acute myocardial infarction and the results of others with

Table 7-13 *RVR and Cardiac Death or Symptomatic Ventricular Tachycardia in 1 Year*[84]

	Death or VT		
RVR	Present	Absent	Total
Present	15	4	19
Absent	4	25	29
TOTAL*	19	29	48

* Mortality with RVR, 79%; without RVR; 14%; $P < .001$; odds ratio, 19.5.

patients who have chronic coronary artery disease[79–81] may reflect real differences between the two phases of coronary artery disease. Our data suggest that this is not the case, however. We studied 24 patients 10–24 days after an acute myocardial infarction, using A1V2 and V1V2 stimulation and made the following observations:

1. With A1V2, only 1 of 24 patients (4%) had intraventricular RVR, compared with 19 of 48 patients (40%) reported by Greene, Reid, and Schaefer.
2. With V1V2, only 5 of 24 patients (20%) had RVR.
3. Of 7 patients who had spontaneous ventricular tachycardia or ventricular fibrillation 1–2 weeks after infarction and who underwent complete electrophysiologic study as a guide to antiarrhythmic management, none of the 7 had RVR with A1V2. In a population similar to that of Greene, Reid, and Schaeffer, we found the prevalence of intraventricular RVR to be very low using A1V2 stimulation.

Ventricular Tachycardia and Fibrillation

If RVRs are not a useful endpoint in electrophysiologic studies to identify patients at risk for ventricular tachycardia or cardiac death in the year after acute myocardial infarction, might ventricular tachycardia induction be a more useful marker? Although the answer to this question is not yet certain, the early impression is yes. Studies by Hamer et al.[85,86] and Richards et al.[87,88] from Australia are quite striking. Hamer et al.[85,86] studied 70 patients surviving acute myocardial infarction complicated by heart failure or arrhythmias 7–20 days after the infarction. In each patient, 24-hour ambulatory ECG recordings and electrophysiologic studies were performed off of antiarrhythmic medications had been administered. The electrophysiologic studies included stimulation of the right ventricular apex in all 70 patients, V2 stimulation during A1 pacing (at paced cycle lengths of 500 and 600 msec) in 35 patients, V2 stimulation during V1 pacing (at paced cycle lengths of 500 and 400 msec) in all 70 patients, high-current V2 and V2V3 stimulation in 33 patients, and V1V2 stimulation at a second right ventricular site in 50 patients. Of the 37 patients who underwent the entire electrophysiologic protocol (Table 7-14), RVR or ventricular tachycardia was present in 20, with 12 having either sustained ventricular tachycardia (8 patients) or unsustained ventricular tachycardia of greater than 5 beats (4 patients) and 8 patients having less than 5 RVR. Of the 12 patients with inducible, sustained ventricular tachycardia or unsustained ventricular tachycardia of greater than 5 beats, 5 (42%) died in the next 12 months, 4 suddenly. Of the 25 with no RVR or less than 5 RVR, 1 (4%) died over the same period. Interestingly, only 5 of the 12 patients with 5 or more RVR to programmed ventricular stimulation had spontaneous ventricular arrhythmias in Holter ECG recordings that "suggested a need for treatment." We have performed predischarge electrophysiologic tests in patients with myocardial infarction and have found that ventricular tachycardia or ventricular fibrillation can be elicited during programmed ventricular stimulation in patients who have very few or no spontaneous VPD on 24-hour ECG recordings. Hamer, et al. concluded that although ventricular function is a major determinant of prognosis after myocardial infarction, the mechanism of sudden death is usually a ventricular tachyarrhythmia, and

Table 7-14 *Mortality at 1 year in Patients with Inducible Ventricular Tachycardia (VT) before Discharge after Myocardial Infarction*[85,86]

Inducible VT (> 5 VPDs)	Death in 1 year		
	Present	Absent	Total
Present	5	7	12
Absent	1	24	25
TOTAL*	6	31	37

* Mortality with VT, 42%; without VT, 4%; $P < .05$; odds ratio 12.0.

the assessment of ventricular electrical stability is a useful direct approach to examining this problem.

Similar to the study of Hamer et al. are the results of Richards et al.[87,88] (Table 7-15). V1V2 and V2V2V3 stimulation were applied at the right ventricular apex and right ventricular outflow tract at both low- and high-current intensities in 165 patients 6–28 days after myocardial infarction and in 111 control patients who did not have ischemic heart disease. All patients with inducible ventricular tachycardia that lasted greater than 10 seconds or ventricular fibrillation were defined as "unstable," and those with ventricular tachycardia of less than 10 seconds or no ventricular tachycardia were defined as "stable." All control patients were stable. Of the infarct survivors, 23% were unstable, although there was no difference in

Table 7-15 *Mortality at 1 year in Patients with Inducible Ventricular Tachycardia and Ventricular Fibrillation (VT/VF) after Myocardial Infarction*[84]

	Death in 1 Year		
Inducible VT/VF	Present	Absent	Total
Present	10	28	38
Absent	7	120	127
TOTAL*	17	148	165

* Mortality with VT/VF, 26%; without VT/VF, 6%; $P < .01$; odds ratio, 5.9.

age or clinical status from the stable postmyocardial infarction patients. The cumulative 1-year mortality was 26% in unstable postmyocardial infarction patients and 6% in stable postmyocardial infarction patients ($P < .001$). This difference was independent of medical or surgical therapy during the year. In the unstable patients, 80% of the deaths were instantaneous and ventricular tachyarrhythmias were documented in 63%, whereas none of the deaths in stable patients were instantaneous. Richards et al. concluded that about 20%–25% of infarct survivors have electrically unstable ventricles at 6–24 days after myocardial infarction and that these patients have a high risk of sudden cardiac death by 1 year. Most interestingly, the patients in this study were "hemodynamically stable," unlike the high-risk group of patients studied by Hamer et al.

Uther et al.[88] did not compare electrophysiologic studies to ambulatory ECG recordings, but they did compare electrophysiologic studies and exercise tests in 74 patients. In patients with no inducible ventricular tachycardia and no ST depression in stress testing, there was no 1-year mortality. In those with inducible ventricular tachycardia (independent of stress test results), the 1-year mortality was 29% compared to 4% without ventricular tachycardia, whereas in those with ST depression (independent of electrophysiologic results) the 1-year mortality was 13% compared to 6% in those without ST depression. As a result of these studies, Richards et al. suggested that programmed ventricular stimulation is a more potent identifier of sudden cardiac death risk in the year after myocardial infarction than is exercise testing, but that both together could identify all first-year mortality. Since both of the reports by the Richards et al. were in abstract form, and the description of the patients studied is scanty (i.e., inclusion and exclusion criteria are not available), further details from their group and confirmation by others will be necessary before this conclusion can be regarded as a certainty.

Although the specific role and utility of electrophysiologic studies after acute myocardial infarction awaits further delineation, several small series suggest that electrophysiologic studies may be more sensitive indicators of arrhythmic risk after myocardial infarction than either ambulatory ECG recording or exercise testing. Moreover, these studies suggest that electrophysiologic evaluation may be of benefit both in the subgroups already known to be at high risk because of poor ventricular function and/or complex ventricular ectopy, as well as in survivors of myocardial infarction who are hemodynamically stable and have infrequent VPDs.

ISCHEMIC JEOPARDY AFTER MYOCARDIAL INFARCTION

Postinfarction ischemic risk is the most difficult of the functional risk variables to recognize and quantitate by noninvasive means. It is useful to divide postinfarction patients into two groups when considering ischemic risk: (1) those manifesting ischemia early after infarction and (2) those without clinically apparent ischemia after infarction.

Angina after Myocardial Infarction

The precise frequency of early postinfarction ischemia is not known. The prevalence of predischarge chest pain is as high as 35%,[32] but some patients with symptoms may not have ischemia. Angina accompanied by ischemic ST changes occurred in 18% of postinfarction patients at the Johns Hopkins Hospital.[89] The latter figure may be high because of the high frequency of complex cases referred to that institution. Schuster and Bulkley[89] classified postinfarction angina as ischemia at a distance defined as ST or T wave abnormalities in ECG leads remote from those ECG leads containing the changes of the original infarction or ischemia in the infarct zone, that is, transient ST or T wave abnormalities in the same ECG leads as the original infarction. As a group, patients with either form of ischemia had good left ventricular function (mean LVEF = 52% ± 17%), triple-vessel coronary artery disease (85%), and the onset of angina a mean of 35 days after infarction. Those with ischemia at a distance usually had occlusion of the vessel supplying the site of infarction and a second critically stenosed vessel supplying the distant ischemic zone. Those with ischemia in the same area as the infarct usually had a tightly stenotic but still patent coronary artery that supplied the region of the infarct, and 44% (12/27) had non-Q wave infarcts. The 6-month mortality was 72% in the ischemia at a distance group and 33% in the ischemia within the infarct zone group. These mortality risks indicate primarily ischemic risk. Most patients in these two groups are not at high risk because of LVEF or ventricular arrhythmias. Cardiac catheterization with coronary angiography is indicated in all of these patients to define their anatomy in order to select a therapy, including coronary bypass surgery or angioplasty, when indicated. Those patients with poor left ventricular function (LVEF < 30%) who manifest postinfarction angina present a more difficult problem but probably also should be studied to define anatomy and attempt to identify potentially reversible ischemic dysfunction.

Reciprocal ST Changes—A Marker of Ischemia at a Distance?

It is now recognized that patients with inferior myocardial infarction have a high incidence of significant left anterior descending coronary artery disease.[90–91] Patients with acute inferior infarction and acute midprecordial ST segment depression have a higher mortality than patients who lack this finding.[92] In earlier studies it was postulated that precordial ST segment changes represent ischemia at a distance and reported that ST segment depression in leads V_1 to V_4 has a predictive value of 95% for significant left anterior descending coronary heart disease.[92–93] More recent studies utilizing coronary angiography, radionuclide ventriculography, and thallium-201 scintigraphy demonstated that these precordial ST changes are markers for larger infarct size and that the incidence of concomitant left-system coronary artery disease is similar in patients with or without reciprocal ST segment depression.[94–96] Nevertheless, it can be aruged that because of the high incidence of concomitant left anterior descending coronary artery and left circumflex artery disease, regardless of the presence or absence of precordial ST changes, all patients with inferior myocardial infarction, especially those with good left ventricular function, should be considered as candidates for cardiac catheterization and coronary angiography.

Nontransmural Infarction–A Marker for Ischemic Risk

Until recently, nontransmural myocardial infarction was believed to be a benign hospital course with a good long-term prognosis. Now, nontransmural myocardial infarction is recognized as a marker for ischemic jeopardy, and pathophysiologically, nontransmural myocardial infarction is more akin to preinfarction angina than transmural myocardial infarction. Although there is enzymatic evidence of necrosis, this is an incomplete event; the necrosis is attributed to prolonged ischemia due to transient occlusion or a sudden increase in myocardial oxygen requirements in the area of myocardium supplied by a critically stenosed vessel.[97,98] These patients are at high risk for subsequent reinfarction. In the retrospective study of Hutter et al.[97] 20% of the patients with nontransmural myocardial infarction had a subsequent myocardial infarction within 9 months of their index infarction, and by 54 months nearly 60% of the patients with nontransmural myocardial infarction suffered recurrent myocardial infarction.

In a prospective study of 200 patients with myocardial infarction, Marmor, Sobel, and Roberts[98] obtained serial MB-creatine kinase measurements, ECGs, and radionuclide ventriculograms for at least 14 days after infarction. Using these sensitive and specific indices of infarction, they found that 43% of the patients with index nontransmural myocardial infarction suffered early recurrent infarction compared to only 8% of the patients whose index infarction was transmural. Patients with nontransmural myocardial infarction have low in-hospital and early postdischarge mortality.[97,98] This is not surprising, since in the absence of reinfarction these patients have a nearly normal LVEF. By about 4 years the mortality in patients with nontransmural myocardial infarction approaches that of those with transmural myocardial infarction.[97] Current practice at our institution is to perform coronary angiography during the hospitalization for subendocardial infarctions to define coronary anatomy and jeopardized myocardium. Management of these patients may then include angioplasty, coronary bypass surgery, or pharmacologic therapy where appropriate.

Predischarge Evaluation of Ischemic Risk

Exercise Electrocardiography

In an effort to detect myocardial ischemic risk in the convalescent phase of acute myocardial infarction, several institutions have studied exercise testing before hospital discharge. Studies of the relationship of exercise ST segment depression of 0.1 mV or more in at least one ECG lead to posthospital death are summarized in Table 7-16. The data shown in Table 7-16 are quite variable. The odds ratio for death during follow-up of 1–2 years in patients with ST segment depression during exercise ranged from 0.3:1 to 19:1. Exercise ST depression

Table 7-16 *Prognostic Significance of Exercise-Induced ST Depression ≥ 0.1 mV before Hospital Discharge after Myocardial Infarction*

Investigator	Exercise ST Depression ≥ 0.1 mV	Number of Patients	Cardiac Deaths	Nonfatal Reinfarctions	Odds Ratio*	P
Kaku et al.[90]	Yes	14	0	—		
	No	31	3	—	0.3	> .05
Weld et al.[31]	Yes	52	7	3		
	No	183	14	7	1.9	> .05
Starling et al.[63]	Yes	42	4	6		
	No	88	6	6	2.0	> .05
Sami, Kraemer, and DeBusk[57]	Yes	18	4	2		
	No	67	0	8	3.6	> .05
Smith et al.[62]	Yes	20	4	2		
	No	42	1	1	7.3	< .05
Srinivasan et al.[99]	Yes	18	6	—		
	No	136	7	—	9.0	< .05
Theroux et al.[61]	Yes	64	16	—		
	No	146	2	—	19.7	< .05

* Odds of experiencing cardiac death and/or recurrent acute myocardial infarction when exercise ST depression is present versus absent.

was the most important prognostic factor in the study of Theroux et al.[61] but had no prognostic significance in the study by Kaku et al.[100]

There are many reasons why such divergent data have been obtained. First of all, exercise ST segment depression after myocardial infarction is used as a rationale for performing coronary angiography and revascularization surgery in many institutions, and this intervention probably alters outcome in many patients. This is especially true of marked ST segment depression and may be the reason that marked ST depression carries no more prognostic significance than ST depression of 0.1 mV.[31] The studies in Table 7-16 do not differentiate between positive ST segment responders who have been surgically revascularized and those who have not. Second, there are important differences in enrollment criteria among these studies. Some authors enrolled only patients who had uncomplicated myocardial infarction, whereas others exercised any patient who was ambulatory and about to be discharged from the hospital. A patient with severe left ventricular failure usually will perform less exercise than a patient without failure, and ischemia is less likely to be revealed at low exercise levels. Third, many of the patients who participated in studies of postinfarction exercise were taking cardioactive drugs, which can affect the exercise ST segment response (e.g., digoxin and propranolol). We think that it is undesirable to exclude patients taking digoxin from analysis, since the death rate is high in this group. Propranolol decreases the pressure-rate product at the end of a low-level predischarge exercise test, thereby decreasing the likelihood of exposing ischemia. We recommend that all patients who take the low-level exercise test to detect ischemia should not be receiving beta-blocker therapy. Fourth, there are significant differences between the exercise protocols. One significant difference is the number of ECG leads in which ST segment depression is measured. Another is the maximum energy expenditure permitted in the test. Still another is the use of 70% of the predicted maximum heart rate or ventricular arrhythmias as a criterion for stopping. Fifth, the ST segments should be read by an investigator who is ignorant of outcome; there is a subjective element to ST segment measurement that easily can be affected by knowledge of outcome.

Combining all of the studies in Table 7-16, 41 of 228 patients (18%) with ST segment depression died, compared to 33 of 693 patients (5%) without exercise ST segment depression. This gives an overall impression of a highly significant difference. Pooling of data from such heterogenous studies is not a valid statistical procedure, however.

Rarely, patients with exercise ST segment will develop ventricular tachycardia or ventricular fibrillation, indicating an ischemic etiology of the lethal arrhythmia. The ischemia must be treated effectively in order to control the malignant arrhythmia. Since the maximum exercise expenditure in the low-level protocol can be readily reproduced at home soon after discharge, exercise ventricular tachycardia or fibrillation proceded by ischemia requires aggressive intervention just as it does in chronic ischemic heart disease.[101,102] In such patients, the therapy of choice is surgical revascularization. After surgery, exercise testing should be repeated to confirm the absence of exertional ischemia and ventricular tachycardia or fibrillation. Patients with ischemia and malignant ventricular arrhythmias who are poor candidates for bypass surgery should be treated vigorously with antianginal or antiarrhythmic therapy.

Exercise Testing with Thallium-201 Scintigraphy or Radionuclide Ventriculography

Low-level exercise electrocardiography in the predischarge phase of acute myocardial infarction establishes prognosis and is useful in prescribing postdischarge physical activity. The identification of high-risk patients by exercise electrocardiography is multifactorial, with ST segment depression, exercise duration, and exercise arrhythmias all identified as prognosticators.[31,57,61–63] The sensitivity of exercise electrocardiography to identify ischemic risk after infarction is reduced, especially in patients with left ventricular dysfunction.[103,104] Although exercise-induced ST segment depression is specific in identifying additional coronary artery disease and jeopardized myocardium, it is sensitive only in patients with inferior or subendocardial infarctions and not in patients with anterior infarctions or severe left ventricular dysfunction.[103,104]

The use of thallium-201 scintigraphy and radionuclide ventriculography has proven to increase significantly the sensitivity of exercise testing in detecting coronary artery disease with little or no loss in specificity.[105–107] These radionuclide techniques complement exercise electrocardiography and can be used in patients in whom exertional ST segment depression is of little or no use (left bundle-branch block and digitalis therapy).

In the past few years these radionuclide techniques have been used on conjunction with exercise tests to identify multivessel disease and jeopardized myocardium after myocardial infarction. In a study of 65 patients with documented transmural myocardial infarction, Dunn et al.[108] found that exercise thallium-201 scintigraphy identified 84% of the patients with JEP-70. Exercise thallium-201 scintigraphy was slightly more sensitive and much more specific than exercise electrocardiography in detecting multivessel coronary artery disease. The patients in this study were selected largely for angina and were studied a mean of 30 months after infarction.

Turner et al.[109] performed exercise tests with thallium-201 scintigraphy in 32 patients, 2½–3 weeks after infarction and also obtained left ventriculograms and coronary angiograms in these patients before discharge. They defined jeopardized (JEP) myocardium as hypokinetic or normally contracting regions of myocardium supplied by a stenotic coronary artery. Regions supplied by a vessel with 50%–69% stenosis were defined as JEP-50, and regions supplied by a vessel with greater than or equal to 70% stenosis were defined as JEP-70. Exercise electrocardiography and exercise thallium-201 scintigraphy were more sensitive than exercise electrocardiography in identifying patients with greater than 70% stenosis of the left anterior descending coronary artery, but less than half of the patients with anterior myocardial infarctions and 70% stenosis of a right or left circumflex coronary artery could be identified by either test. Rigo et al.[110] also found that exercise thallium scintigraphy was sensitive and specific in identifying multivessel coronary artery disease in patients with inferior myocardial infarction but not in patients with anterior myocardial infarction.

Submaximal exercise testing with radionuclide ventriculography has been used after myocardial infarction to evaluate the response of global LVEF and regional wall motion abnormalities.[28,111–113] Corbett et al.[11] recently demonstrated that failure to increase LVEF by at least five points, an increase in end systolic volume of more than 5%, and failure of the systolic blood pressure–end systolic volume ratio to increase by more than 35% with submaximum exercise were all more sensitive and specific in predicting cardiac events after infarction than either exercise electrocardiography or the resting LVEF. Because this study was small (60 patients) and highly selective (patients with unstable angina and severe congestive heart failure were excluded) and had a high proportion (40%) of subendocardial myocardial infarction, these results will have to be confirmed in larger trials.

Upton et al.[112] studied 42 patients with exercise electrocardiography and ventriculography 3 and 8 weeks after infarction. Only 21% of their patients developed exercise-induced ST segment depression of at least 0.1 mV at 3 or 8 weeks, and all of these patients also demonstrated a decrease in EF or new wall motion abnormalities with exercise. Exercise ventriculography was more sensitive, and 53% of their patients had either a decrease in EF or an increase in wall motion abnormalities with exercise at 3 and 8 weeks. In addition, no patients with resting EF below 35% developed ST segment depression with exercise, but 55% of these patients developed an exercise-induced decrease in EF or new wall motion abnormalities. As these authors pointed out, however, an exercise-induced decrease in global LVEF has been demonstrated to be a nonspecific marker of coronary artery disease.[112,114,115]

In the only study designed to evaluate the sensitivity and specificity of exercise radionuclide ventriculography to detect multivessel coronary artery disease after infarction, the results were similar to those with exercise electrocardiography and thallium-201 scintigraphy.[113] An exercise-induced decrease in global EF by at least five points had a sensitivity of 64% and a specificity of 92% in detecting multivessel disease in patients with inferior myocardial infarctions but could not distinguish single from multivessel disease in patients with anterior infarctions. Exercise-induced regional wall motion abnormalities were highly specific in detecting multivessel disease in inferior and anterior myocardial infarction but had a sensitivity of only 30%.[113]

In summary, radionuclide techniques and electrocardiography are reasonably sensitive and specific in identifying multivessel coronary artery disease in patients with inferior or subendocardial infarctions, but none of these modalities are reliable in detecting multivessel disease and jeopardized myocardium in patients with anterior myocardial infarction or severe left ventricular dysfunction.

Coronary Angiography

Coronary angiography can be safely preformed in patients with acute myocardial infarction before hospital discharge.[24,116–120] The major role of early coronary angiography in patients with nontransmural myocardial infarction and postinfarction angina has been discussed in a previous section. The role of coronary angiography to evaluate the presence of multivessel coronary artery disease and jeopardized myocardium after infarction is not established. Certainly it can be argued that noninvasive methods are sufficiently sensitive and specific in identifying jeopardized myocardium in patients with inferior myocardial infarction and good left ventricular function and that coronary angiography should be limited to those patients with evidence of jeopardized myocardium on predischarge noninvasive testing. The high prevalence (50%–80%) of significant left coronary artery disease and jeopardized myocardium in these patients means that at least one half of these patients will ultimately have coronary angiography. In the patients with anterior myocardial infarction and left ventricular dysfunction, it is difficult to establish the presence of additional jeopardized myocardium with noninvasive methods. Patients with transmural anterior myocardial infarctions have a somewhat lower incidence of multivessel disease than patients with transmural inferior myocardial infarctions, but the prevalence of significant triple-vessel disease is about 50% even in these patients, and these are the patients who can least afford to lose any more myocardium.[24,116] Although left ventricular dysfunction is the major determinant of mortality in patients with anterior myocardial infarctions, the presence of triple-vessel disease appears to add an independent risk.[19] In the study of Sanz et al.[19] patients with an EF of 21%–49% and triple-vessel disease had a higher mortality than patients with single- or double-vessel disease and a similar EF. Studies in symptomatic patients with triple-vessel disease and left ventricular dysfunction demonstrate significantly improved survival with surgical treatment.[121,122] One cannot extrapolate from these studies to asymptomatic patients after infarction, but in view of the poor outlook for postinfarction patients with left ventricular dysfunction and triple-vessel disease who are treated medically, a randomized trial of surgical versus medical therapy appears warranted. Coronary bypass surgery would be primarily aimed at alleviating ischemic jeopardy in these patients but may also result in improved left ventricular function,[123,124] perhaps due to revascularization of stunned myocardium.[21] Because of the poor prognosis of patients with severe left ventricular dysfunction and the lack of sensitivity or specificity of noninvasive methods to determine ischemic jeopardy in these patients, it is reasonable to perform coronary angiography in patients with an EF less than 30% after infarction to identify ischemic jeopardy. It remains to be determined whether recognition and treatment of ischemic jeopardy will result in improved survival in some subsets of patients with severe left ventricular dysfunction.

EVALUATION AND MANAGEMENT OF PATIENTS AFTER MYOCARDIAL INFARCTION

The previous discussion in this chapter has provided evidence that left ventricular dysfunction, ventricular arrhythmias, and ischemic jeopardy each *independently* contribute to the risk of dying in the year after acute myocardial infarction. Because LVEF is a very potent risk predictor and provides information independently of clinical assessment, this test is useful for all postinfarction patients. In nearly all patients, the LVEF stabilizes by the second or third day after infarction and remains constant for the next 6 months or longer. The optimum time to measure LVEF is at about the time of discharge from the CCU. Radionuclide ventriculography is the method of choice for measuring LVEF unless the patient has an ischemic problem that dictates predischarge coronary angiography. In these cases, the radionuclide ventriculogram can be omitted, since LVEF will be measured by dye ventriculography done at cardiac catheterization. Even though more than half of the patients have essentially no risk attributable to ventricular arrhythmias after myocardial infarction, we recommend a 24-hour Holter ECG recording in all patients before discharge. When we learn how to predict significant ventricular arrhythmias from clinical variables, which patients are most likely to have, we can use this test more selectively. Ventricular arrhythmias detected in the CCU are not useful predictors of long-term mortality or who will have significant ventricular arrhythmias at the time of discharge. The frequency and complexity of ventricular arrhythmias falls to a minimum at about 3–6 days after infarction and then rises to a maximum at about 6–12 weeks. The best time to record a 24-hour ECG therefore is between 10 days and discharge. Programmed ventricular stimulation appears to be more sensitive for picking up life-threatening ventricular arrhythmias than 24-hour ECG recordings. Until more data are available on the use of programmed ventricular stimulation early after acute myocardial infarction, we recommend that this technique be used clinically in patients who have a LVEF less than 40% on radionuclide ventriculography or those who show repetitive ventricular arrhythmias in a 24-hour ECG recording. Ischemic jeopardy is the most controversial postinfarction risk factor. Exercise ST segment changes or exercise radionuclide assessment of left ventricular function or perfusion studies have limited utility for detecting ischemic jeopardy. All three are reasonably good for detecting anterior ischemia after a first inferior myocardial infarction. None of the three has much use in detecting inferior ischemia after a first anterior infarction, however. A few authors recommend coronary angiography for all patients before discharge after myocardial infarction. Although this proposal has some merit, most cardiologists use coronary angiography in selected subgroups of patients. Patients who continue to have angina pectoris in the hospital after myocardial infarction and those with nontransmural myocardial infarction should have coronary angiography before discharge. Also, many cardiologists favor coronary angiography for all patients who have a first inferior myocardial infarction within 3 months if not before discharge. This recommendation is based on the high likelihood of significant lesions in the left anterior descending coronary artery of these patients. At present there is no consensus about whether to perform early coronary angiography in patients with anterior infarction and poor left ventricular function (< 40%. Some cardiologists argue that these patients should not be studied unless they develop angina pectoris, because their surgical mortality is so high. Others aruge for early angiography because these patients can ill afford to lose any additional myocardium to the ischemic process and because of the chance that left ventricular function may improve after aggressive medical or surgical treatment to ameliorate ischemia.

The functional approach to the assessment of risk after myocardial infarction is proving useful, and new information on the sources of risk is generating many new hypotheses about approaches to management. Most of these ideas about therapy await formal testing in future therapeutic trials.

REFERENCES

1. Bigger JT Jr: New directions and new uses for risk stratification in the post-hospital phase of acute myocardial infarction. Am J Med 67:1, 1979
2. Peel AAF, Semple T, Wang I, et al: A coronary prognostic index for grading the severity of infarction. Br Heart J 24:745, 1962
3. Pell S, and D'Alonzo CA: Immediate mortality and five year survival of employed men with a first myocardial infarction. N Engl J Med 270:915, 1964
4. Weinblatt E, Shapiro S, Frank CW, et al: Prognosis of men after first myocardial infarction: mortality and first recurrence in relation to selected parameters. Am J Public Health 58:1329, 1968
5. Badger GF, Liebow IM: Myocardial infarction in the practices of a group of private physicians. IV. Factors related to the longevity of patients with myocardial infarction during the first five years. J Chronic Dis 21:473, 1968
6. Norris RM, Caughey DE, Mercer CJ, et al: Coronary prognostic index for predicting survival after recovery from acute myocardial infarction. Lancet 2:485, 1970
7. Moss AJ, Davis HT, DeCamilla J, et al: Ventricular ectopic beats and their relation to sudden and nonsudden cardiac death after myocardial infarction. Circulation 60:998, 1979
8. Page DL, Caulfield JB, Kastor JA, et al: Myocardial changes associated

with cardiogenic shock. N Engl J Med 185:133, 1971

9. Schelbert HR, Henning H, Ashburn WL, et al: Serial measurements of left ventricular ejection fraction by radionuclide angiography early and late after myocardial infarction. Am J. Cardiol 38:407, 1976
10. Reduto LA, Berger HJ, Cohen LS, et al: Sequential radionuclide assessment of left and right ventricular performance after acute transmural myocardial infarction. Ann Intern Med 89:441, 1978
11. Shah PK, Pichler M, Berman DS, et al: Left ventricular ejection fraction determined by radionuclide ventriculography in early stages of first transmural myocardial infarction: Relation to short-term prognosis. Am J Cardiol 45:542, 1980
12. Wolk MJ, Scheidt S, Killip T: Heart failure complicating acute myocardial infarction. Circulation 45:1125, 1972
13. Killip T, Kimball JT: Treatment of myocardial infarction in a coronary care unit: A two-year experience with 250 patients. Am J Cardiol 20:457, 1967
14. Bigger JT Jr, Heller CA, Wenger TL, et al: Risk stratification after acute myocardial infarction. Am J Cardiol 42:202, 1978
15. Battler A, Karliner JS, Higgins CB, et al: The initial chest x-ray in acute myocardial infarction: Prediction of early and late mortality and survival. Circulation 61:1004, 1980
16. Shell WE, DeWood MA, Peter T, et al: Comparison of clinical signs and hemodynamic state in the early hours of transmural myocardial infarction. Am Heart J 104:521, 1982
17. Ramanathan K, Bodenheimer MM, Banka VS, et al: Natural history of contractile abnormalities after acute myocardial infarction in man: Severity and response to nitroglycerin as a function of time. Circulation 63:731, 1981
18. Kostuk WJ, Ehsani AA, Karliner JS, et al: Left ventricular performance after myocardial infarction assessed by radioisotope angiocardiography. Circulation 47:242, 1973
19. Morrison J, Coromilas J, Munsey D, et al: Correlation of radionuclide estimates of myocardial infarction size and release of creatine kinase MB in man. Circulation 62:277, 1980
20. Rogers WJ, McDaniel HG, Smith LP, et al: Correlation of angiographic estimates of myocardial infarct size and accumulated release of creatine kinase MB in isoenzyme in man. Circulation 56:199, 1977
21. Braunwald E, Kloner RA: The stunned myocardium: Prolonged, postischemic ventricular dysfunction. Circulation 66:1146, 1982
22. Schulze RA Jr, Strauss HW, Pitt B: Sudden death in the year following myocardial infarction—Relation to ventricular premature contractions in the late hospital phase and left ventricular ejection fraction. Am J Med 62:192, 1977
23. Coromilas J, Ong L, Eisenberg S, et al: Radionuclide descriptors of myocardial infarction and long-term prognosis. Circulation 62(suppl 3):126, 1980
24. Taylor GJ, Humphries JO, Mellits ED, et al: Predictors of clinical course: Coronary anatomy and left ventricular function after recovery from acute myocardial infarction. Circulation 62:960, 1980
25. Mukharji J, Rude RE, Poole K, et al: Late sudden death following acute myocardial infarction, importance of combined presence of repetitive ventricular ectopy and left ventricular dysfunction. Clin Res 30:108A, 1982
26. Wackers FJ, Berger HJ, Weingerg MA, et al: Spontaneous changes in left ventricular function over the first 24 hours of acute myocardial infarction: Implications for evaluating early therapeutic interventions. Circulation 66:748, 1982
27. Nemerovski M, Shah PK, Pichler M, et al: Radionuclide assessment of se-

quential changes in left and right ventricular function following first acute transmural myocardial infarction. Am Heart J 104:709, 1982

28. Borer JS, Rosing DR, Miller RH, et al: Natural history of left ventricular function during 1 year after acute myocardial infarction: Comparison with clinical, electrocardiographic and biochemical determinations. Am J Cardiol 46:1, 1980
29. Snaford CF, Corbett, J, Nicod P, et al: Value of radionuclide ventriculography in the immediate characterization of patients with acute myocardial infarction. Am J Cardiol 49:637, 1982
30. Feild BJ, Russell RO, Moraski RE, et al: Left ventricular size and function and heart size in the year following myocardial infarction. Circulation 50:331, 1974
31. Weld FM, Chu K-L, Bigger JT Jr, et al: Risk stratification with low-level exercise testing 2 weeks after acute myocardial infarction. Circulation 64:306, 1976
32. Moss AJ, Bigger JT Jr, Case RB, et al: Risk stratification and prognostication after myocardial infarction. J Am Coll Cardiol 1:716, 1983.
33. Moss AJ, Schnitzler R, Green R, et al: Ventricular arrhythmias 3 weeks after acute myocardial infarction. Ann Intern Med 75:837, 1971
34. Kotler MN, Tabatznik B, Mower MM, et al: Prognostic significance of ventricular ectopic beats with respect to sudden death in the late postinfarction period. Circulation 47:959, 1973
35. Vismara LA, Amsterdam EA, Mason DT: Relation of ventricular arrhythmias in the late hospital phase of acute myocardial infarction to sudden death after hospital discharge. Am J Med 59:6, 1975
36. Luria MH, Knoke JD, Margolis RM, et al: Acute myocardial infarction: Prognosis after recovery. Ann Intern Med 85:561, 1976
37. Wenger TL, Bigger JT Jr, Merrill GS: Ventricular arrhythmias in the late hospital phase of acute myocardial infarction. Circulation 51-52(suppl 2):110, 1975
38. Rehnqvist N: Ventricular arrhythmias prior to discharge after acute myocardial infarction. Eur J Cardiol 4:63, 1976
39. Moss AJ, DeCamilla JJ, Davis HP, et al: Clinical significance of ventricular ectopic beats in the early posthospital phase of myocardial infarction. Am J Cardiol 39:635, 1977
40. Rehnqvist N, Sjogren A: Ventricular arrhythmias prior to discharge and one year after acute myocardial infarction. Eur J Cardiol 5:425, 1977
41. Schulze RA Jr, Rouleau J, Rigo P, et al: Ventricular arrhythmias in the late hospital phase of acute myocardial infarction: Relation of left ventricular function detected by gated cardiac blood pool scanning. Circulation 52:1006, 1975
42. Bigger JT Jr, Weld FM: Analysis of prognostic significance of ventricular arrhythmias after myocardial infarction: Shortcomings of Lown grading system. Br Heart J 45:717, 1981
43. Florenz MK, Rolnitzky LM, and Bigger JT Jr: A rapid ECG processing computer program using the finite state machine approach, in Computers in Cardiology, IEEE Computer Society, Long Beach Calif., 1975, p 145
44. Birman KP, Rolnitzky LM, Bigger JT Jr: A shape-oriented system for automated Holter ECG analysis, in Computers in Cardiology, Long Beach, Calif., IEEE Computer Society, 1978, p 217
45. Ruberman W, Weinblatt E, Goldberg JD, et al: Ventricular premature beats and mortality after acute myocardial infarction. N Engl J Med 179:750, 1977
46. Lown B: Sudden cardiac death: The major challenge confronting contemporary cardiology. Am J Cardiol 43:313, 1979
47. Fleiss JL: Statistical Methods for Rates and Proportions. New York, John Wiley & Sons Inc, 1973

48. Anderson KP, DeCamilla J, Moss AJ: Clinical significance of ventricular tachycardia (3 beats or longer) detected during ambulatory monitoring after myocardial infarction. Circulation 57:890, 1978
49. Kleiger RE, Miller JP, Thanavaro S, et al: Relationship between clinical features of acute myocardial infarction and ventricular runs 2 weeks to 1 year after infarction. Circulation 63:64, 1981
50. Bigger JT Jr, Weld FM, Rolnitzky LM: The prevalence and significance of ventricular tachycardia detected by ambulatory ECG recording in the late hospital phase of acute myocardial infarction. Am J Cardiol 48:815, 1981
51. Pantridge JF, Webb SW, Adgey AAJ: Arrhythmias in the first hours of acute myocardial infarction. Prog Cardiovasc Dis 23:265, 1981
52. Califf RM, Burks JM, Behar VS, et al: Relationships among ventricular arrhythmias, coronary artery disease, and angiographic and electrophysiologic indicators of myocardial fibrosis. Circulation 57:725, 1978
53. Gang ES, Bigger JT Jr, Livelli FD Jr: A model of chronic ischemic arrhythmias: The relationships among electrically inducible ventricular tachycardia, ventricular fibrillation threshold, and myocardial infarct size. Am J Cardiol 50:469, 1982
54. Calvert A, Lown B, Gorlin, R: Ventricular premature beats and anatomically defined coronary disease. Am J Cardiol 39:627, 1977
55. Sharma SD, Ballantyne F, Goldstein S: The relationship of ventricular asynergy in coronary artery disease in ventricular premature beats. Chest 66:358, 1974
56. Califf RM, Wagner GS, Rosati RA: Prognostic value of ventricular arrhythmias (abstract). Am J Cardiol 47:397, 1981
57. Sami M, Kraemer H, DeBusk RF: The prognostic significance of serial exercise testing after myocardial infarction. Circulation 60:1238, 1979
58. Granath A, Sodermark T, Winge T, et al: Early work load tests for evaluation of long-term prognosis of acute myocardial infarction. Br Heart J 39:758, 1977
59. Ericsson M, Granath A, Ohlsen P, et al: Arrhythmias and symptoms during treadmill testing three weeks after myocardial infarction in 100 patients. Br Heart J 35:787, 1973
60. Sivertssen E, Bay G, Hansen G, et al: The prognostic value of arrhythmias at rest and in connection with an exercise stress test in the late hospital phase of acute myocardial infarction. J Oslo City Hosp 28:23, 1978
61. Theroux P, Waters DD, Halphen C, et al: Prognostic value of exercise testing soon after myocardial infarction. N Engl J Med 301:341, 1979
62. Smith JW, Dennis CA, Gassman A, et al: Exercise testing three weeks after myocardial infarction. Chest 75:12, 1979
63. Starling MR, Crawford MH, Kennedy GT, et al: Exercise testing early after myocardial infarction: Predictive value for subsequent unstable angina and death. Am J Cardiol 46:909, 1980
64. Horowitz LN, Farshidi A, Spielman SR, et al: Predictions of drug efficacy in ventricular tachycardia by electrophysiologic study. Circulation 58(suppl 2):155, 1978
65. Scheinman MM: Induction of ventricular tachycardia: A promising new technique or clinical electrophysiology gone awry (editorial). Circulation 58:998, 1978
66. Wellens HJJ, Lie KI, Durrer D: Further observations on ventricular tachycardia as studied by electrical stimulation of the heart: Chronic recurrent ventricular tachycardia and ventricular tachycardia during acute myocardial infarction. Circulation 49:647, 1974
67. Fisher JD, Cohen HL, Mehra R, et al: Cardiac pacing and pacemakers. II. Serial electrophysiologic—pharmacologic testing for control of re-

current tachyarrhythmias. Am Heart J 93:658, 1977

68. Wellens HJJ, Schuilenberg RM, Durrer D: Electrical stimulation of the heart in patients with ventricular tachycardia. Circulation 46:216, 1972
69. Josephson ME, Horowitz LN, Farshidi A, et al: Recurrent sustained ventricular tachycardia. I. Mechanism. Circulation 57:437, 1978
70. Fisher JD: Ventricular tachycardia—practical and provocative electrophysiology (editorial). Circulation 58:1000, 1978
71. Denes P, Wu D, Dhingra RC, et al: Electrophysiological studies in patients with chronic recurrent ventricular tachycardia. Circulation 54:229, 1976
72. Horowitz LN, Josephson ME, Farshidi A, et al: Recurrent sustained ventricular tachycardia. III. Role of the electrophysiological study in selection of antiarrhythmic regimens. Circulation 58:986, 1978
73. Mason JW, Winkle RA: Electrode catheter induction of ventricular tachycardia: Observations on the technique and its use in choosing and assessing the efficacy of antiarrhytymic drugs in patients with recurrent ventricular tachycardia. Circulation 58:971, 1978
74. Spielman S, Farshidi A, Horowitz LN, et al: Ventricular fibrillation during programmed ventricular stimulation: Incidence and clinical implications. Am J Cardiol 42:913, 1978
75. Ruskin JN, DiMarco JP, Garan H: Out-of-hospital cardiac arrest: Electrophysiologic observations and selection of long-term antiarrhythmic therapy. N Engl J Med 303:607, 1980
76. Ruskin JN, Garan H, DiMarco JP, et al: Electrophysiologic testing in survivors of prehospital cardiac arrest. Am J Cardiol 49:958, 1982
77. Kehoe RF, Moran JM, Zheutlin T, et al: Electrophysiological study to direct therapy in survivors of pre-hospital ventricular fibrillation. Am J Cardiol 49:928, 1982
78. Benson DW Jr, Hession WT, Zavoral JH, et al: Sudden cardiac arrest in young adults: Clinical and electrophysiological findings. Am J Cardiol 49:928, 1982
79. Livelli FD Jr, Bigger JT Jr, Reiffel JA, et al: Response to programmed ventricular stimulation: Sensitivity, specificity, and relationship to heart disease. Am J Cardiol 50:451, 1982
80. Farshidi A, Michelson EL, Greenspan AM, et al: Repetitive responses to ventricular extrastimuli: Incidence, mechanism, and significance. Am Heart J 100:59, 1980
81. Ruskin JN, DiMarco JP, Garan H: Repetitive responses to single ventricular extrastimuli in patients with serious significance. Circulation 63:767, 1981
82. Vandepol CJ, Farshidi A, Spielman SR, et al: Incidence and significance of induced ventricular tachycardia. Am J Cardiol 45:725, 1980
83. Fisher JD: Role of electrophysiologic testing in the diagnosis and treatment of patients with known and suspected bradycardias and tachycardias. Prog. Cardiovasc Dis 24:25, 1981
84. Greene HL, Reid PR, Schaeffer AH: The repetitive ventricular response in man: A predictor of sudden death. N Engl J Med 299:729, 1978
85. Hamer A, Vohra J, Hunt D, et al: Prediction of sudden death by electrophysiologic studies in high-risk patients surviving acute myocardial infarction. Circulation 64(suppl 4):84, 1982
86. Hamer A, Vohra J, Hunt D, et al: Prediction of sudden death by electrophysiologic studies in high-risk patients surviving acute myocardial infarction. Am J Cardiol 50:223, 1982
87. Richards DA, Cady DV, Denniss AR, et al: Ventricular electrical instability during the first year following myocardial infarction (abstract). Am J Cardiol 49:929, 1982
88. Uther JB, Cady DV, Denniss AR, et al: Ventricular programmed stimulation and exercise ST segment depres-

sion as prediction of postinfarction mortality (abstract). Am J Cardiol 49:902, 1982
89. Schuster EH, Bulkley BH: Early post-infarction angina: Ischemia at a distance and ischemia in the infarct zone. N Engl J Med 305:1101, 1985
90. Miller RR, DeMaria AN, Vismara LA, et al: Chronic stable inferior myocardial infarction: Unsuspected harbinger of high-risk proximal left coronary arterial obstruction amenable to surgical revascularization, Am J Cardiol 39:954, 1977
91. Chaitman BR, Waters DD, Corbara F, et al: Prediction of multivessel disease after inferior myocardial infarction. Circulation 1085, 1978
92. Shah PK, Pichler M, Berman DS, et al: Noninvasive identification of a high-risk subset of patients with acute inferior myocardial infarction. Am J Cardiol 46:915, 1980
93. Salcedo JR, Baird MG, Chambers RJ, et al: Significance of reciprocal ST-segment depression in anterior precordial leads in acute inferior myocardial infarction: Concomitant left anterior coronary artery disease? Am J Cardiol 48:1003, 1981
94. Goldberg HL, Borer JS, Jacobstein JG, et al: Anterior ST segment depression in acute inferior myocardial infarction: Indicator of posterolateral infarction. Am J Cardiol 48:1009, 1981
95. Gibson RS, Crampton RS, Watson DD, et al: Precordial ST segment depression during acute inferior myocardial infarction: Clinical, scintigraphic and angiographic correlations. Circulation 66:732, 1982
96. Ong L, Valdellon B, Coromilas J, et al: Precordial ST-segment depression in inferior myocardial infarction: Evaluation by quantitative thallium-201 scintigraphy and technetium^{99m} ventriculography. Am J Cardiol 51:734, 1983
97. Hutter AM, DeSanctis RW, Flynn T, et al: Non-transmural myocardial infarction: A comparison of hospital and late clinical course of patients with that of matched patients with transmural anterior and transmural inferior myocardial infarction. Am J Cardiol 48:595, 1981
98. Marmor A, Sobel BE, Roberts R: Factors presaging early recurrent myocardial infarction ("extension"). Am J Cardiol 48:603, 1981
99. Srinivasan M, Young A, Baker G, et al: The value of postcardiac infarction exercise stress testing: Identification of a group at high risk. Med J Aust 1:466, 1981
100. Kaku R, DeMaria AN, Salmon D, et al: Pre-discharge exercise testing following acute myocardial infarction: Value and limitations. Clin Res 26:242A, 1978
101. Thomson PD, Kelemen MH: Hypotension accompanying the onset of exertional angina: A sign of severe compromise of left ventricular blood supply. Circulation 52:28, 1975
102. Codini MA, Sommerfeldt L, Eybel CE, et al: Efficacy of coronary bypass grafting in exercise-induced ventricular tachycardia. J Thorac Cardiovasc Surg 81:502, 1981.
103. Castellanet MJ, Greenberg PS, Ellestad MH: Comparison of ST segment changes in exercise testing with angiographic findings in patients with prior myocardial infarction. Am J Cardiol 42:29, 1978
104. Paine, TD, Dye, LE, Roitman DI, et al: Relation of graded exercise test findings after myocardial infarction to extent of coronary artery disease and left ventricular dysfunction. Am J Cardiol 42:716, 1978
105. Ritchie JL, Zaret BL, Strauss HW, et al: Myocardial imaging with thallium-201: A multicenter study in patients with angina pectoris or acute myocardial infarction. Am J Cardiol 42:345, 1978
106. Borer JS, Kent KM, Bacharach SL, et al: Sensitivity, specificity, and predictive accuracy of radionuclide cineangiography during exercise in patients with coronary artery disease:

Comparison with exercise electrocardiography. Circulation 60:572, 1979
107. Bodenheimer MM, Banka VS, Fooshee CM, et al: Comparative sensitivity of the exercise electrocardiogram, thallium imaging and stress radionuclide angiography to detect the presence and severity of coronary heart disease. Circulation 60:1270, 1979
108. Dunn RF, Freedman B, Bailey LK, et al: Noninvasive prediction of multivessel disease after myocardial infarction. Circulation 62:726, 1980
109. Turner JD, Schwartz KM, Logic JR, et al: Detection of residual jeopardized myocardium 3 weeks after myocardial infarction by exercise testing with thallium-201 myocardial scintigraphy. Circulation 61:729, 1980
110. Rigo P, Bailey IK, Griffith LSC, et al: Stress thallium-201 myocardial scintigraphy for the detection of individual coronary arterial lesions in patients with and without previous myocardial infarction. Am J Cardiol 48:209, 1981
111. Corbett JR, Dehmer GJ, Lewis SE, et al: The prognostic value of submaximal exercise testing with radionuclide ventriculography before hospital discharge in patients with recent myocardial infarction Circulation 64:535, 1981
112. Upton MT, Palmeri ST, Jones RH, et al: Assessment of left ventricular function by resting and exercise radionuclide angiocardiography following acute myocardial infarction. Am Heart J 104:1232, 1982
113. Wasserman AG, Katz RJ, Cleary P, et al: Noninvasive detection of multivessel disease after myocardial infarction by exercise radionuclide ventriculography. Am J Cardiol 50:1242, 1982
114. Port S, Cobb FR, Coleman RE, et al: Effect of age on the response of the left ventricular ejection fraction to exercise. N Engl J Med 303:1133, 1980
115. Osbakken MD, Boucher CA, Okada RD, et al: Spectrum of global left ventricular responses to supine exercise limitations in the use of ejection fraction in identifying patients with coronary artery disease. Am J Cardiol 51:28, 1983
116. Bertrand ME, Lefevre JM, Laisne CL, et al: Coronary arteriography in acute transmural myocardial infarction. Am Heart J 97:61, 1979
117. DeWood MA, Spores J, Notske R, et al: Prevalence of total coronary occlusion during the early hours of transmural myocardial infarction. N Engl J Med 303:897, 1980
118. Turner SD, Rogers WJ, Mantle JA, et al: Coronary angiography soon after myocardial infarction. Chest 77:58, 1980
119. Sanz G, Castañer, Betriu A, et al: Determinants of prognosis in survivors of myocardial infarction: A prospective clinical angiographic study. N Engl J Med 306:1065, 1982
120. Betriu A, Castañer A, Sanz GA, et al: Angiographic findings 1 month after myocardial infarction: A prospective study of 159 survivors. Circulation 65:1099, 1982
121. European Coronary Surgery Study Group: Prospective randomised study of coronary bypass surgery in stable angina pectoris: Second interim report. Lancet 2:491, 1980
122. DeRouen TA, Hammermeister KE, Dodge HT: Comparison of the effects of survival after coronary artery surgery in subgroups of patients from the Seattle Heart Watch. Circulation 63:537, 1981
123. Hellman C, Schmidt DH, Kamath ML, et al: Bypass graft surgery in severe left ventricular dysfunction. Circulation 62(suppl 1):103, 1980
124. Freeman MR, Gray RJ, Berman DS, et al: Improvement in global and segmental left ventricular function after coronary bypass surgery. Circulation 64(suppl 2):34, 1981

Edward L.C. Pritchett

8

AMBULATORY ELECTROCARDIOGRAPHY AND PROGRAMMED ELECTRICAL STIMULATION IN A CLINICAL TRIAL OF SUDDEN CARDIAC DEATH

Rising interest in the problem of sudden cardiac death will eventually culminate in a clinical trial of its prevention. Ambulatory electrocardiography and programmed electrical stimulation may be helpful in the execution of such a trial, since both tools have been used productively to study many different arrhythmias. This chapter considers the evidence that either technique could be an important component of a clinical trial of prevention of sudden cardiac death.

SETTING UP THE CLINICAL TRIAL

Since a clinical trial is a scientific experiment in therapy using human beings as subjects, the usual rules of scientific studies apply: methods must be standardized and reproducible; treatment groups must be assigned randomly; and outcome variables in treatment groups must be compared with the same variables in control groups. A sudden death trial is likely to follow the pattern of other recent large trials. Initially, the trial will seek to identify a population with relatively increased risk of sudden death based on some gross clinical finding (e.g., an abnormal ECG, acute myocardial infarction, or coronary artery stenosis identified by angiography). Since the problem of sudden cardiac death is largely the problem of ischemic heart disease, it is likely that these gross observations will indicate the presence of coronary artery disease.[1] The population at risk then will be screened by more rigorous methods to identify a homogeneous cohort with the highest possible risk.

SUDDEN CARDIAC DEATH
0-8089-1725-0

This refinement of risk makes a trial more efficient. Recruiting and following up patients in a clinical trial is an expensive business.[2] Subjects with little or no risk of developing an index event (in our case, sudden cardiac death) add substantially to the cost of such a trial. The most efficient study would include only patients certain to have an event if left untreated during the observation period.

Once a high-risk group is identified, patients will be randomized to one of two "treatments." One treatment will be a placebo, or "conventional therapy"; the other will be a test regimen. Patients will then be followed up prospectively at regular intervals. The times at which patients die will be noted, and survival will be measured as the elapsed time (in days, weeks, or months) between entrance into the trial and death. Cumulative survival curves for each treatment are constructed using life-table methods, and treatment differences are tested by comparing curves.

CLINICAL TRIAL METHODOLOGY

Clinical trial methodology has evolved rapidly in the past decade based on experience gained from several large trials.[3] The statistical methods, which have become very sophisticated, can be used to determine if the baseline characteristics of patients have influenced apparent treatment effects. The cost of these trials has also risen, and the cost of a sudden death trial will be high. Hundreds to thousands of subjects will need to be enrolled in a sudden death trial to prove clinically important treatment effects in a reasonable follow-up period.[4] Methods incorporated in such a trial must be carefully selected so that conclusions are not weakened or confounded by methodologic errors.

It is easy to see that ambulatory electrocardiography and programmed stimulation might be directly applied to a clinical trial of sudden death prevention in two ways: (1) to identify the cohort with highest risk and (2) as a device to select therapy. For example, treatment in a clinical trial might be an algorithm for selecting an optimum drug regimen instead of a single, simple regimen for every patient. Such an algorithm might depend on information about ventricular arrhythmias on an ambulatory ECG or findings at electrophysiologic testing. The succeeding sections of this chapter discuss the suitability of ambulatory electrocardiography and programmed stimulation for the complementary functions of identifying high-risk patients and devising individualized treatment regimens for a clinical trial of sudden cardiac death.

Identifying High-Risk Patients

Ambulatory Electrocardiography

Ambulatory electrocardiography can be used to identify those patients with acute myocardial infarction who are at higher risk of dying from coronary artery disease or recurrent infarction. Moss et al.[5] studied 193 survivors of myocardial infarction who were younger than 66 using 6-hour ambulatory ECGs recorded immediately before they were discharged from the hospital. More than 20 prema-

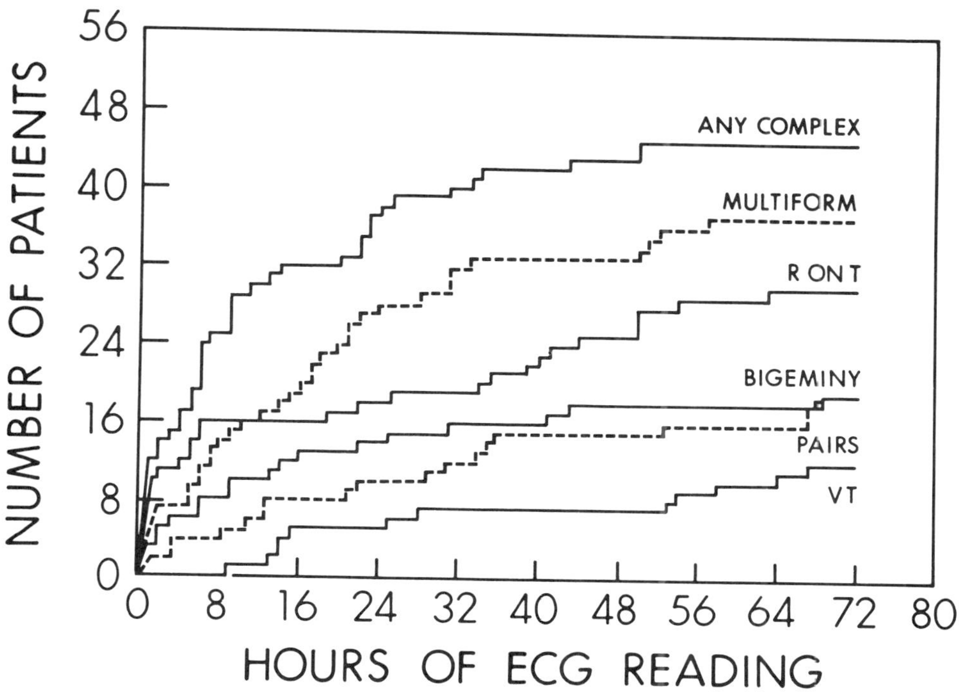

Fig. 8-1. Incidence of ventricular arrhythmias detected by various recording times. (From Winkle RA, Peters F, Hall R: Characteristics of ventricular tachyarrhythmias on ambulatory ECG recordings in postmyocardial infarction patients, Am Heart J 102:162, 1981. With permission.)

ture ventricular beats (VPBs) per hour, multiform VPBs, or ventricular bigeminy carried an ominous prognosis. A subsequent study of 272 patients from this same department seemed to confirm this finding.[6]

Neither of these two studies can escape criticism based on current practices. Six hours of ambulatory ECG recording is short by today's standards. Winkle, Peters, and Hall[7] studied the cumulative incidence of ventricular arrhythmias as a function of recording time in 57 patients 8–11 days after acute myocardial infarction. Ambulatory ECGs were analyzed with a computer-assisted method that accurately identified and counted all ventricular arrhythmias. The prevalence of more serious arrhythmias increased as the length of monitoring increased (Figure 8-1).

Neither report of Moss et al.[5,6] used contemporary life-table methods to analyze survival, and the ambulatory ECGs were interpreted by technicians without the aid of contemporary computer methods for quantitating arrhythmias. Despite these technical reservations, the conclusions have been corroborated in other studies, and it is likely that ambulatory ECG recording could be used to identify a higher risk population among those patients recovering from acute myocardial infarction.[8]

Patients undergoing cardiac catheterization for ischemic heart disease were found to have an increased risk of death if ventricular arrhythmias were found on

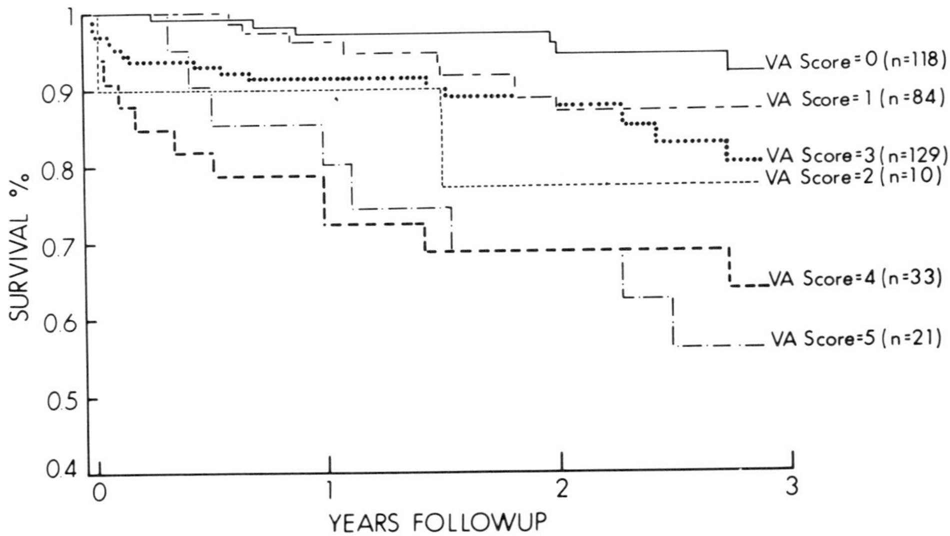

Fig. 8-2. Survival of 395 patients with significant coronary artery disease according to ventricular arrhythmia (*VA*) score. Higher scores were associated with a worse prognosis. (From Califf RM, McKinnis RA, Burks J, et al: Prognostic implications of ventricular arrhythmias during 24-hour ambulatory monitoring in patients undergoing cardiac catheterization for coronary artery disease, Am J Cardiol 50:23, 1982. With permission.)

an ambulatory ECG done shortly after they were catheterized.[9] The authors of the study proposed the following ventricular arrhythmia scoring system: 0, no VPBs; 1, less than 30 VPBs/hr, maximum; 2, greater than or equal to VPBs/hr, uniform; 3, multiform VPBs; 4, two consecutive VPBs; and 5, ventricular tachycardia. Advanced scores were associated with a progressively poorer prognosis during follow-up (Figure 8-2).

Ambulatory electrocardiography also can identify high-risk patients in relatively unselected populations. Follansbee, Michelson, and Morganroth[10] reviewed retrospectively the ambulatory ECGs of 518 consecutive patients, many of whom had no known heart disease. Three or more consecutive VPBs ("triplets") were associated with a high risk of sudden cardiac death. Of the 37 patients with this finding, 10 died suddenly during a mean 19-month follow-up period. Risk was highest for patients with congestive heart failure; 9 of 19 died during the follow-up period.

Programmed Electrical Stimulation

In contrast to ambulatory electrocardiography, programmed electrical stimulation has not been extensively tested as a screening tool to identify patients at high risk of cardiac death. Programmed stimulation has been used far more commonly to study the mechanisms of arrhythmias.[11] The most provocative report using programmed stimulation as a prognostic tool came from Greene, Reid, and Schaeffer[12] who studied the repetitive ventricular response (RVR) in patients with acute myocardial infarction. The RVR was defined as 2 or more VPBs in response to a single electrical stimulus. Patients were studied within 8–85 days after acute myocardial infarction. Of the 48 patients, 19 had RVRs, and 15 of the 19 had ventricular tachycardia or sudden death within 1 year of follow-up. Only 4 of the remaining 29 patients had ventricular tachycardia or sudden death in the follow-up period.

The study of Greene, Reid, and Schaeffer was exciting, but also subject to some criticism. The stimulation sequence used was unusual because ventricular extrastimuli were coupled to an atrial paced beat rather than a ventricular paced beat, which is more common. There were, therefore, few published data with which comparisons could be made. Also, survival data were not analyzed using life-table methods. Nevertheless, this study remains a provocative report that has been neither confirmed nor sufficiently contested.

Selection of Drug Therapy

Ambulatory Electrocardiography

Whether ambulatory electrocardiography can be used as a guide to selecting therapy for paroxysmal arrhythmias has not been tested rigorously. In general, it has been assumed that this is *not* an appropriate use of ambulatory electrocardiography in the clinical setting, and it is unlikely that it would be applicable in the setting of a clinical trial. According to Winkle[13]:

> Although there is probably an incompletely understood relation between suppression of asymptomatic ectopic beats and control of more severe arrhythmias, showing efficacy of a drug for asymptomatic ventricular arrhythmia reduction is not a direct substitute for demonstrating its capacity to prevent recurrent symptomatic ventricular tachycardia or sudden death.

There is only fragmentary evidence to suggest that ambulatory electrocardiography can be used as a guide to choosing specific therapy for individual patients.

The best evidence that suppression of PVBs can be used as a guide to selecting a drug for suppression of symptomatic ventricular tachycardia was contained in a study of propranolol by Woosley et al.[14] Of 32 patients with frequent VPBs, 11 had symptomatic ventricular tachycardia. A greater than 70% reduction in VPBs occurred in 8 of 11 subjects during propranolol therapy, and all 8 had relief from symptomatic tachycardia. This correlation between suppressing VPBs during acute testing and preventing symptomatic ventricular tachycardia has not been demonstrated for other therapies.

Programmed Electrical Stimulation

There is now great enthusiasm for using programmed stimulation as a tool to select drug therapy for select patients with ventricular arrhythmias, including some who appear at high risk for sudden cardiac death. For example, serial electrophysiologic studies have been used as a method to select drug therapy in patients who have already suffered one cardiac arrest. The best-known study, by Ruskin, DiMarco, and Garan,[11] included 31 survivors of out-of-hospital cardiac arrest. Twenty-five patients had inducible ventricular arrhythmias, and chronic antiarrhythmic therapy was based on suppression of inducible arrhythmias during acute testing with programmed stimulation. Complete suppression was achieved in 19 patients, none of whom died during follow-up. The remaining 6 patients continued to have inducible ventricular arrhythmias on all tested drug regimens; 3 of them died during follow-up. The authors concluded that programmed stimulation could be used to select antiarrhythmic therapy in sudden death survivors.

Despite the excitement caused by the report of Ruskin et al., the study should be considered with some reservation before it is applied to a large clinical trial. There was no control group for whom therapy was selected by any other method. The 19 patients with "suppressible" arrhythmias might have done well on any therapy. Only 6 patients had "nonsuppressible" arrhythmias, a small group on which to base sweeping conclusions. Moreover, follow-up data were not analyzed using more appropriate life-table methods. Not in this study nor in any other study has serial electrophysiologic testing been subjected to the rigid controlled trials required of other new treatment modalities.

A particularly disturbing aspect of using programmed stimulation to select antiarrhythmic therapy is that "inducibility" is apparently related to the enthusiasm (or endurance) of the operator. Ruskin, DiMarco, and Garon,[11] for example, contrast their methods with those used by Myerberg, Conde, and Sung[15] in a study of similar patients. Myerberg, Conde, and Sung[15] used single premature ventricular stimuli, whereas Ruskin, DiMarco, and Garon[11] used double premature stimuli and had a much higher yield of ventricular arrhythmias. Reddy and Gettes[16] added isoproterenol infusion to aid in the induction of ventricular arrhythmias after double extrastimuli had failed in their patients with a history of ventricular tachycardia. Fisher et al.[17] have suggested that some patients need to be "primed" using prolonged pacing, pacing at rates greater than 100 beats/min, or exercise. There is a desperate need for standardization of stimulation protocols between laboratories before the technique can be adapted to use in a multicenter clinical trial.

SUMMARY

Both ambulatory electrocardiography and programmed stimulation have been used productively in the study of cardiac arrhythmias. Neither, however, appears ideally adaptable for use in a clinical trial of sudden cardiac death. Ambulatory electrocardiography may have a role to play in assigning risk to some subject populations; its value as a method to select therapy is doubtful. Programmed electrical stimulation appears to be best suited to study mechanisms of arrhythmias. Lack of standardized stimulation protocols and lack of controlled studies of its value in planning therapy render it unproven for use in a large clinical trial.

Acknowledgment

The author much appreciates the efforts of Mrs. Ann Clayton, who typed this manuscript.

REFERENCES

1. Schwartz CJ, Gerrity RG: Anatomical pathology of sudden unexpected cardiac death. Circulation 51-52(suppl 3):18, 1975
2. Levy RI, Sondik EJ: Large scale clinical trials: Are they worth the cost? in Greenberg HM, Dwyer EM Jr (Eds): Sudden Coronary Death, Ann NY Acad Sci 382:411, 1982
3. Friedewald WT, Schoenberger JA: Overview of recent clinical and methodological advances from clinical trials of cardiovascular disease. Controlled Clin Trials 3:259, 1982
4. Biometrics Research Branch: National Heart Institute sample size estimates for medical trials. Circulation 37-38(suppl 1):279, 1969
5. Moss AJ, DeCamilla JJ, Mietlowski W, et al: Prognostic grading and significance of ventricular premature beats after recovery from myocardial infarction. Circulation 51-52(suppl 3):204, 1975
6. Moss AJ, DeCamilla JJ, Davis HP, et al: Clinical significance of ventricular ectopic beats in the early posthospital phase of myocardial infarction. Am J Cardiol 39:635, 1977
7. Winkle RA, Peters F, Hall R: Characteristics of ventricular tachyarrhythmias on ambulatory ECG recordings in postmyocardial infarction patients. Am Heart J 102:162, 1981
8. Coronary Drug Project Research Group: Prognostic importance of premature beats following myocardial infarction: Experience in the Coronary Drug Project. JAMA 223:1116, 1973
9. Califf, RM, McKinnis RA, Burks J, et al: Prognostic implications of ventricular arrhythmias during 24-hour ambulatory monitoring in patients undergoing cardiac catheterization for coronary artery disease. Am J Cardiol 50:23, 1982
10. Follansbee WP, Michelson EL, Morganroth J: Nonsustained ventricular tachycardia in ambulatory patients: Characteristics and association with sudden cardiac death. Ann Intern Med 92:741, 1980
11. Ruskin JN, DiMarco JP, Garan H: Out-of-hospital cardiac arrest. N Engl J Med 303:607, 1980
12. Greene HL, Reid PR, Schaeffer AH: The repetitive ventricular response in man: A predictor of sudden death. N Engl J Med 299:729, 1978
13. Winkel RA, Measuring antiarrhythmic drug efficacy by suppression of asymptomatic ventricular arrhythmias. Ann Intern Med 91:480, 1979
14. Woosley RL, Kornhauser D, Smith R, et al: Suppression of chronic ventricular arrhythmias with propranolol. Circulation 60:819, 1979
15. Myerburg RJ, Conde CA, Sung RJ: Clinical electrophysiologic and hemodynamic profile of patients resuscitated from prehospital cardiac arrest. Am J Med 68:568, 1980
16. Reddy CP, Gettes LS: Use of isoproterenol as an aid to electric induction of chronic recurrent ventricular tachycardia. Am J Cardiol 44:705, 1979
17. Fisher JD, Cohen HL, Mehra R, et al: Cardiac pacing and pacemakers. II. Serial electrophysiologic testing for control of recurrent tachyarrhythmias. Am Heart J 93:658, 1977

Dan M. Roden
Raymond L. Woosley

9

ELECTROPHARMACOLOGY AND PHARMACODYNAMICS OF ANTIARRHYTHMIC DRUGS

The pharmacologic properties of drugs that affect cardiac rhythm can be divided into two broad areas: electropharmacologic properties, which affect initiation and propagation of normal and abnormal cardiac impulses, and ancillary pharmacologic properties. Suppression of cardiac arrhythmias by these drugs is probably related to their electropharmacologic actions, although the nature of this link remains controversial. In practice, the use of antiarrhythmic drugs is frequently limited by their ancillary pharmacologic properties. These properties may include well-defined effects on cardiac contractility or autonomic tone, either of which may indirectly effect rhythm disturbances. Noncardiac pharmacologic effects, such as diarrhea with quinidine or induction of the lupus syndrome with procainamide, frequently limit therapy with antiarrhythmic drugs. Hence, although an understanding of the electropharmacology of these agents can lead to insights into their mechanisms of action in suppressing rhythm disturbances, it is the nonelectrophysiologic properties of these agents that frequently limit therapy.

Factors that affect the relationship between a given dose of a drug and the effect it produces can be divided into two major groups: the first is the relationship between drug dose and plasma concentration, and the second is the relationship between drug concentration (in plasma or tissue) and the effect that the presence of a given amount of drug produces. Variability in either of these two factors can account for interindividual variability in response to drug therapy. Study of the relationship between drug dose and plasma concentrations is termed *pharmacokinetics,* and the evaluation of the relationship between plasma or tissue drug concentrations and drug effects is termed *pharmacodynamics*. Methods for evaluating interindividual variability in pharmacokinetics are fairly well established and will be outlined below; pharmacodynamics, which may be viewed as "individual

SUDDEN CARDIAC DEATH
0-8089-1725-0

sensitivity to a drug," are much less standardized, but are of at least equal importance in characterizing the effect that a given drug produces.

ELECTROPHARMACOLOGY

Classification Schemes

The effects that an antiarrhythmic drug produces in single-cell studies, animal models, and humans define its electropharmacology. A number of schemes have been posed in an attempt to classify these agents according to their effects on cardiac tissue. The ultimate utility of such a classification system would lie in its ability to predict antiarrhythmic responses in patients based on electrophysiologic characterization in preclinical models. Since the ancillary pharmacologic properties of antiarrhythmic agents vary widely and are often multiple, no classification scheme will be perfect. Nevertheless, grouping these agents by electrophysiologic properties may be helpful as in the following examples:

1. Patients who develop torsades de pointes during quinidine therapy probably should not be given the closely related agent disopyramide
2. Patients with ventricular arrhythmias responsive to intravenous lidocaine are more likely to respond to therapy with the oral lidocaine analog tocainide than those whose arrhythmias are lidocaine resistant.[1,2] There are indications for both tocainide and mexiletine,[3] another lidocaine analog, however, that this predictive relationship is imperfect. Tocainide and mexiletine may have electropharmacologic differences from lidocaine, such as in the kinetics of recovery from use-dependent block.[4]
3. It appears likely that a subset of chronic ventricular arrhythmias respond to beta-blockade; almost any beta-blocker will suppress arrhythmias unless its ancillary effects cause intolerance. Similarly, paroxysmal atrioventricular nodal tachycardia probably will respond equally well to calcium channel blockade with either verapamil or diltiazem, although these agents have not yet been formally compared to each other.
4. Multiple reports suggest that antiarrhythmic efficacy may be enhanced by combinations of agents with different electropharmacologic properties;[5] conversely, arrhythmias may be unaffected or exacerbated by combinations of agents with similar electrophysiologic properties.[6] The general applicability of this combination hypothesis remains untested, however.
5. In vitro characterization of apparently desirable electropharmacologic effects can lead to development of agents with similar electropharmacologic properties and fewer side effects. For instance, the properties of a number of agents have been intensively investigated because their electropharmacologic properties resemble those of amiodarone or bretylium. Although both amiodarone and bretylium are effective in appropriate circumstances, side effects are a problem. The development of drugs with similar electropharmacologic properties and fewer side effects might offer better therapy.

A number of major variables have been examined in in vitro and animal models in an attempt to characterize the electropharmacology of these agents, including the effects on resting membrane potential, action potential amplitude, action potential duration, phase 0 slope, refractoriness, membrane responsiveness, normal and abnormal automaticity, early and late afterdepolarizations, recovery from frequency dependent depression of maximal phase 0 slope ($\dot{V}max$), and alterations in impulse propagation. This list is not all inclusive, and the fact that it is so long reflects an incomplete understanding of the factors responsible for the arrhythmia leading to sudden cardiac death and how drugs might modify them.

Sodium Channel Blockers

The conventional antiarrhythmic agents have frequently been subdivided into two general classes, of which lidocaine and quinidine are the prototypes. Quinidine-like drugs, which include disopyramide and procainamide, slow phase 0 upstroke, slow conduction, prolong refractoriness and action potential duration as well as the ratio between the two, decrease membrane responsiveness, decrease excitability, and slow normal automaticity. Lidocaine-like drugs (which include tocainide, mexiletine, and phenytoin), on the other hand, generally shorten the action potential duration and effective refractory period (although they also prolong the ratio of the two) and have less effect on phase 0 slope, conduction velocity, or membrane responsiveness. It is quite clear however, that lidocaine may exert effects that resemble those of quinidine in the presence of ischemia. It now appears that the common effect of all these drugs at the cellular level is to interfere with the entry of sodium into cells. It has been proposed that the difference between quinidine and lidocaine lies primarily in the rate of recovery from use-dependent block and that antiarrhythmic drugs therefore can be classified according to their sodium channel blocking properties. The time constant for recovery of $\hat{V}max$ is probably a continuum, with some drugs having long time constants (e.g., quinidine) and some drugs having short time constants (e.g., lidocaine). Furthermore, quinidine-like drugs may prolong the action potential by interfering with plateau potassium currents,[7] whereas lidocaine, which lacks this action, probably shortens the action potential by blocking the plateau inward sodium (''window'') current.[7]

Over the last 4 years clinical trials have shown that several agents appear to depress phase 0 upstroke velocity to a relatively greater degree than the extent to which they alter refractoriness. These agents, all of which have long time constants for the development of use-dependent block,[8] include encainide, (and its metabolite O-demethyl encainide), flecainide, and lorcainide. Although these drugs appear to be extremely effective in decreasing sporadic ventricular arrhythmias in patients and spontaneous ventricular arrhythmias 24 hours after coronary occlusion in dogs, they appear to be far less effective in preventing sustained reentrant ventricular tachycardia in patients and dog models. Whether this dichotomy of response holds up remains to be evaluated with further testing.

Beta Adrenergic Receptor Blockers

The major electropharmacologic effects of the beta-adrenergic recetor blocking drugs is blunting of the catecholamine-induced increase in normal automaticity. Catecholamines may play a critical role in the genesis and propagation of abnormal action potentials (e.g., during ischemia); blockade of such effects might help explain some of the effects of beta-adrenergic blocking drugs in the prevention of sudden death, although this is by no means the only possible explanation. A number of beta-adrenergic blocking drugs, including propranolol, acebutolol, alprenolol, pindolol, and oxprenolol, display quinidine-like slowing of phase 0 upstroke velocity at high concentrations in vitro.[9] Whether this "membrane-stabilizing effect" is ever present at clinically achieved concentrations remains uncertain. It is fairly certain that propranolol can shorten the action potential duration, both in vitro[10] and in patients.[11] This effect appears to be independent of propranolol's beta-adrenergic receptor blocking properties, since it is also produced by the weakly beta-blocking *d*-isomer (in vitro[10] and in humans[12]) and is also produced after chemical sympathectomy by 6-hydroxydopamine.[13] The ionic mechanism responsible for these changes is not known, although blockade of the plateau inward sodium ("window") current is one reasonable possibility. Sotalol, a beta-adrenergic receptor blocking drug devoid of membrane-stabilizing qualities, has been shown to prolong the action potential duration and effective refractory period in vitro[14,15] and in humans.[16] This "amiodarone-like" effect was present at higher concentrations in vitro than those required to produce substantial beta-blockade.[14] Preliminary evidence in humans suggests that sotalol is a far more effective agent in suppressing chronic ventricular arrhythmias than most beta-blocking drugs, and dose-response data suggest that significant prolongation of the QT interval occurs at concentrations higher than those required to produce substantial beta-blockade.[17]

Slow Current Blockers

Agents whose major effect is to interfere with the slow calcium channel have their major clinical application in rhythm disturbances based in atrioventricular node. This is not surprising, since atrioventricular nodal conduction is largely slow-channel dependent. These drugs, which include verapamil and diltiazem, convert paroxysmal atrioventricular nodal tachycardia to sinus rhythm and slow the ventricular response during atrial flutter or atrial fibrillation. Since calcium channels are believed by some to be important in ischemia-induced ventricular fibrillation, it has been speculated that these agents might be helpful in the prevention of sudden cardiac death. Multicenter trials are currently under way in an attempt to address this question, but to date there is no convincing evidence to suggest that the routine use of calcium channel blockers decreases the incidence of sudden cardiac death.

Action Potential Prolongation

Drugs that have received considerable attention recently are those whose primary electrophysiologic action is to prolong the effective refractory period and action potential duration, while leaving the ratio between the two unchanged. The two prototype agents are bretylium and amiodarone. In the case of bretylium, fairly convincing evidence has been presented that the prolongation of action potential duration and effective refractory period occurs primarily in normal tissues[18]; hence, the reduction of disparities between normal and infarcted tissue may be responsible for its antiarrhythmic actions. Electrophysiologic effects of amiodarone are actually less well characterized, despite more extensive investigation. Inconsistencies in the reported effects of amiodarone may partly be due to the following: the intravenous form is delivered in a vehicle that may have elctrophysiologic properties of its own,[19] the drug probably requires some time before its effects become apparent,[20] and different test systems (several in vitro models and patients) have been used to study its effects. Nevertheless, the predominant electrophysiologic effect of amiodarone appears to be prolongation of the action potential duration.[21] AH interval prolongation is also seen, which may reflect its sympatholytic activity. During chronic therapy, HV prolongation has been reported, as has the prolongation of the ventricular effective refractory period.[25] In vitro studies are more difficult to carry out, since the drug must be administered for some period of time prior to study before the effects can be seen. Prolongation of the action potential duration is the predominant electrophysiologic effect of this drug[23]; noncompetitive beta-blockade and sodium and calcium channel blockade in Purkinje fibers and ventricular muscle also have been reported.[24] Because of the side effects with bretylium or amiodarone therapy, attempts are currently being made to evaluate the basic and clinical pharmacology of a number of other agents that appear to have this action potential–prolonging effect as their primary electropharmacologic action: meobentine, clofilium, sotalol, and N-acetylprocainamide. This last agent, the major metabolite of the quinidine-like drug, procainamide, appears in vitro[25] and in vivo[26,27] to exert much less effect on maximum phase 0 dV/dt or conduction velocity than procainamide, whereas it does prolong the action potential in vitro and effective refractory period in vivo. The ionic mechanism responsible for the electropharmacologic attributes of these agents is not known.

Although the grouping just presented forms a convenient framework in which to consider the antiarrhythmic drugs, it is not all inclusive. Digitalis, which may be antiarrhythmic in some circumstances, does not fall readily into any of these groups. Similarly, others have proposed that blockade of the movement of other ions across cell membranes may in appropriate circumstances be "antiarrhythmic." The agent alinidine (*N*-allyl-clonidine), for instance, specifically slows sinus rate in a fashion not related to beta-blockade or calcium channel blockade. It has been speculated that this effect is produced by blockade of chloride ion movement and that alinidine may therefore represent a new class of antiarrhythmic drugs.[28]

As mentioned previously, the relationship between electropharmacologic properties in vitro in animal systems or even in humans and arrhythmia suppression is not clear, and the potential ability of these agents to prevent sudden cardiac death through electropharmacologic actions is even less clear. One can speculate that a decrease in automaticity might be antiarrhythmic or that a decrease in dispersion of refractoriness or repolarization (as seen with amiodarone-like drugs) may interrupt reentrant circuits. Similarly, an appropriate degree of conduction slowing coupled with changes in refractoriness could abolish reentry, whereas conduction slowing without comparable changes in refractoriness might actually enable reentrant circuits.

DOSE-RESPONSE RELATIONS

Pharmacokinetics

The description of dose-dependent relationships between plasma concentrations of a drug and time comprises its pharmacokinetic properties. These can be evaluated in normal persons and in individuals with ventricular arrhythmias, cardiac failure, and renal or hepatic failure. Several parameters are often calculated to describe the relationship between plasma concentration and dose: clearance, half-lives (both distribution half-life and elimination half-life), volume of distribution.

Clearance

Clearance, usually expressed as volume of plasma per unit of time is simply the amount of plasma from which a drug could be considered to be completely removed in any given unit of time. This can be further subdivided into renal clearance and hepatic clearance. The ultimate plasma concentration achieved during dosing to steady state depends only on the dose administered and clearance (and not on volume of distribution or elimination half-life). This can be expressed in the relationship

$$\text{Plasma concentration} = \text{dose administered per unit time} \div \text{clearance.}$$

Drug Half-lives

Most processes in drug disposition are assumed to proceed at a rate proportional to the amount of drug present, that is, in a first-order manner. In this case, such processes (elimination, absorption, distribution, etc.) can be described by the rate constant, or more usually, a half-life (half-life = ln 2/rate constant). Since any of these processes are half completed in one half-life and 75% are completed in two half-lives, they can be regarded as essentially complete in four or five half-lives. Distribution of a drug from plasma to tissues thus is nearly complete in four or five *distribution* half-lives, and elimination of a drug from the body is nearly complete in four or five *elimination* half-lives. During constant drug administration (either during long-term oral therapy or constant intravenous infusion), the amount of drug in plasma will reach its ultimate steady state value in four or five *elimination* half-lives. Note that the magnitude of the ultimate steady state value is determined only by dose and clearance, but the time required to achieve steady state is determined by elimination half-life. Furthermore, the use of large initial doses (loading doses) may shorten the time to onset of pharmacologic effect, but does not alter the time required to attain steady state.

Some drugs, notably phenytoin, aspirin, and ethanol, are eliminated in a "zero-order" fashion; in other words, the amount of drug eliminated is independent of the amount present. In the case of phenytoin, elimination at low concentrations is a first-order process dependent on the amount of drug present; however, as concentration rises, this elimination process becomes saturated and elimination then proceeds as a zero-order process, that is, a fixed amount of drug for each unit of time, regardless of the plasma concentration. This can lead to large increments in plasma concentration with small increases in dose.

Volume of Distribution

The third important term that can be used to describe the disposition of a drug once it enters the body is volume of distribution. Since drugs undergo a distribution process after intravenous injection, several types can be described: the volume of distribution of the "central" compartment (which usually includes the plasma, heart, brain, and other highly perfused organs) and the volume of distribution at steady state, which describes the total volume within which the drug is distributed (central plus peripheral sites). These volumes of distribution are convenient for pharmacokinetic calculations but actually correspond to no known physiologic site, and because of tissue binding, they may actually exceed the volume of the body several-fold. Knowledge of the size of the various volumes of distribution may be helpful in determining the size of bolus doses required to achieve a given plasma concentration.

Plasma Protein Binding

Another important concept in pharmacokinetics is consideration of plasma protein binding. The pharmacologically active fraction of drugs generally is that portion which is not bound to plasma protein. For a drug that is highly bound to plasma protein, the free portion therefore is quite small. In this setting, changes in plasma protein binding may cause large changes in the amount of free (pharmacologically active) drug. For instance, phenytoin is generally 90% bound to plasma protein. With renal disease, however, this fraction drops to 80%[29]; as a result, at any given total plasma concentration of phenytoin, the amount of pharmacologically active drug is doubled in a patient with renal failure. A total plasma concentration of 20 μg/ml, which would be at the upper limits of the usual therapeutic range in a normal individual, would correspond to a free concentration twice the usual upper limits in a patient with renal failure. Some drugs, such as disopyramide, may display concentration-dependent binding,[30] which further confounds interpretation of plasma concentration monitoring when only total levels are measured. In the case of disopyramide, optical isomers that have different electrophysiologic properties in vitro[31] and in vivo[32] also may interfere with each other's plasma protein binding.[33]

Drug Disposition Associated with Disease States

Once the parameters describing drug disposition are known in relatively normal individuals, studies can be carried out in patients with cardiac failure, renal failure, hepatic failure, and other disease states to determine if disposition is altered. If this is the case, the specific alteration then can be characterized and appropriate changes in loading or maintenance regimens suggested. Similarly, no changes in dosing regimens may be required, but changes in plasma concentration monitoring guidelines may be required (e.g., for renal failure). In virtually all studies to date, antiarrhythmic drug disposition in patients with chronic ventricular arrhythmias (without other obvious organ dysfunction) is not the same as that observed in normal individuals.[34-37] Almost inevitably, the elimination half-life is prolonged in these patients; whether this reflects an effect of age, subtle cardiac dysfunction, or an unknown influence of ventricular arrhythmias on drug disposition is not known.

Pharmacodynamics

Although extensive methods have been developed for characterizing pharmacokinetics, such is not the case for describing the relationship between plasma or tissue concentrations of drugs and their effects. In general, it has been assumed that plasma drug concentrations or concentrations at a site in equilibrium with those in plasma produce the effect seen. A difficulty may arise in attempting to relate drug effect to plasma concentration before steady state is achieved (that is, before the time when tissue and plasma concentrations rise and fall in parallel). There is good evidence for some antiarrhythmic drugs that effect is actually a function of concentration in some peripheral site (e.g., the myocardium).[38] If this is true, a dissociation between plasma concentration and effect may be observed early during therapy, simply because distribution has not yet occurred. For example, this may be the case for the antifibrillatory effects of bretylium, which are reported to reach maximum values only several hours after a bolus plasma injection, at the time of peak myocardial concentrations.[38]

Variability in Plasma Concentration-effect Relations

Once steady state is achieved, extreme variability in the relationship between plasma concentration and effect may have one of several explanations: assay variability, the presence of one or more active drug metabolites, or the mediation of drug effects by cellular alterations that can persist long after drug elimination has occurred (e.g., antineoplastic drugs).

Quinidine

Sokolow and Edgar[39] reported in 1950 that there was a reasonable correlation between plasma levels of quinidine and conversion from atrial fibrillation to sinus rhythm. Their assay was nonspecific, however, and subsequent developments in assay methodology, including double extraction, enzyme immunoassay, and high-performance liquid chromatography have rendered assays of drugs in plasma or urine increasingly specific. The amount of quinidine actually measured by each of these assays has successively fallen. It has been held that the correlation observed by Sokolow and Edgar was actually due to the fact that their assay was nonspecific, and therefore measured active quinidine metabolites.[40] More recently, Holford et al.[41] demonstrated a greater increase in rate-corrected QT interval (QTc) after oral quinidine administration than after intravenous quinidine administration; they suggested that this discrepancy was due to the generation of active quinidine metabolites during oral administration. The activity of several quinidine metabolites has been studied, and one, 3-hydroxyquinidine, was found to worsen arrhythmias in one model.[42]

Procainamide

A similar dissociation between the dose administered and achieved concentration on the one hand and the effect observed on the other hand was noted when small doses of procainamide controlled ventricular arrhythmias in patients with renal failure.[43] This observation led to the examination of plasma concentrations of ^{N}-acetylprocainamide, the major metabolite of procainamide. It was found that high plasma concentrations of this metabolite accumulated in patients with renal failure, since its elimination depends almost entirely on renal clearance. It was thus postulated that this metabolite might have antiarrhythmic activity. Furthermore, it has been recognized that the rate of formation of the metabolite is genetically determined by the level of hepatic *N*-acetyltransferase. In patients who are genetically rapid metabolizers, that is, those who form large amounts of *N*-acetylprocainamide, the lupus syndrome is much less common during therapy with procainamide than in those who are genetically slow metabolizers.[44] Therapy with *N*-acetylprocainamide therefore might be both effective and less likely to produce the lupus syndrome. Subsequent studies in humans have shown that this metabolite is antiarrhythmic but produces troublesome side effects in over half the patients treated.[45-47] Nevertheless, it can suppress arrhythmias during chronic therapy and does not appear to induce antinuclear antibodies or the lupus syndrome.[45-47]

Encainide

A striking example of the participation of active drug metabolites in the production of drug effects has been provided by the investigational antiarrhythmic agent encainide. The earliest studies of oral efficacy in patients with chronic stable ventricular arrhythmias noted that a wide range of dosages and plasma concentrations was required to suppress arrhythmias.[48] A single patient whose arrhythmias did not respond to therapy also failed to demonstrate typical ECG effects during therapy and was the single patient in an early study who failed to generate significant quantities of O-demethyl encainide, a major metabolite in the responders. Subsequent in vitro[49] and animal work[50,51] has confirmed that O-demethyl encainide is actually 10–50 times more active than the parent drug. Hence, it is likely that in the 90%-95% of patients who are able to generate this substance, it is the form that mediates most of the effects seen in humans. On the other hand, in the small number of patients (6%–10%) who are less able to metabolize encainide to O-demethyl encainide, plasma encainide may accumulate to very high plasma concentrations and, in this setting, has been reported to be antiarrhythmic.[52] Confirmation and further characterization of the effects of O-demethyl encainide in humans obviously awaits its direct administration to patients. A similar investigational agent, lorcainide, also has a dealkylated metabolite that, in indirect evidence in humans, appears to be active. Norlorcainide has been administered to one patient and has shown antiarrhythmic activity.[53]

"Deep" Effector Sites

If the effects of a drug depend on a persistent cellular alteration that it induces or on its "penetration" into a "deep" pharmacokinetic compartment (which can conceptually be regarded as a similar phenomenon), then it is likely that plasma concentrations may not always reflect the effects seen. Some of the dissociation between dose and effect described for the drug amiodarone may be due to such an action.[54]

Assessments of Drug Efficacy

In the broadest sense, "pharmacodynamic analysis" describes the relationship between dose and pharmacologic effect. Two effects are most often quantified: a beneficial effect and an adverse effect. For a beneficial effect, it is important to recognize that the dose-response relationship will vary, depending on the pharmacologic end point used to characterize the response. For instance, higher plasma concentrations are generally required to completely suppress all ventricular arrhythmias than those required for many drugs to suppress all complex forms of arrhythmias (couplets or episodes of ventricular tachycardia).[1,48,55] Similarly, the dose-response relationships for suppression of recurrent sustained ventricular tachycardia or prevention of sudden cardiac death are generally much less well defined but are not necessarily the same as those for suppression of stable ventricular arrhythmias. Some drugs may be effective in suppressing chronic stable arrhythmias but ineffective in suppressing sudden cardiac death; conversely, some drugs might be effective in preventing sudden cardiac death but relatively ineffective in changing the frequency of stable ventricular arrhythmias.

Assessment of Drug Toxicity

In terms of the relationships between dose and adverse effects, two general types of responses exist: those which are fairly clearly related to dose or plasma concentrations and those which occur in an apparently nondose-related fashion. In the latter case, variable drug metabolism can occasionally be invoked as a factor influencing the occurrence of adverse drug effects. For instance, it has been fairly well established that the lupus syndrome develops earlier in slow acetylators of procainamide and more frequently during therapy than in those who are rapid acetylators.[44] Other apparently idiosyncratic actions such as aprindine-induced agranulocytosis, amiodarone-induced pulmonary fibrosis, or quinidine-induced torsades de pointes, may have their genesis in similar genetically dependent patterns of drug disposition. Alternatively, the relationships among patterns of drug disposition and underlying disease states may interact to generate adverse drug reactions.

Although the incidence of so-called idiosyncratic reactions may frequently limit therapy, it is the margin, or therapeutic ratio, between plasma concentrations generally regarded as effective and those plasma concentrations which predictably produce dose-related side effects that ultimately determines the likelihood of successful therapy. For drugs with wide therapeutic ratios, infrequent dosing may be feasible with few side effects, whereas a narrow therapeutic ratio mandates frequent dosing and suggests that frequent side effects will be more likely to occur. Hence, the frequency of dosing is a function of both the width of the therapeutic window and the rate of drug elimination.

Concentration-Response Relationships

Examination of the relationship between plasma concentration and effect can therefore yield useful information about (1) tissue sensitivity, (2) the presence of a "deep" effector site, or (3) the presence of active metabolites. Systematic examination of the dose-response relationship can also yield insights into the relationship between electropharmacology and arrhythmia suppression. For instance, when the relationship between plasma concentration of propranolol and response was examined in a group of patients with ventricular arrhythmias, it was noted that approximately 40% had arrhythmia suppression at plasma concentrations under 100 ng/ml; this is the range usually associated with a high degree of beta-blockade. An additional 30% of patients had ventricular arrhythmia suppression at plasma concentrations of 200–1000 ng/ml, however, suggesting that a non-beta-mediated effect might be operative in these individuals.[55] This observation then led to studies that have demonstrated non-beta-mediated electrophysiologic effects of propranolol in humans.[11,12]

SUMMARY

Scrutiny of the relationship between drug dose and the effects produced thus can yield insights into both pharmacokinetic and pharmacodynamic phenomena. In the former group, mechanisms of drug disposition, alteration in drug distribution, and changes required in loading or maintenance dosing regimens can be derived. Examination of concentration-effect relationships can suggest assay nonspecificity, the presence of a drug in a deep pharmacokinetic compartment, or the presence of one or more active drug metabolites, thus giving insights into the mechanism of drug action.

Although much work has been done to characterize the electrophysiologic and other pharmacologic properties of antiarrhythmic drugs, the essential link between their pharmacologic actions and their arrhythmia-suppressing capabilities remains obscure. Even with a greater understanding of the relationship between electropharmacology and suppression of chronic stable arrhythmias, the potential for these drugs to prevent sudden cardiac death is at this time undefined. Obviously, greater understanding of their electropharmacologic and pharmacodynamic properties will enable design of studies to answer this crucial issue.

REFERENCES

1. Roden DM, Reele SB, Higgins SB, et al: Tocainide therapy for refractory ventricular arrhythmias. Am Heart J 100:15, 1980
2. Winkle RA, Mason JW, Harrison DC: Tocainide for drug-resistant ventricular arrhythmias: Efficacy, side effects, and lidocaine responsiveness for predicting tocainide success. Am Heart J 100:1031, 1980

3. Campbell NPS, Chaturvedi NC, Shanks RG, et al: The development of mexiletine in the management of ventricular dysrhythmias. Postgrad Med J 53:114, 1977
4. Frame L, Gintant G, Hoffman B: Mexiletine and tocainide differ from lidocaine in their use-dependent kinetics. Circulation 66(suppl 2):292, 1982
5. Duff HJ, Roden DM, Primm K, et al: Mexiletine in the treatment of resistant ventricular arrhythmias: Enhancement of efficacy and reduction of dose-related side effects by combination with quinidine. Circulation 67:1124, 1983
6. Duffy E, Swiryn S, Bauernfiend R, et al: Sustained ventricular tachycardia refractory to individual class I drugs: Effect of a second class I drug. Circulation 64(suppl 4): 136, 1984
7. Colatsky TJ: Mechanisms of action of lidocaine and quinidine on action potential duration in rabbit cardiac Purkinje fibers: An effect on steady state sodium currents? Circ Res 50:17, 1982
8. Campbell TJ: Kinetics of onset of rate-dependent effects of class I antiarrhythmic drugs are important in determination of their effects on refractoriness in guinea pig ventricle and provide a theoretical basis for their subclassification. Cardiovasc Res 17:352, 1983
9. Singh BN: Anti-arrhythmic actions of beta-adrenergic receptor antagonists: Review of fundamental aspects. NZ Med J 76:333, 1972
10. Pruett JK, Walle T, Bagwell EE: Association of in vivo and in vitro propranolol levels in canine Purkinje fibers with antiarrhythmic effects. J Pharmacol Exp Ther 202:45, 1977
11. Duff HJ, Roden DM, Brorson L, et al: Electrophysiologic actions of high plasma concentrations of propranolol in human subjects. J Am Coll Cardiol 2:1134, 1983.
12. Duff HJ, Wood AJJ, Dawson AK, et al: *d*-Propranolol: Non-adrenergically mediated electrophysiologic actions in man. Circulation 66(suppl 2) 372, 1982
13. Harrison LA, Wittig J, Wallace AG: Adrenergic influence on the distal Purkinje system in the canine heart. Circ Res 32:329, 1973
14. Strauss HC, Bigger JT, Hoffman BF: Electrophysiological and beta-receptor blocking effects of MJ1999 on dog and rabbit cardiac tissue. Circ Res 26:661, 1970
15. Singh BN, Vaughan Williams EM: A third class of anti-arrhythmic action: Effects on atrial and ventricular intracellular potentials, and other pharmacological actions on cardiac muscle of MJ1999 and AH3474. Br J Pharmacol 39:675, 1970
16. Echt D, Berte LE, Clusin WT, et al: Prolongation of the human cardiac action potential by sotalol. Am J Cardiol 50:1082, 1982
17. Wang T, Bergstrand RH, Siddoway LA, et al: Dissociation of antiarrhythmic and beta-blocking actions of sotalol. Circulation 68 (suppl 3):279, 1983
18. Cardinal R, Sasyniuk BI: Electrophysiological effects of bretylium tosylate on subendocardial Purkinje fibers from infarcted canine hearts. J Pharmacol Exp Ther 204:159, 1978
19. Sicart M, Besse P, Choussat A, et al: Action hemodynamique de l'amiodarone intra-veineuse chez l'homme. Arch Mal Coeur 70:219, 1977
20. Heger JJ, Prystowsky EN, Jackman WM, et al: Amiodarone: Clinical efficacy and electrophysiology during long-term therapy for recurrent ventricular tachycardia or ventricular fibrillation. N Engl J Med 305:539, 1981
21. Olsson SB, Brorson L, Varnauskas E: Class 3 antiarrhythmic action in man: Observations from monophasic action potential recordings and amiodarone treatment. Br Heart J 35:1255, 1973
22. Finerman WB, Hamer A, Peter T, et al: Electrophysiologic effects of chronic amiodarone therapy in patients with ventricular arrhythmias. Am Heart J 104:987, 1982
23. Singh BN, Vaughan Williams EM: The effect of amiodarone, a new anti-

anginal drug, on cardiac muscle. Br J Pharmacol 39:657, 1970

24. Rosenbaum MB, Chiale PA, Halpern MS, et al: Clinical efficacy of amiodarone as an antiarrhythmic agent. Am J Cardiol 28:934, 1976
25. Dangman KH, Hoffman BF: In vivo and in vitro antiarrhythmic and arrhythmogenic effects of *N*-acetylprocainamide. J Pharmacol Exp Ther 217:851, 1981
26. Jaillon P, Winkle R: Electrophysiologic comparative study of procainamide and *N*-acetylprocainamide in anesthetized dogs: Concentration-response relationships. Circulation 60:1385, 1979
27. Jaillon P, Rubenson D, Peters F, et al: Electrophysiologic effects of *N*-acetylprocainamide in human beings. Am J Cardiol 47:1134, 1981
28. Millar JS, Vaughan Williams EM: Anion-antagonism—A fifth class of antiarrhythmic action? Lancet 1:1291, 1981
29. Reidenberg MM, Odar-Cederloff I, Von Bahr C, et al: Protein binding of diphenylhydantoin and desmethylimipramine in plasma from patients with poor renal function. N Engl J Med 285:264, 1971
30. Lima JJ, Boudoulas H, Blanford M: Concentration-dependence of disopyramide binding to plasma protein and its influence on kinetics and dynamics. J Pharmacol Exp Ther 219:741, 1981
31. Mirro MJ, Watanabe AM, Bailey JC: Electrophysiologic effects of the optical isomers of disopyramide and quinidine in the dog: Dependence on stereochemistry. Circ Res 48:867, 1981
32. Pollick C, Giacomini KM, Blaschke TF, et al: The cardiac effects of *d*- and *l*-disopyramide in normal subjects: A noninvasive study. Circulation 66:447, 1982
33. Valdivieso L, Blaschke T, Giacomini K: Disopyramide enantiomers bind stereoselectively to human plasma protein. Proceedings of the Second World Conference on Clinical Pharmacology, Washington, D.C. 1983, p 116
34. Lalka D, Meyer MB, Duce BR, et al: Kinetics of the oral antiarrhythmic lidocaine congener, tocainide. Clin Pharmacol Ther 19:757, 1976
35. Klein MC, Levine PA, Ryan TJ: Antiarrhythmic efficacy, pharmacokinetics and clinical safety of tocainide in convalescent myocardial infarction patients. Chest 77:726, 1980
36. Prescott LF, Clements JA, Pottage A: Absorption, distribution and elimination of mexiletine. Postgrad Med J 53:50, 1977
37. Vozeh S, Katz G, Steiner V, et al: Population pharmacokinetic parameters in patients treated with oral mexiletine. Eur J Clin Pharmacol 23:445, 1982
38. Anderson JL, Patterson E, Conlon M, et al: Kinetics of antifibrillatory effects of bretylium: Correlation with myocardial drug concentrations. Am J Cardiol 46:583, 1980
39. Sokolow M, Edgar AL: Blood quinidine concentrations as a guide in the treatment of cardiac arrhythmias. Circulation 1:576, 1950
40. Guentert TW, Upton RA, Holford NHG, et al: Divergence in pharmacokinetic parameters of quinidine obtained by specific and nonspecific assay methods. J Pharmacokinet Biopharma 4:303, 1979
41. Holford NHG, Coates PE, Guentert TW, et al: The effect of quinidine and its metabolites on the electrocardiogram and systolic time intervals: Concentration-effect relationships. Br J Clin Pharmacol 11:187, 1981
42. Drayer DE, Lowenthal DT, Restivo KM, et al: Steady-state serum levels of quinidine and active metabolites in cardiac patients with varying degrees of renal function. Clin Pharmacol Ther 24:31, 1978
43. Drayer DE, Lowenthal DT, Woosley RL, et al: Cumulation of *N*-acetylprocainamide, an active metabolite of procainamide, in patients with impaired renal function. Clin Pharmacol Ther 22:63, 1977
44. Woosley RL, Drayer DE, Reidenberg MM, et al: Effect of acetylator pheno-

type on the rate at which procainamide induces antinuclear antibodies and the lupus syndrome. N Engl J Med 298:1157, 1978

45. Roden DM, Reele SB, Higgins SB, et al: Antiarrhythmic efficacy, pharmacokinetics and safety of *N*-acetylprocainamide in human subjects: Comparison with procainamide. Am J Cardiol 46:463, 1980
46. Lahita R, Kluger J, Drayer DE, et al: Antibodies to nuclear antigens in patients treated with procainamide or acetylprocainamide. N Engl J Med 301:1382, 1979
47. Stec GP, Lertora JJL, Atkinson AJ, et al: Remission of procainamide-induced lupus erythematosus with *N*-acetylprocainamide therapy. Ann Int Med 90:799, 1980
48. Roden DM, Reele SB, Higgins SB, et al: Total suppression of ventricular arrhythmias by encainide: Pharmacokinetic and electrocardiographic characteristics. N Engl J Med 302:877, 1980
49. Elharrar V, Zipes DP: Effects of encainide and metabolites (MJ14030 and MJ9444) on canine cardiac Purkinje and ventricular fibers. J Pharmacol Exp Ther 220:440, 1981
50. Roden DM, Duff HJ, Altenbern D, et al: Antiarrhythmic activity of the O-demethyl metabolite of encainide. J Pharmacol Exp Ther 221:522, 1982
51. Duff HJ, Dawson AK, Roden DM, et al: Electrophysiologic actions of O-demethyl encainide: An active metabolite. Circulation 68:385, 1983
52. Carey EL, Duff HJ, Roden DM, et al: Relative electrocardiographic and antiarrhythmic effects of encainide and its metabolites in man. J Clin Invest 73:539, 1984
53. Meinertz T, Kasper W, Kersting F, et al: Lorcainide: Plasma concentration-effect relationship. Clin Pharmacol Ther 26:187, 1979
54. Siddoway LA, McAllister CB, Wilkinson GR, et al: Amiodarone dosing: A proposal based upon its pharmacokinetics. Am Heart J 106:951, 1983
55. Woosley RL, Kornhauser D, Smith R, et al: Suppression of chronic ventricular arrhythmias with propranolol. Circulation 60:819, 1979

Kenneth M. Kessler
Robert J. Myerburg

10

SAFETY AND EFFICACY OF CURRENTLY AVAILABLE ANTIARRHYTHMIC AGENTS FOR THE PREVENTION OF SUDDEN DEATH

During the past decade, information about the efficacy and safety of antiarrhythmic agents for prevention of sudden death has evolved faster than new drugs have been developed or studies to confirm new hypotheses have been completed. Earlier concepts that focused on the endpoint of the suppression of premature ventricular contractions (PVCs) for prevention of sudden death represented an oversimplification. Therapeutic concepts have evolved as the result of multiple complementary developments in pharmacology and epidemiology. Key initial developments were in the fields of drug analysis and the statistical approach to PVC suppression.[1,2] Easier and more rapid methods for drug analysis became available, which helped improve interpretation of drug responses and allowed more appropriate study design and individualization of therapy. With the recognition of the significant spontaneous variability in PVC frequency, studies of antiarrhythmic efficacy became more precise; however, proof of consistent sudden death prevention by antiarrhythmic has not been obtained.

The key to modernization of drug therapy for sudden death prevention is recognition of the need to individualize therapy and to concentrate on identified high-risk subgroups. The PVC theory (i.e., quantitative PVC suppression) began to be questioned when it was not confirmed by appropriate clinical studies. Except with acute ischemia, the relationship of PVC suppression to sudden death prevention is incompletely studied, and a direct cause-and-effect relationship has

---

Supported in part by a grant from the National Institutes of Health, National Heart Lung & Blood Institute, HL 28130-01 and a Grant-in-Aid from the American Heart Association of Greater Miami.

SUDDEN CARDIAC DEATH
0-8089-1725-0

never been confirmed. Furthermore pro-arrhythmic drug effects became increasingly evident,[3,4] risk-benefit concepts began to be reassessed and treatment was directed primarily at high-risk subgroups in an effort to avoid therapeutic risk in low-risk subjects. Concurrently, the possible dissociation of anti-PVC and antifibrillatory effects of antiarrhythmic agents became increasingly evident.[5,6] With these refinements, investigators began to recognize the necessity of more precisely defining and subcategorizing the clinical setting, arrhythmia form, and drug intervention when dealing with sudden death prevention. As a consequence, current therapy for the prevention of sudden cardiac death has become endpoint oriented and directed to high-risk subgroups (e.g., sudden death survivors). Current therapeutic endpoints include (1) suppression of ventricular ectopy, especially complex forms; (2) suppression of inducible arrhythmias; and (3) blood-level monitoring. Although investigations tend to concentrate on only one concept at a time, these endpoints are potentially complementary, not mutually exclusive. We are now at a stage when therapeutic algorithms can be applied to selected subsets of patients at high risk for fatal ventricular arrhythmias for the purpose of testing their influence on clinical outcomes.

ANTIARRHYTHMIC AGENTS FOR SUPPRESSION OF SIMPLE VENTRICULAR ECTOPY

The PVC theory is based on data accumulated in the 1950s and 1960s. Sudden cardiac death appeared to be directly related to the evolution of ventricular tachyarrhythmias associated with ischemic heart disease.[7-9] Since the terminal event was arrhythmic and control of ischemic heart disease did not necessarily alleviate the risk of a fatal arrhythmia, prevention of sudden death focused on drug therapy with antiarrhythmic agents. This simplistic approach was reinforced by earlier workers who identified PVCs as (1) warning arrhythmias in the acute infarction setting[10] and (2) as a chronic risk factor for mortality, particularly in the presence of ischemic heart disease.[11-13] The use and development of antiarrhythmic agents thus focused on risk factor (PVC) suppression, which could be accomplished reasonably well, but the real mystery, the relationship of this risk factor to the clinical outcome of sudden death, remained largely ignored.

Quinidine

Quinidine is the oldest of the antiarrhythmic agents commonly used today. The drug was first described in 1848 by Heyningen and "modern" usage began at the turn of this century. Sokolow's review in 1951[14] is characteristic of early studies on quinidine; the drug was judged effective for ventricular arrhythmias in 80%–90% of the patients. More recent studies have added several theoretic and practical advantages, including assay techniques that separately measure the parent drug, inactive and active metabolites, and recognition of the spontaneous variability in PVC frequency.[1,2]

A recent study by Carliner et al.,[15] using a newer assay technique, showed at least 90% suppression of PVCs in 12 of 14 patients treated with 800–1800 mg of quinidine daily. Correlations of PVC frequency to serum levels were suggestive but inconclusive for individual patients and poor for the group as a whole. A therapeutic response was noted at levels ranging from 0.72–5.92 μg/ml. Similarly, Winkle et al.[16] showed a 90% reduction in PVC frequency in 62% of patients receiving 1.8 g/day of quinidine. Jelinek, Lohrbauer, and Lown[17] were less successful; using 1.2 and 1.8 g/day of quinidine, PVCs were suppressed in only 7 of the 23 patients treated, and side effects occurred in 6 patients. They therefore questioned the safety of this drug. On the other hand, an article 2 years later from the same institution[18] reported that oral drug testing with quinidine (a 600 mg loading dose) was successful in 9 of 18 patients, acutely; 7 of whom showed good long-term results. Pro-arrhythmic effects in 4 of the 18 again suggested that the risk/benefit ratio must be carefully scrutinized and therapy should be directed to high-risk patients. Of special interest is a study by Krone et al.[19] wherein subtherapeutic doses of quinidine decreased the number of PVCs with short coupling intervals. This is one of the few studies that examined the effect of antiarrhythmic agents at subtherapeutic levels, with therapeutic defined in terms of PVC suppression. The results are of interest in view of the potential dichotomy of anti-PVC and antifibrillatory effects of the membrane-active antiarrhythmic agents, especially since the effective antifibrillatory threshold may be lower than the anti-PVC threshold, at least in some patients.[20]

In terms of more advanced forms, or postinfarction arrhythmias, quinidine is rarely, if ever, used today for the conversion or prevention of ventricular tachycardia. In recent studies focusing on the three newer endpoints for the prevention of sudden cardiac death, quinidine has been shown effective in preventing recurrent life-threatening arrhythmias in selected patients.

Procainamide

Procainamide was developed as a consequence of the observed antiarrhythmic properties of the anesthetic agent procaine, and its clinical effectiveness was reported in 1951.[21] Early, frequently uncontrolled, studies considered procainamide effective for the treatment of PVCs in 90% of patients and ventricular tachycardia in 80% of patients.[22] More recent, better-controlled studies have been more conservative with respect to the percentage of patients responding to procainamide with 90% or greater PVC suppression on a 3g/day dosage regimen.[23] On the other hand, some investigators have advocated higher doses and consequently higher levels of procainamide for resistant arrhythmias in high-risk patients who manifest tolerable or no side effects.[20,24]

Giardina et al.[25] used doses of sustained-release procainamide that achieved peak and through plasma levels of 10.4 and 6.4 μg/ml and found a greater than 75% reduction in PVC frequency in 75% of patients. As with quinidine, only a few studies have addressed the electrophysiologic effects that may occur at a concentration level below that needed for PVC suppression. In one study both antiarrhythmic (increasing the cycle length of fixed coupled PVCs before their abolishment) and proarrhythmic effects (greater prolongation of conduction than refractoriness with facilitation of reentry) have been documented.[26]

Procainamide has been reintroduced recently for ventricular arrhythmia prevention and treatment in the acute ischemic setting.[27] Long-term studies using procainamide for chronic PVC suppression and improving mortality have been largely disappointing, often because of a high dropout rate due to side effects.[28]

Disopyramide

Disopyramide is a relatively new antiarrhythmic agent that was released for the treatment of ventricular arrhythmias in 1977. Several larger, well-designed trials have shown efficacy for PVC suppression. Smith et al.[29] showed significant PVC suppression with 400–800 mg/day of oral disopyramide. Ventricular ectopic beats were reduced from a control value of 177 beats/hr to 30 beats/hr as assessed by 10-hour Holter monitoring. Other trials have appraised disopyramide as equal or superior to either quinidine or procainamide with respect to PVC suppression and relatively fewer side effects.[30]

Many studies have used intravenous disopyramide, which is not currently available in the United States, for the treatment of ventricular tachycardia, ventricular fibrillation, and postmyocardial infarction arrhythmias. Jennings et al.[31] found that oral administration of disopyramide within 36–48 hours of the onset of symptoms of acute myocardial infarction was effective in reducing the frequency of PVCs and ventricular tachycardia but not in preventing ventricular fibrillation. Controlled comparisons to standard therapy with lidocaine and/or procainamide have not been carried out. Vismara et al.[32] have demonstrated the efficacy of oral disopyramide for the treatment of refractory ventricular tachycardia in 6 of 7 patients undergoing electrophysiologic testing and subsequently treated orally.

Phenytoin

Phenytoin was found to be an effective antiarrhythmic in 1938. It was not until 1950 that its antiarrhythmic potential was realized, however, and its use in the treatment of digoxin-induced tachyarrhythmias established. Investigation into the potential use of phenytoin in life-threatening arrhythmias has been limited, since ventricular arrhythmias not due to digitalis excess show only a limited response to phenytoin.[33] Nevertheless, efficacy in clinical arrhythmias associated with congenital or acquired QT prolongation has been documented.[34] Phenytoin is also successful in preventing ventricular arrhythmias after surgery for congenital heart disease. A study by Kavey, Blackman, and Sondheimer[35] showed the suppression of ventricular ectopy, including complex forms, in 19 of 19 patients who had undergone repair of congenital lesions (16 tetralogy of Fallot repairs and 3 aortic valve surgeries). Complete suppression was noted in 15 of the 19 patients. The studies by Stone, Klein, and Lown[36] and Lovell et al.[37] in adults failed to show that disopyramide prevented sudden death associated ischemic heart disease.

Bretylium

Bretylium was first introduced as an antihypertensive agent, but has gained acceptance for the treatment of resistant ventricular tachyarrhythmias, particularly ventricular fibrillation. Results have been impressive, since the report by

Bacaner,[38] who successfully suppressed a variety of ventricular arrhythmias in 30 patients, including ventricular fibrillation in 9 patients, ventricular tachycardia unresponsive to standard agents in 4 patients, and ventricular ectopy in 12 patients. Other studies have confirmed the efficacy of bretylium, including the dramatic results of Arcidiacono,[39] who noted medical defibrillation 10–20 minutes after administration of 300–400 mg of bretylium during continuous cardiopulmonary resuscitation in 10 of 17 patients, and successful DC conversion in 4 others.

Bretylium offers a different mechanism of action as a type III agent, which tends to produce uniform refractoriness of the ventricle. As such, it has an antifibrillatory potential that is not evident in group I agents. Definition of this agent's full therapeutic potential has been hindered by its routine intravenous route of administration; the inability to develop it as a first-line agent because of side effects, particularly hypotension; and the ethical problems of controlled research in patients with life-threatening arrhythmias for which standard effective therapy (lidocaine, procainamide, and defibrillation) has been established. In one of the rare recent studies with an adequate number of patients and a minimum of confounding issues, Paddu, Jouve, and Torresani[40] administered bretylium for the prevention of life-threatening arrhythmias in the acute infarction setting. Of 1225 patients studied, 412 treated with conventional therapy had an incidence of ventricular fibrillation of 5.09%, whereas 843 patients prophylactically treated with bretylium tosylate (10 mg/kg/day for 5 days) had a ventricular fibrillation rate of 1.30% ($P < .001$). These suggestive data will need further support.

Development of oral bretylium-like agents is under way. How these agents and other type III antiarrhythmics such as amiodarone conform or do not conform to current concepts of sudden death therapy will be detailed in the discussion of suppression of induced forms as a clinical endpoint.

CLINICAL CONTEXT

Life-threatening arrhythmias occur most frequently in association with ischemic heart disease, but not exclusively so. Left ventricular dysfunction is often present in these patients and further confounds the issues of treatment subsets. Unfortunately, even less is known about life-threatening arrhythmias in most other clinical settings, including sudden death associated with aortic stenosis, mitral valve prolapse, cardiomyopathy, infectious and infiltrative diseases, cardiac trauma, and tumors. Ventricular arrhythmias associated with hypertrophic cardiomyopathies indicate a poor prognosis, particularly for patients and family members who have septal hypertrophy, an abnormal ECG, and a familial history of sudden death.[41] Although much rarer, the poor prognosis for individuals with idiopathic QT prolongation is well documented. Schwartz[42] showed that 78% of the patients who had a ventricular tachyarrhythmia were dead within 4 years. In the various subsets of patients prone to sudden cardiac death, the prognosis appeared most closely related to their underlying heart disease. Although standard antiarrhythmic therapy may be used for some subsets, such therapy may aggravate the problem (e.g., quinidine in idiopathic QT prolongation) or be less than optimum (e.g., beta-blocking drugs are better for some patients with mitral valve prolapse or hypertrophic cardiomyopathy) in other subsets. Control for the clinical subset is a key determinant to successful evaluation of sudden death prevention in both ischemic and nonischemic cardiac disease.

RATIONALE FOR CURRENT APPROACHES

Antiarrhythmic therapy for chronic ventricular arrhythmias in patients at risk for potentially lethal arrhythmias must consider (1) the manifest form of the chronic and potentially lethal arrhythmia, (2) the clinical setting in which the arrhythmia occurs, and (3) the validity of the clinical endpoints that are used to monitor the effectiveness of therapy. When therapeutic effectiveness is defined in terms of sudden death prevention, one has a statistically secure endpoint for epidemiologic and longitudinal drug trials, but an endpoint that does not predict the risk in an individual patient. Other endpoints of therapy are needed to ensure that our treatment is effective in preventing mortality. Despite an ever-increasing body of information on this topic, the complex interaction between the three factors described above has made interpretation of data most difficult and to date no uniformly accepted approach for management of patients at risk for sudden death exists. The eventual key must be understanding the mechanisms of the interactions of these variables, such that they can be adequately controlled for or weighted during clinical trials. Meanwhile, what has evolved in recent years has been three relatively separate lines of investigation for the use of antiarrhythmic agents in patients at risk for potentially lethal arrhythmias. Each has a superficially different therapeutic endpoint: (1) suppression of ventricular ectopy, in specific, complex forms; (2) therapy guided by the results of programmed electrical stimulation, and (3) empiric therapy using drug levels as an index of protection.

SUPPRESSION OF VENTRICULAR ECTOPY

Acute Ischemia

Historically, suppression of ventricular ectopy has meant the eradication of PVCs. This approach was later amended to take into account the spontaneous variability in the rate of ventricular ectopic beats.[1,2] The endpoint of PVC suppression has been applied to both acute and chronic ischemic settings, although these probably represent different subsets. A clear distinction between sudden death prevention and the associated therapeutic goals in acute ischemia or infarction versus chronic heart disease has not been developed.

In acute ischemia, experimental electrophysiologic changes occur quickly, particularly in the form of slowed conduction, which sets the stage for reentrant arrhythmias.[43] Clinical experience and epidemiologic studies support a similar hypothesis.[44] Prevention of acute arrhythmias has focused on prevention of so-called warning arrhythmias, which were often forerunners of ventricular fibrillation.[10] When ventricular fibrillation was documented in the relative absence of such warning arrhythmias,[45] routine, immediate prophylactic antiarrhythmic therapy with lidocaine was advocated for all acute myocardial infarction patients.[46] Although ventricular fibrillation was indeed prevented by moderate-dose lidocaine prophylaxis, hospital mortality was not necessarily improved when a protected environment and defibrillation were available.[46] The risks of the side effects, including central nervous system effects, hypotension, respiratory failure; probability of dosage error; and change in drug kinetics (due to congestive heart failure or shock) must be weighed against the benefits (ventricular fibrillation and potential mortality prevention) and individualized to the patient and clinical setting (e.g., the patient already in a CCU or a patient with an expected delay in arrival to an appropriately monitored setting).

Although enhanced automaticity forms the basis for some arrhythmias in the acute ischemic setting, it is generally the complex, frequent, or potentially lethal ventricular arrhythmias, assumed to be reentrant in mechanism, that must be treated aggressively. Lidocaine, in a 75–100 mg bolus or repeat 50–75 mg boluses, followed by a 2–4 mg/min drip, is frequently effective. If lidocaine fails or there are side effects, intravenous procainamide, 20 mg/min with a loading dose of up to 500–1000 mg, followed by a 3–4 mg/min infusion, will be sufficient to control most arrhythmias.[47] Bretylium is another alternative for arrhythmias resistant to first-line drugs. In all cases, antiarrhythmic therapy should be combined with optimum clinical management.

In the absence of continued hemodynamic compromise, conducting system involvement, and infarct extension or aneurysm formation, acute electrical instability generally disappears within the first 72 hours of the onset of myocardial infarction. The frequency and complexity of ventricular ectopy dramatically declines, frequently disappearing altogether. Indeed, the occurrence of early-hospital arrhythmias does not predict the occurrence of late-hospital or posthospital arrhythmias,[13] and early arrhythmias alone are not an indication for long-term therapy. This information underscores the need to appropriately subcategorize the forms, clinical settings, and endpoints for therapy.

Subacute Ischemic Heart Disease

The convalescent stage of acute myocardial infarction provides a unique subset of patients in which to examine the efficacy of endpoints in sudden death prevention. Lie et al.[48] found that among 30 patients who manifested late-hospital ventricular fibrillation after myocardial infarction 14 (47%) occurred in a subset of patients who had bundle-branch block accompanying anteroseptal myocardial infarction. These 14 represented 35% of a total of 40 patients who had acute myocardial infarction and bundle-branch block. A follow-up report[49] suggests that this risk is present for 6 weeks after infarction and then resolves. The therapeutic implications from these observations, although resulting from a small data base, are that prophylactic treatment with antiarrhythmic agents for at least 6 weeks would seem advisable in patients who have anteroseptal myocardial infarction with bundle-branch block. Subsequent therapy would depend on other clinical risk factors. This therapy would then represent only empiric therapy, with no measurable premorbid clinical endpoint, selected for an extremely high-risk subset of patients.

A second group at high risk, but with a more demonstrable premorbid endpoint, are patients with symptomatic sustained ventricular tachycardia occurring during the convalescent phase after acute myocardial infarction, usually with an anterior location.[50] Symptomatic ventricular tachycardia within the first 2 months of infarction was associated with an 83% (25/30 patients) short-term mortality, compaired to a 47% (18/38 patients) mortality in patients who have an arrhythmia beyond 2 months after the index myocardial infarction. [50] The prognosis was poor, and often there was associated left ventricular dysfunction. Management strategies included therapy guided by electrophysiologic testing.

Chronic Ischemic Heart Disease

Therapeutic efforts to prevent sudden death have long focused on postinfarction ventricular ectopy with PVC prevention, again dominating earlier thinking, therapy, and clinical trials. The fact that patients who manifest frequent PVCs in the late hospital or early posthospital phase of recovery from acute myocardial infarction are at increased risk for sudden cardiac events has been established[11], with "frequent" being defined variably at 10, 20, or 30 PVCs/hr.[51]. Sudden death after infarction was particularly evident 6 months to 4 years after the index event and typically occurred in those patients who had left ventricular dysfunction in the acute setting combined with ventricular ectopy on late Holter monitor recordings.[52] The risk of electrical instability was shown to be further complicated by the frequent coexistence of left ventricular dysfunction.[53] Left ventricular dysfunction has been and will remain a complicating factor for the treatment of ventricular arrhythmias and for the adequate interpretation of studies dealing with populations of varying levels of left ventricular function.

Antiarrhythmic therapy to improve mortality in survivors of acute myocardial infarction is a goal not easily achieved. First, in terms of PVC theory, there are no data available to confirm that chronic PVC suppression alters risk.[55] Interpretation of long-term arrhythmia treatment for sudden death prophylaxis with the membrane-active antiarrhythmic agents has been thwarted by (1) changing guidelines for therapy, (2) drugs that function through multiple mechanisms (e.g., beta-blocking agents), (3) concurrent interventions (e.g., coronary bypass surgery), and (4) the potential dissociation of anti-PVC and antifibrillatory effects of groups I and III agents.[6,56]

Empiric studies during the last decade have left the question of sudden death prevention after myocardial infarction unanswered. A study by Kosowsky et al.[28] using procainamide, 500 mg tid or qid, was randomized and placebo controlled; 78 patients were studied, with 4 deaths in the control group. Unfortunately, since this was not of statistical significance and because of a relative high incidence of side effects, usage of procainamide therapy was discouraged.

Although the therapeutic endpoints have changed in recent years, no subsequent examination of procainamide (or the other type I agents disopyramide and quinidine) in large trials for sudden death prevention are forthcoming. Other studies on phenytoin have also proven dissappointing.[37,57] and attention is focused onto the newer agents.[58] These agents often are developed along the lines of PVC theory, which is a potential shortcoming. Ryden et al.[59] and Bastian et al.[60] failed to show a protective effect of tocainide. Both studies were limited by elimination of higher risk groups from the study. Chamberlain et al.[61] again limited by a complex inclusion/exclusion schema, failed to show a change in mortality using oral mexiletine. Only in the study by Hugenholtz et al.,[62] which used aprindine, were complex forms of ventricular arrhythmias taken into account. Although the study was limited by its short duration, a small but statistically insignificant difference in mortality was noted. The clinical usefulness of even the newer antiarrhythmic agents for sudden death prevention after myocardial infarction thus remains unclear. Furthermore, the applicability of several of the agents to long-term sudden death prevention trials has been critiqued and seriously questioned.[63]

Monitoring patients after infarction has led to one of the major steps forward in conceptualizing risk associated with ventricular arrhythmias. Monitoring has demonstrated the high-risk implication of complex, rather than simple, ectopic forms as forerunners of potentially lethal arrhythmias. In a 3-year study using 1-hour Holter tapes, Ruberman et al.[64] showed a 15.5% sudden death risk in patients with complex forms, a 4.2% risk in patients with simple forms, and 4.3% risk in those free of PVCs. In these studies, frequency paralleled complexity, since more than 75% of the patients with complex ventricular arrhythmias had a PVC frequency of greater than 10 beats/hr, whereas 75% of the patients with simple forms had a PVC frequency less than 10 beats/hr. This would suggest that simple PVCs may represent more of a marker for potentially lethal ventricular arrhythmias and complex forms are forerunners.

Subsequently, Ruberman et al.[65] showed a 5-year sudden death mortality of 25% in patients with Lown grades 4 and 5 ectopy compaired to a 6% cumulative mortality in those free of ventricular ectopy. Runs of ectopic beats occurring on either of two 1-hour Holter monitor recordings (taken at 6-month intervals) were just as significant as runs occurring on both Holter monitor recordings; however, complex forms occurring on only one Holter monitor recording were far less significant than complex forms occurring on both recordings.[66] These findings are in concert with Bigger and Weld,[67] who found that specific advanced forms, particularly salvos or runs of nonsustained ventricular tachycardia, were important predictors of sudden death. Unfortunately, none of these excellent epidemiologic studies, which refine our concept of the risk factor (complex ventricular ectopy) give us perspective as to the value of antiarrhythmic therapy in altering the incidence of sudden cardiac death in postmyocardial infarction patients.

In 1977 Lown and Graboys[68] proposed a therapy aimed specifically at the eradication of advance forms rather than total ventricular ectopy. Although this approach did not prove uniformly successful, early findings suggested that complexity rather than frequency constituted a valid and more reliable endpoint in preventing potentially lethal ventricular arrhythmias. Their current work is even more provoking.[69] Survival among 123 patients with malignant ventricular arrhythmias treated with individualized antiarrhythmic therapy was assessed for an average of 29.6 months. Only 6 sudden deaths (an annual mortality of 2.3%) occurred in the 98 patients in whom the advanced ventricular forms (Lown grades 4B and 5) were successfully abolished; 17 of the 25 patients in whom advanced forms could not be controlled died. Arrhythmia control was the major factor influencing survival even in patients with left ventricular dysfunction. In patients with control of complex forms, sudden death was more frequent in individuals in whom effective agents had been discontinued or reduced in dosage, underscoring stable therapy as an important variable in effective sudden death prevention.

Of the nine antiarrhythmic agents tested, four were beta-blockers and two are not currently available for general use. Graboys et al.[69] did not describe in detail the individual agents chosen for therapy. Lown [70] has reported the use of 14 different agents in 197 trials to control malignant arrhythmias in 72 patients and included the details of his drug-testing rationale and schema. Most often multiple drug trials using combinations of agents are necessary to control these complex arrhythmias. For example, in their 1977 article, Lown and Graboys[68] described the use of one drug in 2 patients, two drugs in 10 patients, three drugs in 10 patients, four drugs in 3 patients, and five drugs in 1 patient. The currently available antiarrhythmic agents procainamide, quinidine, and disopyramide were variably effective (6/19 patients, 8/21 patients, and 3/8 patients, respectively) and were most often part of a combination of agents rather than being given alone.

Although some features of the study design are of concern, such as patient selection, diffuse etiologies and forms of arrhythmias, and lack of quantification of classes 4B and 5 events, a relationship between suppression of complex forms and survival was convincingly demonstrated. The remaining problem is whether or not the intervention (antiarrhythmic therapy) selected high-risk and low-risk subsets. Indeed, what would the outcome have been if of the patients whose complex forms were suppressed, half were treated and half were not? Furthermore, concepts of risk regarding frequency versus complexity of ventricular ectopic forms have not merged into a unified concept[67] and may need to be combined to eventually prove clinical applicability.

Meanwhile, on a statistical basis, patients with frequent (> 10 PVCs/hr) and complex arrhythmias (Lown grades 4B and 5 and possibly 3 and 4A) appear to be at highest risk. Reduction to less than 10 PVCs/hr and reduction of complex forms, particularly to less than Lown grade 4, seem to be reasonable guidelines until this endpoint is substantiated. This approach, together with monitoring plasma levels and use of programmed stimulation studies in selected patients provide the most rationale approach to sudden death prevention after myocardial infarction.

PROGRAMMED VENTRICULAR STIMULATION

Rationale

Programmed ventricular stimulation during electrophysiologic study of patients with recurrent ventricular tachycardia or survivors of prehospital cardiac arrest has contributed a new therapeutic endpoint. The hypothesis is ventricular arrhythmias that are induced by ventricular stimulation are related to and/or are a specific marker for the clinically manifest life-threatening arrhythmia[71] and that acute drug therapy which will prevent inducible ventricular arrhythmias will serve as appropriate guides to clinical management and thereby predict clinical success—the prevention of life-threatening recurrence.[72-74]

Ventricular Tachycardia

The area of least controversy concerns patients with recurrent symptomatic ventricular tachycardia or prehospital cardiac arrest due to hypotensive sustained ventricular tachycardia. In this subset of patients there is a 70%–80% chance of inducing ventricular tachycardia during programmed ventricular stimulation.[9,75] Achievement of the endpoint (loss of inducibility during drug testing) is generally accepted as a valid predictor of a long-term favorable outcome when the patient is treated with an oral agent or agents to achieve similar levels to those which were suppressive during electrophysiologic study.[72-74,76] The currently available antiarrhythmic agents have been evaluated in this schema. Quinidine was effective in 3 of 14 patients studied by Horowitz et al.,[72] 2 of 7 of the patients treated by Winkle et al.,[16] and 6 of 13 patients treated by Mason and Winkle.[73] Cain and Josephson[77] quote an overall 24% rate of quinidine effectiveness in preventing inducible ventricular tachycardia (18/76 patients) at their institution. DiMarco, Garan, and Ruskin[78] showed that quinidine used alone or in combination with other agents was effective in 40% of their patients. Variability in drug efficacy between studies may be related to differences in populations and drug and stimulation protocols.

Procainamide was effective in 9 of 14 trials by Horowitz et al.,[72,] 0 of 6 trials by Winkle et al.,[16] and 3 of 6 patients treated by Mason and Winkle.[73] Again, interstudy differences make the results difficult to compair. The suppression of inducible responses tends to depend on plasma concentration, with apparently two response patterns.[79] In the minority of patients the arrhythmia simply is progressively more difficult to initiate as the plasma concentration of procainamide rises. A more complex response is seen in the majority of patients, however. As the plasma concentration of procainamide increases in these patients, there is a window where the cycle length increases but the tachycardia is more easily induced. Later suppression of induction becomes manifest. Of the currently available agents, procainamide, in the experience of several investigators, is the single most effective agent for the prevention of ventricular tachycardia.[5,20,80] Higher doses with through levels into the 12–15 μg/ml range are often needed for therapeutic effectiveness[24,30] in patients with resistant ventricular arrhythmias.

Disopyramide also can be used to prevent inducible ventricular tachycardia and was effective in 1 of 14 trials by Horowitz et al.[72] and 3 of 4 trials by Mason and Winkle.[73] Experience provided by Cain and Josephson[81] suggests an overall 36% (14/45 trials) effectiveness rate.

Additive Effects and Interchangeability

The combined administration of two type I agents has been rationalized to minimize side effects, which assumes that low doses of two agents will have fewer side effects than a moderate dose of one agent, and optimize electrophysiologic effects, which assumes improved therapeutic outcome without increased risk of toxicity. Although combined agents are at times useful, both of the assumptions are faulty, and an increased benefit with decreased risk has never been proven. With respect to life-threatening arrhythmias, the results of Ross et al.[82] and Duffy et al.[83] showed no benefit from combining class I agents when each has separately failed during electrophysiologic testing. Moreover, although some concordance of quinidine and procainamide effectiveness can be shown, this does not seem to hold for disopyramide, emphasizing the need to carefully individualize therapy.[84]

Ventricular Fibrillation

Issues and endpoints are less clear with regard to patients who manifest ventricular fibrillation. Attempts to induce sustained ventricular tachycardia or ventricular fibrillation in patients whose clinically manifest arrhythmia was ventricular fibrillation have not been uniformly successful; the inducibility rate is about 30%.[9,85] Both Ruskin, DiMarco, and Garan[85] and Josephson et al.[75] suggest that therapy guided by protection against inducible ventricular arrhythmias may be effective in improving the long-term mortality in this subset of patients.

In the remaining 70% of patients, ventricular tachycardia is either not inducible (30%) or is nonsustained.[86] Although inducible nonsustained forms may constitute a high-risk indicator, suppression of these forms may or may not predict protection. Noninducible patients with grades 4B and 5 ventricular arrhythmias may benefit from antiarrhythmic therapy.[69]

Perspectives

Currently, the major advantage to ventricular stimulation studies is to provide an individualized endpoint for therapy. One can elect to study almost all patients with life-threatening arrhythmias or only patients who do not have suppression of high-grade ectopy with standard therapy.[69] Certain pitfalls in our current approach to programmed stimulation studies must be remembered, however. These include factors of reproducibility of induction to serve as an appropriate baseline for therapy, how aggressive a pacing protocol can be and still remain predicitve, how sustained an induced form must be, the interpretation of nonsustained forms, the predictive value of noninducibility, and whether inducible and spontaneous forms are equivalent.[88] The major pitfall would be to consider the issue closed and accept ventricular stimulation studies as the ultimate answer. Programmed ventricular stimulation is certainly helpful in guiding therapy in patients with recurrent sustained, symptomatic ventricular tachycardia, particularly those quiescent between clinically manifest episodes. Many questions need to be answered, however, before the ultimate role of ventricular stimulation studies in the prevention of potentially lethal ventricular arrhythmias is established.

Type III Agents—Exception or Prototype

Type III agents form an interesting, and potentially crucial, exception to the evaluation of the prevention of potentially lethal ventricular arrhythmias, particularly ventricular fibrillation, by programmed stimulation studies. These drugs may serve as truly antifibrillatory agents because they unify ventricular refractoriness by decreasing the disparity in action potential duration between normal and ischemic regions.[89] Heger et al. [90] demonstrated the lack of correlation between the clinical and electrophysiologic response to amiodarone. Indeed, failure to protect the patient from induced arrhythmia during programmed stimulation studies did not negate a favorable clinical outcome. This has been confirmed by others, including Nademanee et al.,[91] who studied 24 sudden death survivors, 21 of whom had ventricular fibrillation. Suppression of induced forms was inconsistent, whereas suppression of complex ventricular ectopic beats, ventricular tachycardia, and fibrillation better predicted long-term efficacy in preventing recurrent cardiac arrest.

Similar studies have documented that bretylium failed to protect against inducible ventricular arrhythmias.[92,93] Pharmacologic date on both of these drugs show delayed achievement of optimum tissue levels, with tissue rather than plasma levels being predictive of electrophysiologic effectiveness.[94] Since the mechanisms of early (first minutes of ischemia) and late arrhythmias vary, the model in which these drugs are studied may be crucial to their proper evaluation. In an animal model in which ventricular fibrillation was initiated, prior administered bretylium was effective in preventing ventricular fibrillation at a site distant from a previously induced myocardial infarction.[95] Also relevant are the findings of Puddu, Jouve, and Torresani[40] in which bretylium was an effective prophylactic agent in the acute ischemic setting in humans. Although these studies suggest the potential usefulness of bretylium for sudden death prevention, two vexing problems remain. First, programmed stimulation studies will have to be done in a delayed fashion to prove the clinical usefulness of these type III drugs, but this delay makes such an endpoint less useful clinically. The second and most distressing problem is whether the type III agents are a much ignored prototype for sudden death prevention, especially for prevention of ventricular fibrillation. Because of the traditional PVC theory, drug testing and development have always concentrated on PVC suppression. This may be applicable to complex forms and ventricular tachycardia but may have obscured issues vital to the successful prevention of ventricular fibrillation.[96] An open mind with respect to these factors is needed for future research direction.

EMPIRIC THERAPY GUIDED BY ADEQUATE AND STABLE BLOOD LEVEL MONITORING

The empiric approach is limited by the fact that its basis is statistical and therefore cannot provide an individualized endpoint to identify protection in a given patient at risk. Nevertheless, results of this approach in sudden death survivors have been encouraging,[5,97] particularly since other endpoints may be unavailable. Survivors of sudden death often do not have Holter evidence of grades 4B and 5 ventricular arrhythmias, and they often are not inducible during programmed stimulation studies. Yet their risk for recurrent arrest is most real.

Adequate and stable plasma levels of the standard antiarrhythmic agents procainamide and quinidine appeared to protect against recurrent cardiac arrest.[5] Among 16 patients followed up with a dose-adjusted level-monitored program, all 8 patients with recurrent cardiac arrest had unstable plasma levels, whereas 6 of 8 patients without recurrent cardiac arrest had stable plasma levels ($P < .01$). Of further interest was the apparent dissociation of anti-PVC and antifibrillatory effects of these group I agents: prevention of recurrent cardiac arrest was independent of successful PVC suppression. Dissociation of the concentration-response curves for ventricular tachycardia and chronic PVC suppression using procainamide as the index drug also has been demonstrated.[20] A similar dissociation of effects has been observed with the type III antifibrillatory agent bretylium.[6] This information again underscores the limitations of the traditional PVC theroy and broadens our concepts for future approaches to sudden death prevention.

SAFETY

Each of the currently available antiarrhythmic agents has side effects that preclude their usage in a significant number of patients. In high-risk patients some side effects may have to be tolerated if the prescribed agent is effective and no alternative agent of lesser toxicity is available. A partial list of the classic side effects and precautions in prescribing standard arrhythmic agents will be described. Quinidine has both dose-related and idiosyncratic side effects occurring in as many as one third of the patients treated. Gastrointestinal side effects, including nausea, vomiting, and diarrhea; cinchonism; dermatologic manifestations ranging from pruritis to exfoliative dermatitis; febrile reactions; granulomatous hepatitis; and hematologic abnormalities such as thrombocytopenia and hemolytic anemia have been documented. Adverse reactions related to vagolytic activty (e.g., paradoxic tachycardia), QT prolongation, depression of myocardial conduction and contraction at high doses all occur as a direct extension of drug effect.

Procainamide induces ANA conversion and a lupus-like syndrome, particularly in slow acetylators. Since the clinical syndrome occurs only in 20%–30% of ANA converters, a positive ANA titer without associated manifestations does not constitute grounds for discontinuing necessary and effective therapy. Gastrointestinal, febrile, hepatic, and dermatologic adverse effects occur, as well as rare cases of agranulocytosis. Hypotension and myocardial muscle and electrical depression may occur as a direct drug effect, particularly at high doses or with intravenous administration.

Overall, disopyramide is proposed to have side effects in fewer patients; however, a significant number of potential adverse reactions may occur with this agent. Anticholinergic effects, with dry mouth, urinary retention, constipation, blurred vision, and gastrointestinal and dermatologic reactions, are not uncommon. Electrophysiologic effects with QT prolongation and depression of conduction occur as with the other type I agents. Disopyramide appears to have a more significant myocardial depressant effect with precipitation of congestive heart failure, particularly in patients with impaired left ventricular function and a history of cardiac decompensation.[98] Significant drug-drug and drug-disease interaction also occur and must be carefully evaluated when using these agents.

In addition to these standard statements regarding drug therapeutics, a relatively new concept has evolved with respect to antiarrhythmic drug therapy, that of proarrhythmic effects. Since current agents have multiple electrophysiologic effects, which in turn depend on concentration and whether ischemic or nonischemic conditions prevail, it is little wonder that each of the currently available and experimental antiarrhythmic drugs has the potential of aggravating, rather than suppressing, electrical instability. Three recent studies will be reviewed as examples.

Denes, Giabster, and Huang[99] found five episodes of primary ventricular fibrillation during the Holter monitoring of 3307 consecutive patients. In these five patients quinidine was identified as a co-contributor to the potentially lethal arrhythmia. Left ventricular dysfunction, QT prolongation, and an increase in ventricular arrhythmias preceding the ventricular fibrillation, as well as the recent initiation of quinidine therapy, were also documented. These data underscore the rare but real dangers of initiating drug therapy, in this case quinidine, particularly in individuals with preexisting left ventricular dysfunction. These patients must be monitored for early warning signs of drug toxicity (QT prolongation or an increase in the frequency or complexity of ventricular ectopy) during the initiation of therapy. In their evaluation of 83 patients with ventricular tachycardia, Rickenberger et al.[100] detected 11 patients who had more severe ventricular tachycardia initiated during programmed stimulation while they were receiving specific drugs (disopyramide, 2 patients; quinidine, 2 patients; amiodarone, 4 patients; and encainide, 7 patients) than in the absence of these agents.

Velebit et al.,[3] identified proarrhythmic effects in 80 of 772 (11.1%) oral drug trials, representing 53 of 155 patients studied. Aggravation of arrhythmia was rigorously defined as a fourfold increase in ventricular ectopic complexes, a tenfold increase in repetitive forms, or the initiation of sustained ventricular tachycardia for the first time. Blood concentration measurements were in the therapeutic range in each case. In these studies[3,4] proarrhythmic effects were noted with a maximum frequency of 23.3% with encainide and a minimum frequency of 4.8% with ethmozine. Standard type I agents showed proarrhythmic effects in 15.4% of trials using quinidine, 9.1% of trials using procainamide, and 5.9% of trials using disopyramide. In conclusion, significant proarrhythmic drug effects must be added to the standard list of adverse drug reactions when considering antiarrhythmic therapy for potentially lethal ventricular arrhythmias.

SUMMARY

None of the currently available antiarrhythmic agents are uniformly safe or effective for sudden death prevention. Unfortunatley, this is also true for the experimental drugs currently under investigation. With the erosion of the traditional PVC theory, endpoints to guide clinical efficacy are somewhat in disarray, with evidence supporting the potential usefulness of three major approaches: (1) suppression of complex forms, (2) suppression of inducible repetitive forms, and (3) maintenance of adequate and stable blood levels. Proarrhythmic effects have further complicated the issue of safety. Furthermore, the dissociation of anti-PVC and antifibrillatory effects of both types I and III agents needs intensive reevaluation to ensure that the traditional PVC theory had not misled us too far.

Currently patients with potentially lethal ventricular arrhythmias must be treated carefully, but aggressively, with the strengths of the various endpoints of therapy applied to each patient individually. Treatment of the whole patient, combined with careful documentation of anatomy, hemodynamics, and electrophysiology, should be carried out. Ventricular stimulation studies provide the most individualized approach, particularly for patients with sustained ventricular tachycardia. In other cases, suppression of complex forms, especially when combined with adequate and stable blood levels of antiarrhythmic agents, may provide protection for an individual patient. The key to sudden death prevention may well lie in further understanding of the relationship of lethal arrhythmias to the pathophysiologic processes underlying sudden cardiac deaths. This has proven to be the case in idiopathic QT prolongation where therapy aimed at the electrophysiologic anomaly rather than solely arrhythmia prevention has improved clinical prognosis. Although more information is needed, drug therapy must be used as optimally as possible and, when appropriate, in combination with other treatment modalities such as coronary bypass surgery, aneurysectomy, and implantable debrillators. Only with a comprehensive program can we hope to effectively prevent sudden cardiac death.

REFERENCES

1. Winkle RA: Antiarrhythmic drug effect mimicked by spontaneous variability of ventricular ectopy. Circulation 57:1116, 1978
2. Morganroth J, Michelson EL, Horowitz LN, et al: Limitations of routine long-term electrocardiographic monitoring to assess ventricular ectopic frequency. Circulation 58:408, 1978
3. Velebit V, Podrid P, Lown B, et al: Aggravation and provocation of ventricular arrhythmias by antiarrhythmic drugs. Circulation 65:886, 1982
4. Podrid PJ: Aggravation of arrhythmias: A potential complication of therapy. Primary Cardiology:75, 1983
5. Myerburg RJ, Conde C, Sheps DS, et al: Antiarrhythmic drug therapy in survivors of prehospital cardiac arrest: Comparison of effects on chronic ventricular arrhythmias and recurrent cardiac arrest. Circulation 59:855, 1979
6. Durandhar RW, Bakersmith D: Bretylium tosylate, in Gould LA (Ed): Drug treatment of cardiac arrhythmias. Mount Kisco, NY, Futura Publishing Co Inc, 1983, p 299
7. Baum RS, Alvarez H III, Cobb LA: Survival after resuscitation from out-of-hospital ventricular fibrillation. Circulation 50:1231, 1974
8. Schaffer WA, Cobb LA: Recurrent ventricular fibrillation and modes of death in survivors of out-of-hospital ventricular fibrillation. N Engl J Med 293:259, 1975
9. Myerburg RJ, Conde C, Sung RJ, et al: Clinical, electrophysiologic and hemodynamic profile of patients resuscitated from prehospital cardiac arrest. Am J Med 68:568, 1980
10. Lown B, Fakhro AM, Hood WB, et al: The coronary care unit. JAMA 199:156, 1967
11. Moss JA, Schnitzler R, Green R, et al: Ventricular arrhythmias 3 weeks after acute myocardial infarction. Ann Intern Med 75:837, 1971
12. Kotler MN, Tabatznik B, Mower MM, et al: Prognostic significance of ventricular ectopic beats with respect to sudden death in the late postinfarction period. Circulation 47:959, 1973

13. Vismara LA, Amsterdam EA, Mason DT: Relation of ventricular arrhythmias in the late hospital phase of acute myocardial infarction to sudden death after hospital discharge. Am J Med 59:6, 1979
14. Sokolow M: The present status of therapy of the cardiac arrhythmias with quinidine. Am Heart J 42:771, 1951
15. Carliner NH, Fisher ML, Crouthamel WG, et al: Relation of ventricular premature beat suppression to serum quinidine concentration determined by a new and specific assay. Am Heart J 100:483, 1980
16. Winkle RA, Alderman EL, Fitzgerald JW, et al: Treatment symptomatic ventricular tachycardia. Ann Intern Med 85:1, 1976
17. Jelinek MV, Lohrbauer L, Lown B: Antiarrhythmic drug therapy for sporadic ventricular ectopic arrhythmias. Circulation 49: 659, 1974
18. Gaughan CE, Lown B, Laningan J, et al: Acute oral testing for determining antiarrhythmic drug efficacy. Am J Cardiol 38:677, 1976
19. Krone RJ, Miller JP, Kleiger RE, et al: The effectiveness of antiarrhythmic agents on early-cycle premature ventricular complexes. Circulation 63:664, 1981
20. Myerburg RJ, Kessler KM, Kiem I, et al: Relationship between plasma levels of procainamide, suppression of premature ventricular complexes and prevention of recurrent ventricular tachycardia. Circulation 64: 280,1981
21. Mark LC, Kayden HJ, Steele JM, et al: The physiological disposition and cardiac effects of procaine amide. J Pharmacol Exp Ther 102:5, 1951
22. Kayden HJ: The current status of procaine amide in the management of cardiac arrhythmias. Prog Cardiovasc Dis 3:331, 1961
23. Winkle RA, Gradman AH, Fitzgeral JW, et al: Antiarrhythmic drug effect assessed from ventricular arrhythmia reduction in the ambulatory electrocardiogram and treadmill test: Comparison of propranolol, procainamide and quinidine. Am J Cardiol 42:473, 1978
24. Greenspan AM, Horowitz LN, Spielman SR, et al: Large dose procainamide therapy for ventricular tachycardia. Am J Cardiol 46:453, 1980
25. Giardina EGV, Fenster PE, Bigger JT, et al: Efficacy plasma concentrations and adverse effects of a new sustained release procainamide preparation. Am J Cardiol 46:855, 1980
26. Giardina EGV, Bigger JT: Procaine amide against re-entrant ventricular arrhythmias. Circulation 48:959, 1973
27. Kock-Weser J, Klein SW, Foo-Canto LL, et al: Antiarrhythmic prophylaxis with procainamide in acute myocardial infarction. N Engl J Med 281:1253, 1969
28. Kosowsky BD, Taylor J, Lown B, et al: Long-term use of procaine amide following acute myocardial infarction. Circulation 47:1204, 1973
29. Smith WS, Vismara LA, Kalmansohn RB, et al: Clinical studies of Norpace. Angiology 26 (suppl 1:124, 1975
30. Heel RC, Brogden RN, Speight TM, et al: Disopyramide: A review of its pharmacological properties and therapeutic use in treating cardiac arrhythmias. Drugs 15:331, 1978
31. Jennings G, Jones MBS, Besterman EMM, et al: Oral disopyramide in prophylaxis of arrhythmias following myocardial infarction. Lancet 1:51, 1976
32. Vismara LA, Vera Z, Miller RR, et al: Efficacy of disopyramide phosphate in the treatment of refractory ventricular tachycardia. Am J Cardiol 39:1027, 1977
33. Bigger J, Schmidt D, Kutt H: Diphenylhydantoin sodium and its cardiac antiarrhythmic effects. Circulation 38:363, 1968
34. Crampton R: Preeminence of the left stellate ganglion in the long Q-T syndrome. Circulation 59:769, 1979
35. Kavey REW, Blackman MS, Sondheimer HM: Phenytoin therapy for

ventricular arrhythmias occurring late after surgery for congenital heart disease. Am Heart J 104:794, 1982

36. Stone N, Klein MD, Lown B: Diphenylhydantoin in the prevention of recurring ventricular tachycardia. Circulation 43:420, 1971
37. Lovell RRH, Mitchell ME, Prineas RJ, et al: Phenytoin after recovery from myocardial infarction. Lancet 2:1055, 1971
38. Bacaner MB: Treatment of ventricular fibrillation and other acute arrhythmias with bretylium tosylate. Am J Cardiol 21:530, 1968
39. Arcidiacono R: Use of bretylium tosylate in ventricular fibrillation. Clin Ther 84:253, 1978
40. Puddu PE, Jouve R, Torresani J: Bretylium tosylate: A suitable drug in the prevention of primary ventricular fibrillation. Presented at the Eighth European Congress of Cardiology, Paris, June 22-26, 1980
41. Epstein SE, Maron JB: Sudden death in patients with hypertrophic cardiomyopathy, in Kulbertus HE, Wellens WJJ (Eds): Sudden Death. The Hague, The Netherlands, Martinus Nijhoff, 1980, p 347
42. Schwartz PJ: The long QT syndrome, in Kulbertus HE, Wellens HJJ (Eds): Sudden Death. The Hague, The Netherlands, Martinus Nijhoff, 1980, p 358
43. Scherlag BJ, El-Sherif N, Hope R, et al: Characterization and location of ventricular arrhythmias resulting from myocardial ischemia and infarction. Circ Res 35:372, 1974
44. Pantridge JE, Gettes JS: Cardiac arrest after myocardial infarction. Lancet 1:807, 1966
45. El-Sherif N, Myerburg RJ, Schelag BJ, et al: Electrocardiographic antecedents of primary ventricular fibrillation. Br Heart J 38:415, 1976
46. Lie KI, Wellens HJ, van Capelle FJ, et al: Lidocaine in the prevention of primary ventricular fibrillation. N Engl J Med 291:1324, 1974
47. Gianelly R, von der Groeben JO, Spivack PA, et al: Effect of lidocaine on ventricular arrhythmias in patients with coronary heart disease. N Engl J Med 277:1215, 1967
48. Lie KI, Liem KL, Schuilenburg RM, et al: Early identification of patients developing late in-hospital ventricular fibrillation after discharge from the coronary care unit. Am J Cardiol 41:674, 1978
49. Hauer RNW, Lie KI, Kiem KL, et al: Long-term prognosis in patients with bundle-branch block complicating acute anteroseptal infarction. Am J Cardiol 49:1581, 1982
50. Wellens HJJ, Bar FWHM, Vanagt EJDM, et al: Medical treatment of ventricular tachycardia: Considerations in the selection of patients for surgical treatment. Am J Cardiol 49:186, 1982
51. Winkle RA: Detection of patients at high risk for sudden death: The role of electrocardiographic monitoring, in Kulbertus HE, Wellens HJJ (Eds): Sudden Death. The Hague, The Netherlands, Martinus Nijhoff, 1980, p 275
52. Moss AJ, DeCamilla J, David H: Factors associated with cardiac death in posthospital phase of myocardial infarction, in Kulbertus HE, Wellens HJJ (Eds): Sudden Death. The Hague, The Netherlands, Martinus Nijhoff, 1980, p 237
53. Schulze RA, Strauss HW, Pitt B: Sudden death in the year following myocardial infarction. Am J Med 62:192, 1977
54. Moss AJ, Davis HT, DeCamilla J, et al: Ventricular ectopic beats and their relation to sudden and nonsudden cardiac death after myocardial infarction. Circulation 60:998, 1979
55. Blackburn H, de Backer G, Crow R, et al: Epidemiology and prevention of ventricular ectopic rhythms. Adv Cardiol 18:208, 1976
56. Myerburg RJ, Kessler KM, Zaman L, et al: Survivors of prehospital cardiac arrest. JAMA 247:1485, 1982
57. Peter T, Ross D, Duffield A, et al: Effect on survival after myocardial infarction of long-term treatment

with phenytoin. Br Heart J 40:1356, 1978
58. May GS, Eberlein KA, Furberg CD, et al: Secondary prevention after myocardial infarction: A review of long-term trials. Prog Cardiovasc Dis 24:331, 1982
59. Ryden L, Arnman K, Conradson TB, et al: Prophylaxis of ventricular tachyarrhythmias with intravenous and oral tocainide in patients with and recovering from acute myocardial infarction. Am Heart J 100:1006, 1980
60. Bastian BC, Macfarlane PW, McLauchlan JH, et al: A prospective randomized trial of tocainide in patients following myocardial infarction. Am Heart J 100:1017, 1980
61. Chamberlain DA, Julian DG, Boyle DM, et al: Oral mexiletine in high-risk patients after myocardial infarction. Lancet 2:1324, 1980
62. Van Durme JP, Hagenmeijer F, Bogaert M, et al: Chronic antidysrrhythic treatment after myocardial infarction. Design of Gent-Rotterdan apridine study, in Boissel JP, Klimt CR (eds): Multicenter Controlled Trials: Principles and Problems. Paris, INSERM, 1977, p. 43.
63. Woosley RL, Roden DM, Duff HJ, et al: Selection of an antiarrhythmic drug for sudden-death prevention triai. Am Heart J 103:737, 1982
64. Ruberman W, Weinblatt E, Goldberg JD, et al: Ventricular premature beats and mortality after myocardial infarction. N Engl J Med 297:750, 1971
65. Ruberman W, Weinblatt E, Goldberg JD, et al: Ventricular premature complexes and sudden death after myocardial infarction. Circulation 64:297, 1981
66. Ruberman W, Weinblatt E, Frank CW, et al: Repeated 1 hour electrocardiographic monitoring of survivors of myocardial infarction at 6 month intervals: Arrhythmia detection and relation to prognosis. Am J Cardiol 47:1197, 1981
67. Bigger JT, Weld FM: Analysis of prognostic significance of ventricular arrhythmias after myocardial infarction. Br Heart J 45:717, 1981
68. Lown B, Graboys TB: Management of patients with malignant ventricular arrhythmias. Am J Cardiol 39:910, 1977
69. Graboys TB, Lown B, Podrid PJ, et al: Long-term survival of patients with malignant ventricular arrhythmia treated with antiarrhythmic drugs. Am J Cardiol 50:437, 1982
70. Lown B: Sudden cardiac death: The major challenge confronting contemporary cardiology. Am J Cardiol 43:313, 1979
71. Vande Pol CJ, Farshidi A, Spielman SR, et al: Incidence and clinical significance of induced ventricular tachycardia. Am J Cardiol 45:725, 1980
72. Horowitz LN, Josephson ME, Farshidi A, et al: Recurrent sustained ventricular tachycardia. III. Role of the electrophysiologic study in selection of antiarrhythmic regimens. Circulation 58:986, 1978
73. Mason JW, Winkle RA: Electrode-catheter arrhythmia induction in the selection and assessment of antiarrhythmic drug therapy for recurrent ventricular tachycardia. Circulation 58:971, 1978
74. Josephson ME, Horowitz LN: Electrophysiologic approach to therapy of recurrent sustained ventricular tachycardia. Am J Cardiol 43:631, 1979
75. Josephson ME, Horowitz LN, Spielman SR, et al: Electrophysiologic and hemodynamic studies in patients resuscitated from cardiac arrest. Am J Cardiol 46:948, 1980
76. Wellens HJJ, Bar FWH, Lie KI, et al: Effect of procainamide, propranolol and verapamil on the mechanism of tachycardia in patients with chronic recurrent ventricular tachycardia. Am J Cardiol 40:579, 1977
77. Cain ME, Josephson ME: Quinidine, in Gould LA (Ed): Drug treatment of cardiac arrhythmias. Mount Kisco, NY, Futura Publishing Co Inc, 1983, p 33

78. DiMarco HP, Garan H, Ruskin JN: Quinidine for ventricular arrhythmias: Value of electrophysiologic testing. Am J Cardiol 90:90,1983
79. Horowitz LN, Josephson ME, Kastor JH: Intracardiac electrophysiologic studies as a method for optimization of drug therapy in chronic ventricular arrhythmia. Prog Cardiovasc Dis 23:81, 1980
80. Cain ME, Josephson ME: Procainamide, in Gould LA (Ed): Drug treatment of cardiac arrhythmias. Mount Kisco, NY, Futura Publishing Co Inc, 1983, p 73
81. Cain ME, Josephson ME: Disopyramide, in Gould LA (Ed): Mount Kisco, NY, Futura Publishing Co Inc, 1983, p 109
82. Ross DL, Sze DY, Keefe DL, et al: Antiarrhythmic drug combinations in the treatment of ventricular tachycardia. Circulation 66:1205, 1982
83. Duffy CE, Swiryn S, Bauernfeind RA, et al: Inducible sustained ventricular tachycardia refractory to individual class I drugs: Effects of adding a second class I drug. Am Heart J 106:450, 1983
84. Swiryn S, Bauernfeind RA, Strasberg B, et al: Prediction of response to class I antiarrhythmic drugs during electrophysiologic study of ventricular tachycardia. Am Heart J 104:43, 1982
85. Ruskin JN, DiMarco JP, Garan H: Out-of-hospital cardiac arrest. N Engl J Med 303:607, 1980
86. Ruskin JN: Personal communication, 1984.
87. Lown B: Management of patients at high risk of sudden death. Am Heart J 103:689, 1982
88. Ouyang P, Brinker JA, Bulkley BH, et al: Ischemic ventricular fibrillation: The importance of being spontaneous. Am J Cardiol 48:455, 1981
89. Cardinal R, Sasyniuk BI: Electrophysiological effects of bretylium tosylate in infarcted hearts. Proceedings of the Symposium "Bretylium Tosylate: Current Scientific and Clinical Experience," Amsterdam, Excerpta Medica, 1979, p 15
90. Heger JJ, Prytowsky EN, Jackman WN, et al: Amiodarone: Clinical efficacy and electrophysiology during long-term therapy for recurrent ventricular tachycardia or ventricular fibrillation. N Engl J Med 305:539, 1981
91. Nademanee K, Cannom D, Hendrickson J, et al.: Recurrent sudden arrhythmic cardiac deaths prevented by amiodarone: Efficacy predictable by the initial suppression of ventricular tachyarrhythmias (abstract). Circulation 64 (suppl 4):36, 1981
92. Bauernfeind RA, Hoff J, Swiryn S, et al: Electrophysiologic testing of bretylium tosylate in sustained ventricular tachycardia. Am Heart J 105:973, 1983
93. Greene HL, Werner JA, Gross BW, et al: Failure of bretylium to suppress inducible ventricular tachycardia. Am Heart J 105:717, 1983
94. Anderson JL, Patterson E, Conlon M, et al: Kinetics of antifibrillatory effects of bretylium: Correlation with myocardial drug concentrations. Am J Cardiol 46:583, 1980
95. Holland K, Patterson E, Lucchesi BR: Prevention of ventricular fibrillation by bretylium in a conscious canine model of sudden coronary death. Am Heart J 105:711, 1983
96. Patterson E, Lucchesi BR: Bretylium: A prototype for future development of antidysrhythmic agents. Am Heart J 106:426, 1983
97. Myerburg RJ, Zaman L, Kessler KM, et al: Evolving concepts of management of stable and potentially lethal arrhythmias. Am Heart J 103:615, 1982
98. Podrid PD, Schoeneberger A, Lown B: Congestive heart failure caused by oral disopyramide. N Engl J Med 302:614, 1980
99. Denes P, Gabster A, Huang SK: Clinical, electrocardiographic and follow-up observations in patients

having ventricular fibrillation during Holter monitoring. Am J Cardiol 48:9, 1981

100. Rinkenberger RL, Prytowsky EN, Jackman WM, et al: Drug conversion of nonsustained ventricular tachycardia to sustained ventricular tachycardia during serial electrophysiologic studies: Identification of drugs that exacerbate tachycardia and potential mechanisms. Am Heart J 103:177, 1982

Joel Morganroth
Pasquale F. Nestico
Leonard N. Horowitz

11

EXPERIMENTAL ANTIARRHYTHMIC AGENTS

Studies in individuals who have sudden cardiac death while wearing Holter monitors have demonstrated that the mechanism of this condition in approximately 80% of patients is an acute ventricular tachyarrhythmia (ventricular tachycardia and/or ventricular flutter) that leads to fatal ventricular fibrillation.[1] In only a minority is sudden cardiac death due to an acute ischemic episode leading to a bradyarrhythmia and asystole.

Clinical and epidemiologic studies have clearly shown that the two primary risk factors of sudden cardiac death are the presence of left ventricular dysfunction and ventricular electrical instability, such as frequent premature ventricular complexes (PVCs) or repetitive forms. Repetitive PVCs occur in the form of ventricular couplets or ventricular tachycardia.[2]

TYPES OF PREMATURE VENTRICULAR COMPLEXES

Lethal PVCs

PVCs occur in three different clinical settings.[3] The least common of these occur in patients who have ventricular ectopy that manifests itself as paroxysmal sustained ventricular tachycardia. This form is called "lethal ventricular arrhythmias." The vast majority of these patients have serious left ventricular dysfunction (a mean LVEF of approximately 30% or less). Even the presence of nonsustained ventricular tachycardia (usually defined as 30 seconds of a self-terminating rhythm disturbance) in such patients may cause important hemodynamic symptoms. The most important feature of lethal ventricular arrhythmias is that they cause severe hemodynamic consequences, usually syncope, unstable angina, or exacerbation of congestive heart failure.

SUDDEN CARDIAC DEATH
0-8089-1725-0

The indications for treatment of such patients are immediate relief of hemodynamic symptoms and prevention of sudden cardiac death. Treatment almost always must take place in the hospital where monitoring is available. Confirmation, or a precise diagnosis when obscure, is often best obtained by electrophysiologic testing with programmed stimulation that attempts to induce the rhythm disturbance.

Potentially Lethal PVCs

The more common clinical presentation of PVCs, which accounts for the vast majority of the cases of sudden cardiac death occurs in patients in whom the presence of PVCs causes no important hemodynamic consequence. These patients may occasionally feel palpitations or dizziness, but most are unaware of even frequently occurring PVCs (e.g., 2000 beats/hr/day). In patients who have chronic PVCs without important hemodynamic symptoms, the primary indication for therapy is prevention of sudden cardiac death. This form is called "potentially lethal PVCs." Patients with potentially lethal PVCs can be treated as ambulatory outpatients, since their arrhythmia does not cause hemodynamically important symptoms. There is still controversy as to whether therapy directed at this group of patients will have an impact on sudden cardiac death prevalence. Noninvasive methods, using Holter monitoring, are the logical approach for diagnostic and therapeutic decisions in this patient group. Exercise testing is complementary and especially indicated when PVCs are associated with exertion.

Benign PVCs

Frequent PVCs are not common in the normal population, as was once believed. Individuals who have no underlying coronary artery disease by angiography or myopathic or valvular disease by echocardiography have virtually no repetitive PVC forms (ventricular couplets and/or tachycardia) on 24-hour ambulatory monitoring. The PVC frequency usually is fewer than 100 PVCs/day or less than 5 an hour.[4]

Individuals who have frequent (> 5 PVCs/hr) or repetitive PVCs (e.g., nonsustained ventricular tachycardia) without underlying structural heart disease may be considered to have primary electrical cardiac disease or Benign PVCs, since they fall outside the range of normal. No data exist to suggest that these patients have other than a very low risk for the development of sudden cardiac death; therefore therapy is directed toward the elimination of symptoms, such as palpitations or dizziness. Often reassurance or use of a minor tranquilizer is sufficient to delay anxiety and eliminate symptoms. Further data on the natural history of these patients are needed before prognostic and therapeutic implications can be made.

Once ventricular ectopy is identified, one must be certain that it is not secondary to an easily correctable cause, such as a metabolic abnormality (e.g., hypokalemia) or a toxic reaction to a drug (e.g., digitalis toxicity). An associated conduction abnormality (e.g., second-degree heart block) or the presence of a long QT syndrome will influence proper selection of therapy.

About 10% of the patients treated with antiarrhythmic agents may have an adverse reaction in the form of exacerbation of ventricular ectopy ("proarrhythmic event"). It is therefore essential to follow-up antiarrhythmic therapy with quantitative Holter monitoring to determine whether the drug is effective or is causing a adverse reaction.

Antiarrhythmic agents available in the United States have often proved frustrating for both clinicians and patients. Efficacy rates only range from 50%–75%. These drugs require frequent dosing schedules that limit compliance and are associated with a 20%–30% major side effect rate. Antiarrhythmic agents have specific, serious drawbacks that limit their usefulness, particularly in high-risk patients. For example, disopyramide has a severe negative inotropic effect and thus must be avoided in patients with severely a depressed LVEF—the patient group that may most need therapy.

A variety of new, experimental, antiarrhythmic agents in the United States (many have been available abroad for decades) are becoming more widely used and have fewer side effects, improved dosing schedules, and much higher efficacy rates. The class IC antiarrhythmic agents (e.g., flecainide and encainide) appear to eliminate virtually all PVCs in the vast majority of patients, with very minimal side effects. New agents that combine antiarrhythmic effects and beta-blockade are particularly promising. For example, sotalol has beta-blocker properties and a marked effect on repolarization, similar to that of amiodarone. Table 11-1 details a classification of antiarrhythmic agents and includes many new drugs under clinical

Table 11-1 *Antiarrhythmic Drug Classification*

Class	Description	Examples
IA	Moderate depression of phase 0 depolarization; prolonged repolarization	Quinidine, procainamide, disopyramide
IB	Weak depression of phase 0 depolarization; shortened repolarization	Tocainide, mexiletine, aprindine
IC	Strong depression of phase 0 depolarization; littleeffect on repolarization	Encainide, flecainide, indecainide, propafenone
I	Unclassified; combined effects of IA to IC	Moricizine, pirmenol, cibenzoline
II	Beta-blockers	Propranolol,* pindolol, timolol, atenolol, nadolol, metoprolol
III	Prolonged repolarization	Sotalol,† amiodarone, bretylium
IV	Calcium channel blockers	Nifedipine, diltiazem, verapamil

Modified from Morganroth J: Premature ventricular complexes: Diagnosis and indications for therapy. JAMA 252:673, 1984. With permission.

* Released in the United States for treatment of PVCs. The other beta-blockers listed are experimental agents.

† Also has beta-blocker properties.

Table 11-2 Pharmacology of Antiarrhythmic Drugs

Drug	Percentage of protein binding (%)	Elimination Half-Lives (HR)	Effective concentration (μg/ml)	Bioavail-ability (% dose)	Excretion of unchanged drug
Quinidine	60–90	5–9	2–6	60–90	15
Procainamide	20	3–7	4–8	60–80	50
Disopyramide	40–90	6–9	3–6	60–90	40–60
Mexiletine	50–60	12–16	0.75–2.0	90	20
Tocainide	50	12–16	6.15	90	30–50
Encainide	90	2–3	—	80–90	10
Flecainide	40	14–18	0.5–1.0	90	10
Lorcainide	40	13	0.4–1.0	90	30
Propranolol	90	3–6	0.02–0.9	20–50	35
Amiodarone	—	20–100 days	1–2	90	—

investigation. Tables 11-2 and 11-3 compare their electropharmacologic and clinical features. Other new and promising agents such as moricizine do not fit easily into this modified Vaughan Williams classification and are listed under class ID as an "undefined" group. Each discussion in this chapter will address details of the new experimental antiarrhythmic agents. Class IA agents, including the available drugs quinidine, procainamide, and disopyramide, and will not be considered.

CLASS IB ANTIARRHYTHMICS

Tocainide

History

Tocainide hydrochloride (Tonocard) is a primary amine analog with the chemical name 2-amino-*N*-(2,6-dimethylphenyl)propanamide. It is the newest antiarrhythmic agent approved by the Food and Drug Administration for the treatment of ventricular arrhythmias. Tocainide has been actively studied in both its oral and intravenous form; however, this discussion will only include data on oral tocainide.

Mechanism of Action

In animal models, tocainide demonstrated findings similar to those of lidocaine and therefore is considered a class IB antiarrhythmic agent. It reduces membrane responsiveness, shortens the effective refractory period and action

Table 11-3 Electrophysiologic Effects of Antiarrhythmic Drugs

Drug	SNRT	Conduction Interval				Refractory Periods	
		AH	HV	QRS	QT	HP	Ventricular
Quinidine	–	↓	– ↑	↑	↑	– ↑	↑
Procainamide	–	↓	– ↑	↑	↑	– ↑	↑
Disopyramide	–	↓	– ↑	↑	↑	– ↑	↑
Mexiletine	–	– ↓	–	–	– ↑	↑	–
Tocainide	–	– ↓	–	–	↓	–	– ↓
Encainide	↑ –	–	↑	↑	– ↑	–	–
Flecainide	↑	↑	↑	– ↑	↑	↑	↑
Lorcainide	↑	↑	↑	↑	↑	?	–
Propranolol	↑ –	↑	–	–	↓	–	–
Amiodarone	– ↑	↑	– ↑	–	↑	–	– ↑
Bretylium	?	–	–	–	–	↓	– ↑

Symbols: –, Minimal effect; 1, increase; 2, decrease; ?, unknown effect.
SNRT = Sinus Node Recovery Time

potential duration, and reduces the action potential upstroke velocity and amplitude. Tocainide also has been shown to elevate the threshold to ventricular fibrillation.[5,6] In studies of patients with coronary artery disease treated with intravenous tocainide, Horowitz, Josephson, and Farshidi[7] observed no significant effects on sinus node function, effective refractory periods, or intracardiac conduction times. In a similar study, Anderson et al.[8] showed that the effective refractory periods decreased slightly, whereas sinus node function was unaffected and there was no consistent effect on the His-Purkinje system.

In these studies, the QTc interval slightly decreased and there was no significant effect on PR or QRS intervals as measured on the surface ECG. Tocainide, like lidocaine, does not prolong ventricular depolarization or repolarization in normal subjects or in those with coronary artery disease. Studies in patients with the Wolff-Parkinson-White syndrome have demonstrated a prolongation of the refractory period of the accessory pathway.

Hemodynamics

At therapeutic doses, tocainide did not produce any significant change in heart rate during oral or intravenous administration.[9] Effects of tocainide on blood pressure and peripheral vascular resistance have been somewhat variable. In healthy volunteers no significant change was noted, and in patients with coronary artery disease there was a small but significant increase in pulmonary and systemic vascular resistances, arterial pressure, and left ventricular end diastolic pressure.[9]

Pharmacokinetics

Tocainide is a white, odorless, crystalline powder that is sparingly soluble in water and alcohol and has a bitter taste. The shelf life tablets at room temperature of is about 4 years. The tablets are available in strengths of 400 and 600 mg; both forms are yellow and contain 336 and 504 mg, respectively, of free base tocainide.

Tocainide is well absorbed after oral administration with negligible first-pass elimination, giving a bioavailability approaching 100%. Peak concentration after oral administration occurs within 0.5–2 hours and approximately 50% is protein bound. In patients with myocardial infarction who received 400 mg of tocainide tid, the mean plasma concentrations ranged from 5–7 μg/ml, which is similar to those seen in patients who have been treated successfully for ventricular arrhythmias.[10,11] When doses were increased to 600 mg tid, the plasma concentration ranged from 8–10 μg/ml. Tocainide plasma concentrations of 4–10 μg/ml are considered the optimum range for therapy, based on studies using the hydrochloride salt.[11]

Approximately 45% of tocainide's administered dose is excreted unchanged in the urine, and approximately 25% undergoes hepatic biotransformation involving the formation of a glucuronide.[12] Metabolites of tocainide have shown no clear antiarrhythmic activity in animal models. The amount of tocainide excreted in the urine is significantly reduced if the urine is alkalinized, whereas the amount of the drug recovered is not affected by the administration of food or acidification of the urine.

The plasma half-life has been studied in three groups of healthy volunteers and has averaged approximately 13 hours. The plasma half-life in patients has ranged from 9–37 hours with a mean of approximately 15 hours.[10-13] The mean plasma half-life of tocainide is significantly prolonged to about 27 hours in patients with end-stage renal failure with a creatinine clearance of less than 5 mg/min.

Plasma Level and Dosage

Tocainide is approximately half as potent as lidocaine. The dosage ranges from 1200–1800 mg/day or 400–600 mg orally every 8–12 hours. In the presence of renal insufficiency, plasma-level monitoring should help to avoid toxicity. In some patients with resistant arrhythmias, dosages of as much as 3200 mg/day have been used but with a high incidence of side effects.[14]

Efficacy

POTENTIALLY LETHAL VENTRICULAR ARRHYTHMIAS. A total of 10 single-center, short-term, placebo-controlled trials, including 99 patients who were treated with tocainide for chronic PVCs of various etiologies, have been conducted. The dosage received ranged from 200–800 mg every 8 hours or 400–1000 mg every 12 hours. Approximately 50% of the patients have had a greater than 75% suppression in PVC frequency.[11,13,15]

ACUTE MYOCARDIAL INFARCTION. In a double-blind, randomized, placebo-controlled study, Campbell et al.[16] reported on the prophylactic use of tocainide in patients with myocardial infarction to suppress the emergence of ventricular ectopy. Tocainide significantly reduced runs of ventricular tachycardia compared to the placebo, and the frequency of ventricular couplets, multiform ectopic beats, and R-on-T phenomena were lower in the tocainide group, although the results were not statistically different from the placebo group. One patient developed ventricular fibrillation in the placebo group; none who received tocainide developed ventricular fibrillation. In patients given tocainide, there was a statistically less significant number of hours recorded with PVCs greater than 30 beats/hr compared to the placebo. Two sudden cardiac deaths occurred in the placebo group, and no patient died in the tocainide group. This study suggested that arrhythmia prophylaxis with oral tocainide was beneficial in the early stage of acute myocardial infarction. In addition, it appears to be a useful agent to control ventricular arrhythmias after myocardial infarction.

LETHAL VENTRICULAR ARRHYTHMIAS. Roden et al.[17] reported their experience with 19 patients given tocainide in the CCU who had been refractory to conventional drug therapy. The response to tocainide was defined as a greater than 60% reduction in ventricular ectopy and suppression of symptomatic ventricular tachycardia. In the hospital, 15 of the 19 patients (79%) responded to tocainide and all 13 whose arrhythmias were sensitive to lidocaine were in this group; only 2 of 6 patients resistant to lidocaine responded to tocainide ($P < .05$). The authors concluded that tocainide was an effective agent for the short-term suppression of ventricular arrhythmias, particularly ventricular tachycardia, and that the arrhythmia response to lidocaine was found to be an excellent predictor of tocainide response.

Winkle, Mason, and Harrison[18] also studied the effectiveness of tocainide for drug-resistant ventricular arrhythmias in 38 patients, 31 of whom had recurrent sustained ventricular tachycardia or fibrillation. These patients could not be managed with conventional antiarrhythmic agents. The initial dosage of tocainide was 400 mg every 8 hours, and the dose was increased until the arrhythmias were controlled or side effects occurred. Of 38 patients, 22 (61%) were successfully treated; however, there were 4 patients who had late arrhythmia reoccurences and 18 had continued effectiveness. The total daily dose of tocainide ranged from 600–2400 mg. There was no difference in the plasma concentrations of those who responded and those who did not respond to tocainide (the mean values were 8.9 and 9.4 μg/ml, respectively). Tocainide therapy was successful in 63% of the patients in whom lidocaine was considered effective and was successful in only 2 (17%) of the other 12 patients in whom lidocaine was ineffective or in whom it was not evaluated ($P < .01$). In the 13 patients in whom lidocaine was used to test efficacy in the electrophysiologic laboratory, 9 proved successful. Of these 9, 6 were also successfully treated with oral tocainide. Of the 4 patients in whom lidocaine did not demonstrate efficacy in the electrophysiologic laboratory, 3 failed on oral tocainide. Tocainide was tested in 6 patients during the electrophysiologic study and then used for continued treatment. Tocainide appeared to be successful in treating 4 patients who were also successfully treated with oral long-term therapy. The 2 patients in whom tocainide failed in the electrophysiologic laboratory, also failed on oral tocainide therapy.

Comparison of Tocainide with Other Antiarrhythmic Agents

The largest controlled clinical trial using tocainide in the treatment of chronic ventricular arrhythmias was a multicenter trial designed to compare the clinical effectiveness and safety or oral tocainide with oral quinidine. The report of one of these three centers has been published.[19] This multicenter study included 136 patients. The entrance criteria required the presence of chronic ventricular arrhythmias of at least 60 PVCs/hr/day. Efficacy was evaluated in those patients who met the entrance criteria, who did not develop an adverse effect early in the course of the trial, and had adequate data for evaluation. After a 2-week initial placebo period and 48 hours of Holter monitoring, patients underwent random allocation for 8 weeks to either tocainide, 600 mg every 12 hours, or quinidine, 300 mg every 6 hours. A double placebo was used to maintain the double-blind status of the study. The patients had 24 hours of Holter monitoring every 2 weeks during active treatment. Then, the participants entered a 4-week posttreatment placebo period. Efficacy was defined as the reduction by at least 75% of PVC frequency or the abolition of repetitive ventricular arrhythmias. By combining data from all three clinical sites, 37% of the patients demonstrated efficacy with tocainide and 50% with quinidine (P = NS). There were also no significant differences in the response for repetitive ventricular arrhythmias comparing quinidine to tocainide.

Adverse Effects

Adverse reactions from tocainide generally have been transient, dose related, and reversible with a reduction in dosage or by taking the medication with food or discontinuing the drug. Most side effects are neurologic. About 12%–14% of patients complain of lightheadedness, dizziness, or vertigo, and approximately 4%–6% complain of paresthesias, tremor, or altered mood. The second most common type of adverse reaction is gastrointestinal, with approximately 14% of the patients complaining of nausea and 5% of emesis. Other rare gastrointestinal effects are anorexia, abdominal pain, dry mouth, and altered taste. Sweating and headache have been reported in 5% and 4%, respectively. Confusion, nervousness, anxiety, ataxis, hallucinations, altered vision, or tinnitus have been noted in 1%–3% of patients. Other adverse reactions, such as nystagmus, nightmares, constipation, diarrhea, dyspnea, pleurisy, fever, itching, cramps, hiccups, and alopecia, occur in less than 1% of patients. To date only two patients have developed pulmonary fibrosis and one has developed aplastic anemia that may be related to tocainide therapy.

In the combined multicenter trial comparing oral tocainide with oral quinidine there was an insignificant difference in the percentage of patients either discontinuing therapy or experiencing adverse reactions while receiving the two agents. Diarrhea occurred approximately three times more often in the quinidine group, and dizziness occurred approximately three times more often in the tocainide group. Nausea was equally prevalent in the two groups.

In terms of the proarrhythmic effects, or aggravation of ventricular arrhythmia, Velebit et al.[20] have reported that tocainide may increase ventricular ectopy similarly to virtually all other antiarrhythmic agents. This effect was seen in 12 of

76 patients receiving tocainide in doses of 1200–2400 mg for at least 48 hours. Aggravation was defined as a fourfold increase in the frequency of PVCs, a tenfold increase in repetitive forms, or their first emergence. Engler and LeWinter[21] have reported two patients in whom ventricular fibrillation was induced by tocainide and in whom severe underlying structural cardiac disease with recurrent ventricular tachycardia were present. Tocainide is less of a concern in terms of prolongation of the QT interval on the ECG than other class I antiarrhythmic agents. The potential for tocainide to aggravate arrhythmias is unclear at the present time, but there is no evidence of an enhanced propensity; in fact, the electrophysiologic characteristics of tocainide suggest that it is possibly less arrhythmogenic than other class I agents.

Drug Interactions

The time to reach maximum plasma levels and plasma half-lives of metoprolol and tocainide were the same when these two agents were administered concomitantly. This lack of pharmacokinetic interaction between the two drugs is noteworthy. In addition, clinical studies have shown no significant differences in terms of the frequency of adverse reactions in patients who were receiving tocainide alone compared to those receiving tocainide and digoxin. Digoxin concentrations do increase during the concomitant administration of tocainide. No adverse effects of coumadin and tocainide coadministration have been reported.

Summary

The similarity of tocainide to lidocaine and the predictability of its efficacy in patients responsive to lidocaine are important. Its lack of interaction with beta-blockers and digoxin is also a promising feature. Although tocainide has proven to be effective in the prophylaxis and treatment of patients with both refractory and chronic ventricular arrhythmias, its efficacy is somewhat less than class IA agents, such as quinidine, procainamide, and disopyramide. The side effect profile appears to be similar in percentage to that of quinidine, but often these side effects are milder, better tolerated, and respond to dosage alteration. Tocainide will undoubtedly prove to be a useful new antiarrhythmic agent, particularly when compared to those currently available.

Mexiletine

History

Mexiletine (Mexitil) is a new antiarrhythmic agent that has a relatively long half-life and may be administered orally because it does not undergo significant first-pass degradation by the liver. It is a primary amine whose chemical name is 1-methyl-2-(2,6-xylyloxy)ethylamine hydrochloride. Although mexiletine remains an investigational drug in North America, it has been marketed in Europe for the treatment of ventricular arrhythmias since 1976.

Mechanism of Action

Studies in animals[22] and humans[23] have shown mexiletine to closely resemble lidocaine in its local anesthetic and electrophysiologic actions. In isolated tissue preparations this agent produces no change in the resting membrane potential, but it produces a significant decrease in the rate of rise and maximum height of phase I depolarization (V_{max}). There is little or no alteration in the duration of the action potential, but there is consistent shortening of the relative refractory period of the His-Purkinje system.

Electrophysiologic studies performed in patients receiving mexiletine show that the drug has no significant effect on resting sinus rate, atrial conduction, or atrial refractory periods. In addition, atrioventricular conduction and sinus node recovery time are not consistently affected. In patients with sick sinus syndrome there may be a clinically important depression of sinus node function with sinus bradycardia, sinus arrest, or prolongation of atrioventricular conduction, including a reduction in the rate at which Wenckebach block occurs. It is not clear whether the nodal effects are due to a direct action of the drug, alteration in vagal tone, or both.

There is no change in the HV interval after the administration of mexiletine in patients with normal infra-His conduction. Both mexiletine and lidocaine may prolong the effective refractory period of the diseased His-Purkinje system, acting more like type IA antiarrhythmic agents in this setting. The clinical relevance of this finding is unknown.

Hemodynamics

Studies have investigated the effects of an intravenous dose of mexiletine (1–2 mg/kg) on hemodynamics and left ventricular function.[24,25] All reports have shown a small reduction in cardiac performance seen as an increased left ventricular end diastolic pressure and pulmonary artery diastolic pressure or a decreased ejection rate.

Pharmacokinetics

Pharmacokinetic studies suggest that the disposition kinetics of mexiletine are consistent with a three-compartment model of drug distribution.[26] There is an initial fast distribution into highly perfused tissues, such as the brain, liver, lung, myocardium, and kidney (central compartment). Less than 1% of an administered dose is found in the blood after distribution. This is followed by slower uptake into less well-perfused tissues such as the skin, skeletal and heart muscle, and fat, with a large volume of distribution (> 600 L) (peripheral compartments). Absorption of mexiletine begins in the upper small bowel where alkalinization occurs because in the acidic pH of the stomach; mexiletine is completely ionized and therefore not absorbed. A delay in gastric emptying produced by narcotics or atropine-like drugs will slow absorption of an oral dose.[27] Because of alterations in the side chain of mexiletine, in contrast to lidocaine, it does not undergo significant first-pass hepatic degradation; 90% of an oral dose enters the systemic circulation compared to 30% of an oral dose of lidocaine. Mexiletine is a moderately high, protein-bound drug (its whole blood concentration is 15% higher than its plasma concentration), and only a small portion is found in the blood compartment.

In several studies the plasma half-life in healthy individuals ranged from 6–16 hours, with a mean of 10 hours.[28,29] The plasma half-life is not significantly prolonged in patients with renal insufficiency[27] because mexiletine is metabolized to inactive compounds by the liver. It may be prolonged in patients with myocardial infarction due to decreased hepatic blood flow.[26] In these situations, the therapeutic concentrations may be maintained using 8-hour oral dosage schedules.

Because of the large volume of distribution, steady state levels are only achieved in 2–3 days of long-term oral administration.[30] If rapid onset of action is required, as in acute myocardial infarction or life-threatening arrhythmia, it is necessary to administer an initial loading dose of the drug.

Plasma Level and Dosage

A total daily dosage of 600–1200 mg, given in divided doses every 6–8 hours, during long-term oral therapy can maintain therapeutic plasma levels. The therapeutic plasma levels of mexiletine range from 0.5–2 mg/L. As the blood level rises, the therapeutic efficacy and frequency of adverse effects proportionately increase. At plasma levels of 2 mg/L, a significant number of patients will experience side effects. Conversely, patients with levels below 0.5 mg/L are less likely to have a therapeutic response.

Plasma levels serve only as a rough guide as to clinical response, patient tolerance, and toxic reactions. At times, higher doses of mexiletine may be tried until arrhythmia control is achieved or intolerable side effects occur.

Efficacy

POTENTIALLY LETHAL VENTRICULAR ARRHYTHMIAS. Campbell et al.[31] evaluated the use of oral mexiletine in a controlled, randomized study of 60 patients with ventricular arrhythmias after myocardial infarction. These patients received oral mexiletine, procainamide, or a placebo after 36 hours of lidocaine. Both treatment groups had a 65% reduction of arrhythmias, but there was no difference between the response rates of the two drugs, and both were significantly better than the placebo.

This trial was continued in a group of 97 patients randomized within 12 hours of onset of symptoms of acute myocardial infarction to receive mexiletine or a placebo.[32] R-on-T PVCs occurred in 53% of the placebo-treated patients and 14% of the mexiletine-treated patients. Ventricular tachycardia occurred in 74% receiving the placebo and 30% receiving mexiletine. Ventricular fibrillation occurred only in 2 patients receiving the placebo. The efficacy of mexiletine was similar to that of procainamide, with the arrhythmia suppressed in 50%–60% of the patients. Mexiletine has shown consistent efficacy in 50%–60% of patients with chronic ventricular arrhythmias in several long-term studies.[33-35]

Podrid and Lown[36] studied a large group of patients treated with mexiletine for symptomatic ventricular arrhythmias. After an oral loading dose, short-term therapy (3 days) and, if successful, long-term maintenance (up to 32 months) were used. Overall, a therapeutic response was achieved in 60% of the patients. Among 44 patients receiving long-term therapy, 31 were able to continue with long-term mexiletine therapy alone. Side effects in these trials have been frequent, however, often requiring reductions in dosage or patient discontinuation.

LETHAL VENTRICULAR ARRHYTHMIAS. DiMarco, Garon, and Ruskin[37] studied the use of mexiletine in patients with recurrent ventricular tachycardia or ventricular fibrillation who had recurrences with conventional antiarrhythmic agents. Of 35 patients with inducible arrhythmias, 9 (26%) became noninducible with mexiletine. As in the study by Duff et al.[38] the addition of a type IA agent (quinidine, procainamide, or disopyramide) produced a therapeutic response in 4 more patients (37%).

Palileo et al.[39] evaluated 17 patients with inducible sustained ventricular tachycardia. Five patients developed an increase in ventricular tachycardia after 1 (2 doses) to 6 days of mexiletine, suggesting potentiation of the arrhythmia. Of the 11 patients tested, none had suppression of inducible arrhythmias. Similarly, Waspe at al.[40] evaluated 23 patients with inducible sustained arrhythmias and found that mexiletine alone did not prevent inducibility.

Adverse Effects

Among patients treated in most studies, side effects occurred in 30%–50% and usually included gastrointestinal or central nervous system severe side effects.[33-36] Adjustment of dosage or discontinuation of mexiletine therapy became necessary in 20% of the patients.

No significant hemodynamic cardiovascular side effects such as significant hypotension or cardiac dysfunction have been attributed to mexiletine. In fact, the drug is well tolerated by patients with cardiac dysfunction, including patients with a history of heart failure.

Mexiletine produces a number of side effects in the central nervous system: diplopia, dizziness, dysarthria, confusion, drowsiness, tremor, and paresthesias. In the study by Talbot et al.[41] central nervous system side effects were frequent, occurring in 50% of the patients during initial intravenous administration and persisting in 25% even after a steady state plasma concentration was achieved and the dosage reduced.

Summary

Mexiletine is a new antiarrhythmic drug that acts like other type IB agents to shorten the refractory period. Because the drug does not undergo significant first-pass hepatic degradation, it may be administered orally. Mexiletine may be used in patients with renal insufficiency, since it is primarily metabolized by the liver. It has a rapid dissolution into a large volume of distribution. About 30%–50% of the patients have some side effects, and 20% require dosage adjustment or discontinuation of therapy. When mexiletine is used to treat potentially lethal ventricular arrhythmias, approximately 50%–60% of the patients will respond. Fewer patients with lethal arrhythmias will achieve adequate control with mexiletine. Because its different mechanism of action, mexiletine may have an adjunctive role with type IA agents in the therapy of ventricular arrhythmias.

CLASS IC ANTIARRHYTHMICS

Flecainide

History

Flecainide acetate (Tambocor) is one of a series of new antiarrhythmic drugs that have trifluoroethoxy-benzamide structure. It is a single benzamide with two distinctive structural features: two trifluoroethoxy groups in the aromatic portion of the molecule and a piperidine ring in the amide side chain. Both of the features are essential to the unique properties of flecainide.

Mechanism of Action

In patients with sinus node dysfunction, Vik-Mo, Ohm, and Lund-Johansen[42] found that after 1.5 mg of flecainide per kilogram of body weight was given over 15 minutes, the sinus cycle length was not significantly changed. The maximum sinus node recovery time increased in 8 of 11 patients, and the mean maximum corrected sinus node recovery time increased from 875 ± 180 to 1727 ± 507 msec after flecainide administration. Flecainide therefore must be avoided or the individual effects of the sinus node must be carefully assessed in patients with clinical or laboratory evidence of sinus node dysfunction.

Hellestrand et al.[43] assessed the effect of 2 mg of flecainide per kilogram of body weight administered over 5 minutes in 47 patients who underwent electrophysiologic study and measured parameters of conduction, such as the PA, AH (during normal sinus rhythm and atrial pacing), and HV intervals; QRS duration; and QT (during atrial pacing) and QTc intervals. The longest paced cycle length producing retrograde (ventriculoatrial) Wenckebach block was significantly increased. The QT interval during normal sinus rhythm and the longest paced cycle length producing antegrade Wenckebach block were also significantly increased. In contrast, the JT interval was significantly shortened.

Among 39 patients without ventricular preexcitation, the HV interval significantly increased from 44 ± 9 to 61 ± 12 msec, with the maximum change being 40 msec. The increment varied from 0% (2 patients) to 100%, with a mean of 42%; 70% of these patients developed an HV greater than 55% msec. One patient with complete right bundle-branch block and left anterior fascicular block on the surface ECG and a normal HV interval, but a history of complete hear block, developed complete infra-His block during flecainide administration. The QRS duration increased in 44 patients and remained unchanged in 3 patients, and the increment in QRS duration ranged from 0%–79% (mean of 23%).

Flecainide produced complete antegrade accessory pathway block in 2 of 8 patients with overt ventricular preexcitation and significantly increased antegrade refractoriness in 6 of 8. Retrograde conduction in the basal state was shown in 16 accessory pathways; 7 were concealed, and all of these were completely blocked by flecainide. Of the 9 accessory pathways still capable of retrograde conduction after flecainide administration, refractoriness increased in 4 patients and shortened slightly in 2. In 3 cases the ventricular refractory period was longer than the accessory pathway refractory period, preventing deterioration of the latter. There was no significant effect on atrial or atrioventricular nodal refractoriness. Right ventricular refractoriness was significantly prolonged from 220 ± 22 to 229 ± 23 msec (with a mean of 9 msec).

Hemodynamics

Legrand et al.[44] studied the hemodynamic effects of intravenous flecainide (2 mg/kg of body weight over 30 minutes) in 10 patients with coronary artery disease without overt congestive heart failure. There was no significant change in heart rate, systemic arterial blood pressure, and systemic or pulmonary vascular resistances. The pulmonary capillary wedge pressure significantly increased, however. Furthermore, there was a significant decrease in stroke volume, left ventricular stroke work index, ejection fraction (as measured by contrast ventriculography), and mean velocity of circumferential fiber shortening. Intravenous flecainide administration thus appears to have a direct myocardial depressant effect in patients with heart disease, similar to that reported with all class I antiarrhythmic drugs.

Flecainide produced a decrease in the rate of cell depolarization, conduction velocity, and height of the action potential, particularly in the absence of a change in the resting membrane potential, and these effects were characteristic of type IC antiarrhythmic action.

This agent had no antiadrenergic effects, and there was no antagonism to calcium-induced contraction, even at twenty times the effective concentration of verapamil. Flecainide therefore had no class II or IV activity.

Pharmacokinetics

In a study of 16 normal men Conrad et al.[45] noted that single intravenous doses of flecainide acetate ranging from 0.5–2 mg/kg of body weight resulted in a plasma concentration ranging from 70–340 ng/ml, roughly proportional to the dose. Furthermore, single oral doses ranging from 60–240 mg (0.65–3.53 mg/kg of body weight) resulted in peak plasma levels of 69–240 ng/ml proportional to dose, at about 2.5 hours (1.5–3 hours, mean 2.6).

About 95% of the oral dose of flecainide is absorbed and delivered unchanged to the systemic circulation. The drug is 35%–42% bound to plasma proteins. After single doses by either route, the plasma half-life ranges from 7–22 hours (mean, 14), independent of dose.

Plasma Level and Dosage

At steady state, 200 mg of flecainide taken orally twice a day results in a wide range of 3-hour peak plasma levels of 312–1251 ng/ml (a mean of 778) as determined 3 hours after the previous dose; 250 mg taken twice daily results in 622–1425 ng/ml (a mean of 1044). The mean elimination half-life is 20 hours, ranging from 12–27 hours.[46,47]

As far as the effects on the ECG are concerned, at doses that demonstrate chronic arrhythmia suppression, flecainide uniformly increases the PR interval (16%–37%), QRS duration (10%–27%), and QTc interval (5%–14%).[46] Unless extreme, prolongation of ECG intervals do not seem to reflect the arrhythmogenic implications associated with other type I antiarrhythmic agents. The changes in the QTc interval are largely due to changes in QRS duration, with minimum changes in the JT interval. In a large comparative study of flecainide with quinidine, the magnitude of total QT prolongation was similar for the two drugs, but 60% of the QT prolongation among flecainide patients was explained by the increase in QRS duration, whereas 85% was explained by JT prolongation in the quinidine group.[49] In the case of flecainide, it is postulated that QTc prolongation may reflect uniform prolongation of repolarization, rather than dispersion of repolarization. Effective flecainide levels have ranged from 312–1425 ng/ml peak[48] and 163–814 ng/ml through.[46]

In clinical studies reported by Duff et al.[48] the degree of antiarrhythmic effect of flecainide was linearly related to both the extent of QRS prolongation (r = .68) and the plasma concentration of flecainide (r = .70). The oral dose is 100–300 ng, twice a day.

POTENTIALLY LETHAL VENTRICULAR ARRHYTHMIAS. A multiinstitutional, single-blind, placebo-control protocol[46-48] demonstrated 97% PVC suppression in 31 of 33 patients with chronic frequent PVCs by oral flecainide at dosages ranging from 100–300 mg every 12 hours (a mean of 206 mg). At least a third of these patients had been resistant or intolerant to multiple antiarrhythmic agents. In all 31 responders during a 2-week follow-up period, there was a sustained 94% suppression rate. In a chronic long-term study, flecainide maintained PVC suppression in 9 patients for a mean follow-up period of 12 months.

COMPARATIVE TRIAL. A large, double-blind, 16-center trial compared oral flecainide acetate (200–300 mg) given twice daily with quinidine sulfate (300–400 mg) given every 6 hours in 280 patients with chronic PVCs.[29] In this parallel study there was an 80% suppression of PVCs in 85% of the patients receiving flecainide compared with 57% of the patients receiving quinidine. In addition, flecainide completely suppressed couplets and ventricular tachycardia in 68% of the patients, compared to 33% of the patients in the quinidine group. PR and QRS intervals were prolonged 40 and 20 msec, respectively, but were not affected by quinidine. Both drugs prolonged the QT intervals by 30 msec; however, only quinidine significantly prolonged the JT intervals.

LETHAL VENTRICULAR ARRHYTHMIAS. Anderson, Lutz, and Allison[50] studied 6 patients with inducible ventricular tachycardia lasting at least 30 seconds or resulting in symptoms or hemodynamic compromise at initial study. Flecainide was administered to each patient at a dosage of 150 or 200 mg every 12 hours for 4–6 days. After steady state plasma levels were achieved, a repeated electrophysiologic study showed that 3 of 6 patients had no inducible arrhythmia. A fourth patient had persistence of inducible ventricular sustained tachycardia, but the cycle length increased from 325–610 msec (partial response). Another patient had acceleration of the tachycardia rate. The sixth patient, whose tachycardia had terminated spontaneously in the baseline study, required lidocaine and overdrive ventricular pacing for termination of a tachycardia induced while taking flecainide. The 50% success rate indicated in this pilot study is encouraging. Other electrophysiologic studies to be reported in patients with coronary artery disease show a response rate in about 15%–25% of the patients studied.

Adverse Effects

During a multicenter clinical trial[49] of oral administration of flecainide for 2 weeks, 19 of 141 patients (13%) had adverse effects that required cessation of therapy, and 84 of 141 patients (60%) reported at least one side effect. The most common adverse effects were dizziness (30%), blurred vision (28%), headache (9%), and nausea (9%). In a comparable group of 139 patients receiving quinidine (300–400 mg every 6 hours), 15% had side effects requiring discontinuation of therapy, and the overall incidence of adverse effects was 65%. Many side effects are related to peak plasma levels and can be eliminated by reducing the dose slightly and maintaining antiarrhythmic efficacy or by increasing the interval between dosages to 8 hours, thereby blunting the peaks.

PROARRHYTHMIC EFFECT. The proarrhythmic effects may be quite different when patients are categorized according to those who have lethal ventricular arrhythmias and those who have chronic or potentially lethal ventricular arrhythmias with no immediate hemodynamic compromise.[51] The proarrhythmic prevalence was about 12% and 4%, respectively, in these two groups. The prevalence and severity in patients with lethal arrhythmias is markedly reduced with proper attention to dose and changes in dose regimen. The starting dosage should be 100 mg twice a day, and the dose should not be changed for at least 3–4 days. Patients with severe ventricular dysfunction or lethal ventricular arrhythmias should be carefully monitored in the hospital during dose initiation.

Summary

Flecainide is a chemically unique antiarrhythmic agent. It has clinically desirable properties of high efficacy and a long duration of action. The agent has excellent pharmacokinetics, making it a convenient drug for oral or intravenous use. Side effects seem to occur somewhat less frequently than with quinidine. In the attempt to prevent sudden arrhythmic death, flecainide is certainly an asset in the armamentarium of the clinical cardiologist.

Encainide

History

The chemical synthesis of encainide resulted from investigation of a number of open-chain analogs of methylsergide in search of potential prophylactic agents for vascular headache. The chemical structure of encainide is 4-methyoxy-2′[2-1-methyl-2-piperidyl)ethyl] benzanilide.

Mechanism of Action

Encainide at doses carefully titrated for antiarrhythmic effect had no effect on the basic cycle length, sinus node recovery time, or sinoatrial conduction time in patients without previous evidence of sinus node dysfunction.[52,53] In two patients with prolonged sinus node recovery times at baseline, the drug resulted in a further increase and dose-related sinus pauses of less than 3 seconds' duration.[5]

Caution thus must be exercised in elderly patients or in those who have evidence of underlying sinus node disease.

There are discrepancies between the electrophysiologic effects of intravenous and oral encainide. Sami et al.[53] found that in 10 patients with coronary artery disease who were given encainide (0.6–0.9 mg/kg, by intravenous infusion over a 15-minute period), the HV and QRS intervals increased by 31% and 18%, respectively, in proportion to the plasma encainide concentration. There was no significant change in AH interval, corrected sinus node recovery time, Wenckebach cycle length, QT interval, or refractory periods of the right atrium, atrioventricular node, or right ventricle.

After steady state oral dosing, however, the electrophysiologic profile of encainide is different than that resulting from acute single-dose intravenous infusion. Jackman et al.[54] performed intracardiac electrophysiologic studies on 15 cardiac patients before and during long-term encainide therapy (100–300 mg/day, mean 242 ± 66). Oral encainide significantly lengthened intraatrial, atrioventricular nodal, His-Purkinje, and perhaps intraventricular conduction as measured by the PA, AH, HV, and QRS intervals and the shortest atrial pacing cycle length maintaining 1 : 1 atrioventricular nodal conduction. In contrast to the acute small-dose intravenous studies, refractory periods of the right atrium and right ventricle and measures of repolarization were also increased. After larger intravenous doses similar changes may occur, however. There was no correlation between the magnitude of change in any electrophysiologic variables and the plasma encainide concentration obtained at the time of study, logarithm of the encainide concentration, plasma *O*-demethylencainide (ODE) concentration, or sums of the encainide and metabolite concentrations (7 patients).

In patients with preexcitation syndromes, oral encainide completely blocks antegrade conduction in accessory pathways when the minimum cycle length (allowing 1 : 1 antegrade conduction) is greater than 260 msec in the control state. Complete retrograde block over the accessory pathway is produced in about 50% of patients, but cannot be predicted by the control cycle length, allowing retrograde ventriculoatrial conduction. The known increase in atrial refractoriness by encainide correlates with antegrade block, but the importance of atrial refractoriness in producing the block is uncertain.[55,56]

Hemodynamics

In an initial clinical trial that excluded patients with clinical symptoms of the New York Heart Association classes III or IV, Roden et al.[57] found that there was no significant change of mean ejection fraction measured by resting radionuclide ventriculography during therapy with antiarrhythmic doses of encainide. Furthermore, DiBianco et al.[52] found no change greater than 5% in resting or exercise LVEF among 12 patients given antiarrhythmic doses of encainide.

Sami et al.[58] studied 23 patients with repetitive PVCs and depressed left ventricular function (an ejection fraction <45%). Of these patients, 13 had a history of congestive heart failure of New York Heart Association classes III or IV. After 1–2 weeks of oral doses of encainide (75–200 mg/day), titrated for 80% reduction of PVC frequency on 24-hour Holter recordings, no patient had clinical worsening of congestive heart failure, and the mean gated radionuclide ejection fraction was unchanged.

These data suggest that oral encainide has no clinically significant negative inotropic effect, even in patients with an impaired LVEF or a history of dyspnea at rest during short-term follow-up.

Pharmacokinetics

Roden et al.[57] found that the mean elimination half-life was 2.7 ± 0.2 hours (range, 1.9–3.8) after the single 25 mg dose, and it increased to only 3.4 ± 0.3 hours ($P < .05$) under steady state conditions.

Winkle et al.[59] administered a single 75 mg intravenous dose of encainide to 9 patients. The average plasma half-life after intravenous dosing was 3.4 ± 1.7 hours, with a range of 2–6.9. The calculated bioavailability ranged from 7%–82% as compared to concentration-time curves for intravenous dosing. The clearances ranged from 210–1790 ml/min (with a mean of 1157 ± 522). After oral dosing, the serum half-life tended to be shorter than after intravenous dosing in most patients (average, 2.5 ± 0.8 hours).

Wang et al.[60] found bimodal pharmacokinetics among 10 healthy men who received unlabeled encainide, 50 mg every 8 hours, and 54 mCi of ^{14}C-encainide intravenously concomitantly with the first and eighth oral doses. Eight subjects metabolized encainide rapidly, with a mean systemic availability of 26% ± 19%, a plasma encainide level of 19 ng/ml, and a half-life of 2.67 ± 0.93 hours. Two subjects were slow metabolizers, with systemic availability of 89% ± 13%, serum encainide levels that were twenty times higher (a mean of 377 ng/ml), and a mean half-life of 8.7 ± 3.4 hours. Rapid metabolizers produced 3-methoxy-*O*-demethylencainide (MODE). In contrast, the two slow metabolizers produced no detectable MODE but made larger amounts of ODE. In neither group did unmetabolized encainide accumulate significantly.

Both major metabolites, ODE and MODE, are pharmacologically active and have longer plasma half-lives than the parent compound.[61-66] After 6 months of long-term encainide therapy in 13 patients receiving doses titrated to suppress PVCs (100–250 mg/day in divided doses), the elimination half-life was 1 hour, too short to explain the observed clinical duration of the antiarrhythmic effect. Even after 24 hours, the plasma concentration of MODE decreased by less than half and no half-life could be calculated, although it is probably about 1 day.[57] After 1 months of long-term therapy with 90% PVC suppression, the median time for arrhythmia return after drug withdrawal was 12–14 hours in 12 patients, and the pharmacokinetics of encainide and its metabolites remained unchanged.[64]

Plasma Level and Dosage

The minimum plasma level, which results in 90% suppression of chronic PVCs, ranges from 3–170 ng/ml (a mean of 39 ± 19) after a single 75 mg intravenous dose and 1–48 ng/ml (a mean of 14 ± 16) after oral dosing.[57,59] The duration of action, as measured by 90% PVC suppression after a single intravenous dose ranged from 1–36 hours with a mean and median of 8 hours and 3–25 hours after a single oral dose.[59] The dose of encainide orally may range from 10–75 mg, three or four times a day, with most patients responding to 25–50 mg, three times a day

Efficacy

POTENTIALLY LETHAL VENTRICULAR PREMATURE DEPOLARIZATION. In the study by Winkle et al.,[59] a single intravenous dose of 75 mg of encainide, resulted in 90% suppression of PVCs in 7 of 9 patients with frequent ventricular extrasystoles and 80% suppression in 8 of 9 patients for a time interval ranging from 1–36 hours (a mean of 8 hours of 90% suppression for each patient).

In a dose-ranging, double-blind, oral protocol that included both placebo control and washout periods, Roden et al.[57] found almost complete abolition of ventricular ectopy (> 99% reduction) in 10 of 11 patients, 7 of whom had been resistant or intolerant to four or more previous drug regimens. The doses ranged from 25–100 mg every 8 hours, and efficacy persisted for 6–12 months of follow-up.

DiBianco et al.[52] found that oral encainide (a mean dose of 75 mg, every 6 hours) titrated to a Holter monitor response resulted in an 80% reduction in PVC frequency in 20 of 21 patients with PVCs of greater than or equal to 60 beats/hr. There was a reduction in couplets by 99.8% and in salvos of nonsustained ventricular tachycardia by 99%.

Morganroth et al.[67] found that encainide (25–75 mg, every 6 hours) significantly reduced the PVC frequency in 27 of 30 patients, with complete suppression (< 1 PVC/hr) in 13 (48%) of these patients. Repetitive PVCs were abolished in 16 (84%) of 19 patients. At a dosage of less than 50 mg, every 6 hours, that was devoid of any side effects, PVCs were abolished in 10 (77%) of 13 patients, and repetitive forms were abolished in 13 (81%) of 16 patients.

Sami et al.[68] conducted an 8-week, longitudinal, crossover comparative study on fixed oral doses of quinidine and ecainide in 20 men with PVCs. Encainide (50 mg, every 6 hours) suppressed all PVCs recorded on ambulatory electrocardiography in 44% of the patients, reduced the frequency by 80% or more in 88% of the patients, and suppressed complex forms in all patients. On the other hand, quinidine (300 mg, every 6 hours) failed to totally suppress PVCs in any patient, resulted in an 80% reduction in PVC frequency in less than half of the patients, and suppressed complex forms in half of the patients. In this fixed-dose comparative study, encainide was more potent and more efficacious for PVC suppression than quinidine. Encainide was also better tolerated.

LETHAL VENTRICULAR ARRHYTHMIAS. Winkle & Mason[69] evaluated 38 patients with three documented episodes of symptomatic ventricular tachycardia during the 6-month period before enrollment. Adequate suppression could not be achieved with at least two other antiarrhythmic agents; 79% had failed to be controlled with less than 4 other antiarrhythmic agents. Oral encainide (150–250 mg, daily, divided into 4–6 doses) was administered at an individualized dose and frequency based on arrhythmia suppression as recorded on continuous ECG monitoring. The drug completely eliminated recurrence of sustained ventricular tachycardia in 54% of the patients for 6 months and 29% of the patients for 18–30 months of therapy. Few classic electrophysiologic studies in patients with lethal ventricular arrhythmias to define efficacy have been conducted. The rate of efficacy appears to be about 30%–40%.

Adverse Effects

With long-term administration in 119 patients, encainide produced blurring of vision in 23 patients (19%). Dizziness or ataxia occurred in 14 patients (12%), and headache, tremor, nausea, and constipation were seen in less than 3%. Encainide was only discontinued in one patient with preexisting visual impairment because of side effects. The occurrence of adverse effects appears to be determined by the total daily dose and the peak plasma level attained. The incidence of side effects is 67% at doses greater than 50 mg every 6 hours, with only a 14% incidence of side effects at lower doses.[67] Side effects tend to occur within 2 hours of drug administration, when the peak plasma level would be expected to occur.

Since toxicity is related to the time of peak levels, adverse effects are often avoided by giving smaller doses more frequently and avoiding the high peaks and dips in plasma concentration that are associated with less frequent dosing.

Asymptomatic sinus pauses (< 2 sec duration) have also been reported to occur in 3% of cases. This may represent a group of patients with previous borderline abnormal sinus node dysfunction.[52]

Proarrhythmic Effects

Proarrhythmic effects have been seen in 10 (8%) of 119 patients receiving long-term oral encainide therapy. Half of these had a previous history of sustained ventricular tachycardia requiring cardioversion. The proarrhythmic effect depends on the population studied and averages about 2% for those with potentially lethal ventricular arrhythmias and 11% for those treated with lethal ventricular arrhythmias.[69]

Like the neurologic and gastrointestinal side effects, there is evidence that the proarrhythmic effects of encainide are dose related.[70] Although proarrhythmic effects appear to be dose related, they cannot be predicted by QRS interval prolongation, which is usually moderate, or QTc interval prolongation, which is usually minimal.

On the basis of these data it is recommended that patients with known lethal arrhythmias be treated in the hospital with continuous ECG monitoring. At least 48 hours should elapse before a dose is changed, and antiarrhythmic efficacy should be objectively documented.

Drug Interactions

Among 10 patients who received long term maintenance doses of digoxin, 1–2 weeks of therapy with encainide resulted in no significant change in the mean serum digoxin level (1.04 ± 0.43 before, 1.22 ± 0.47 after).[58]

Summary

Encainide is a potent antiarrhythmic agent with a class IC profile of action. Because of wide interpretation variations in bioavailability, the dose must be individually titrated based on antiarrhythmic effect for optimum safety and efficacy. Its toxic/therapeutic ratio is large, and it has been well-tolerated and efficacious in long-term use. The parent compound undergoes rapid hepatic metabolism, and the resulting metabolites have equipotent or greater antiarrhythmic activity and long plasma half-lives. Although it appears to be a nearly ideal antiarrhythmic agent, without adversely effecting depressed left ventricular performance, careful use in patients with sinus node disease and mild to moderate conduction abnormalities is essential.

Lorcainide

History

Lorcainide (Remivox) is an antiarrhythmic drug with local anesthetic activity whose chemical name is *N*-(4-chlorophenyl)-*N*-[1-(1-methylethyl)-4-piperidinyl]benzeneacetamide.

Mechanism of Action

Several studies have reported on the electrophysiologic effects of lorcainide in humans. In normal subjects, lorcainide has no major effects on sinus node function. After intravenous administration, the drug results in a mild increase in heart rate. There is no alteration in sinus node recovery and sinoatrial conduction times. In patients with preexisting sinus node dysfunction, lorcainide must be used with caution. Manz, Steinbeck, and Luderitz[71] noted that after lorcainide administration (2 mg/kg, intravenously) 3 of 7 patients developed heart rates of less than 50 beats/min because of sinus node exit block. There was a marked prolongation of the corrected sinus node recovery time.

Lorcainide tends to prolong the atrial effective refractory period, but most studies have shown no changes in the right ventricular refractory period or the effective refractory period of the atrioventricular node. In patients with the Wolff-Parkinson-White syndrome both retrograde and antegrade refractory periods of accessory pathways were prolonged by lorcainide.[72-74] The effects of lorcainide on the surface ECG consist of prolongation of QRS, PR, and QTc intervals. Oral treatment with lorcainide was found to increase the AH interval and ventricular effective refractory period but did not alter the sinus cycle length.[75-78]

Hemodynamics

In patients with chronic cardiac disease there was a slight decrease in aortic pressure without a change in the systemic vascular resistance or cardiac output.[80] In contrast, in patients with acute myocardial infarction treated with lorcainide (150 mg, intravenously) there was no significant change in blood pressure, but there was a slight increase in peripheral resistance and a small reduction in cardiac index and stroke volume.[81]

Pharmacokinetics

When administered orally, lorcainide is almost completely absorbed. The bioavailability and plasma levels are low with low initial doses (100–150 mg) but are higher when higher initial doses are given.[82,83] At steady state, the bioavailability is approximately 100%. Orally administered lorcainide is metabolized to a pharmacologically active compound, norlorcainide, an *N*-dealkylated form. Metabolites thus may play an additional role in arrhythmia suppression.[75-77]

The distribution half-life of lorcainide is short, approximately 30 minutes in both animals and humans. The volume of distribution at steady state appears to be between 5 and 10 L/kg. This agent is found to be 83% protein bound in normal subjects and 75% in patients with congestive heart failure.[83-85]

In humans, less than 2% of an intravenous dose of lorcainide was recovered unchanged in the urine.[83] The elimination half-life of lorcainide was found to be close to 7.7 hours by some investigators,[82,83] whereas Somani[86] found a longer elimination half-life of 13.1 hours. These different findings may be explained by individual variability in lorcainide pharmacokinetics. Kates, Keefe, and Winkle[87] reported a clearance of 14.4 ml/min/kg in patients with chronic PVCs.

The pharmacologically active metabolite, norlorcainide, accumulates during long-term oral therapy with lorcainide. Kates, Keefe, and Winkle[87] reported an accumulation half-life of 26.8 hours after 1 week of oral lorcainide therapy in patients with chronic ventricular ectopy.

Plasma Level and Dosage

Klotz, Muller-Seydlitz, and Heimburg[84] found the plasma concentration of lorcainide associated with effective suppression of ventricular ectopic beats to be 150–400 μg/L. These concentrations were usually obtained with a dosage schedule of 100 mg, two or three times daily. Morganroth[88] found mean plasma lorcainide concentrations of 200 and 90 μg/L in responders and nonresponders, respectively. Differences in sampling times relative to the last dose are probably responsible for the variation in plasma concentrations between studies.

A log-linear relationship between lorcainide plasma concentrations and QRS interval was noted by Meinertz et al.[77] soon after administration of a single intravenous dose of the agent. A similar effect was noted after oral administration but with lower plasma concentrations required to produce the same degree of QRS prolongation. It therefore has been suggested that the ECG QRS interval is an index of drug effect and therapeutic efficacy. The slow-accumulating pharmacologically active metabolite, norlorcainide, also produced QRS interval prolongation. The plasma concentration required to suppress PVCs during long-term oral treatment may be lower than that required during short-term oral or intravenous lorcainide therapy.[77-79]

Since lorcainide has a wide therapeutic range, individualization of therapy is necessary. The usual starting oral dose is 100 mg, twice daily. Total daily doses greater than 600 mg have occasionally been used, however.[89] Patients should not have their doses increased more often than once a week. This is because the time to reach steady state lorcainide and especially norlocainide concentrations exceeds 4.5 days. QRS prolongation can be used as a rough index of plasma concentration and may be useful in assessing adequacy of dosage. A lower dosage may be required in patients with cirrhosis or congestive heart failure, since these conditions produce decreased hepatic blood flow.[85]

Efficacy

POTENTIALLY LETHAL VENTRICULAR ARRHYTHMIAS. Several open studies have shown a favorable effect of lorcainide on ventricular ectopic beats. A great than 80% suppression of ventricular ectopic beats was found in 23 of 27 patients treated with an average intravenous dose of 139 mg.[90] Furthermore, Meinertz et al.[89] noted suppression of these arrhythmias in 11 of 12 patients treated with oral therapy. Included were 7 of the 8 patients who failed to respond to at least one antiarrhythmic agent. Amery et al.[91] noted a positive response (defined as a > 50% reduction of ventricular ectopic beats) in 84% of the patients treated orally with the drug and in 82% treated intravenously. In a single-blind study, Morganroth[88] treated 12 patients with 100 mg of lorcainide, twice daily, and reported that 8 of them had a greater than 70% suppression of ventricular ectopic beats.

LETHAL VENTRICULAR ARRHYTHMIAS. Intravenous or oral lorcainide has eliminated inducible ventricular tachycardia in a variable proportion of patients ranging from 0%–100%. Sung and Somani[92] studied 5 patients treated with 2 mg/kg of intravenous lorcainide, and all of them had induction of ventricular tachycardia despite treatment. Somberg et al.[93] reported suppression of ventricular tachycardia in all 7 patients treated with 100 mg of intravenous lorcainide. The drug was, however, administered only 9 hours after intravenous procainamide, and plasma concentrations of either drug were not reported.

ACUTE MYOCARDIAL INFARCTION. In a well-designed study,[94] 50 patients with acute myocardial infarction were treated intravenously with either lorcainide (150 mg over 15 minutes, followed by 300 mg/day for 72 hours) or lidocaine (4 mg/min for 30 minutes, followed by 2 mg/min for 72 hours). There was no significant difference between the two groups in episodes of ventricular tachycardia or fibrillation.

Adverse Effects

Although side effects are common during oral lorcainide therapy, they are rarely serious and tend to resolve or diminish with continuation of treatment. The most common side effects are sleep disturbances, which occur in 100% of the patients and often resolve with time if lorcainide is continued; the sleep disturbances usually respond well to a benzodiazepan.[88] Other common side effects include headache, nausea, excessive perspiration, and a hot sensation. Tingling commonly occurs during intravenous administration. Some patients have experienced worsening of preexistent sinus node dysfunction and infranodal conduction problems. These patients should be followed up carefully during lorcainide treatment. Aggravation of arrhythmias has been noted.[95] Frequently, lorcainide had to be discontinued because of side effects.[95]

Summary

Lorcainide is an effective new antiarrhythmic agent in suppressing PVCs. The drug also has significant activity against ventricular tachycardia. Long-term studies are needed to confirm its efficacy and the apparent absence of serious side effects. Lorcainide has a relatively long half-life, which, together with a convenient dosage schedule, may make it more acceptable to patients than other types of antiarrhythmic agents if the initial side effect of insomnia can be eliminated.

Propafenone

History

Propafenone is a new antiarrhythmic agent that was synthesized in 1970 and has been commercially available in Germany since 1977 as Rythmonorm. The chemical name for propafenone is 1-[2-[2-hydroxy-3-(propylamino)-propoxy]-phenyl]-3-phenyl-l-propanone.

Mechanism of Action

Seipel et al.[96] monitored the effects of propafenone, 1–2 mg/kg over 5 minutes, during his bundle evaluation in 25 patients. They found that sinus node frequency was reduced significantly. Significant bradycardia was seen in patients with sinus node disorder. Sinus node recovery time and corrected sinus node recovery time during high-frequency stimulation increased the latter by 46%. Conduction times were increased in a relatively uniform fashion. The sinoatrial and intraatrial conduction times (PA interval) increased significantly as it was the conduction time in the His-Purkinje system (HV interval). The effective refractory period of the atrium and the functional refractory period of the atrioventricular node significantly increased.

In another study[97] 15 patients received 2 mg/kg of propafenone intravenously in 3 minutes. There was a significant increase of the PQ time (16.7%), AH interval (9), HV interval (33%), and width of the QRS complex (13.8%). In contrast to the results of Seipel et al.,[96] the intraatrial conduction time (PA interval), heart rate, and sinus-node recovery time were not influenced. In 6 of 7 patients, the effective refractory period of the atrioventricular node was prolonged, and in one it remained unchanged.

Hemodynamics

Bachour and Hochrein[98] monitored the ECG, cardiac output, and pulmonary and systemic arterial blood pressure in 23 patients with coronary artery disease (15 patients had had acute transmural myocardial infarctions and 16 had previously received digitalis). The administration of 70 mg of intravenous propafenone over 2 minutes increased the mean PCW pressure 2.2 mm Hg, with the maximum increase observed 10 minutes after the injection. Right atrial and pulmonary artery pressure rose significantly between 5 and 20 minutes after the injection, returning to baseline levels during the first hour. The mean arterial pressure fell slightly. Peripheral resistance increased from 12%–22%, and cardiac output decreased by 13%–15% despite abolition of ventricular extrasystoles for at least 15 minutes in 11 of 14 patients. By 45 minutes the extrasystoles recurred, with an accompanying decrease in cardiac output and arterial blood pressure. In 9 control patients with similar medical histories but normal sinus rhythm, propafenone again produced similar changes in cardiac output and mean PCW pressure. Values tended toward normalization by 10 minutes. No pathologic ECG changes were noted.

The hemodynamic effects of 2 mg of intravenous propafenone (given over 5 minutes) were studied in 9 patients with coronary artery disease during cardiac catheterization.[99] Hemodynamic measurements were made in the control state and repeated at fixed intervals during the 20 minutes after infusion. Propafenone caused a moderate decrease in contractility without altering either the heart rate or the aortic pressures. However, 2 patients received a higher dose (3 mg/kg), and severe depression of myocardial contractility, with hypotension and bradycardia, occurred.

During a double-blind, crossover trial, Baker et al.[100] studied the effect of propafenone (450–900 mg/day) on left ventricular function in 14 patients, assessed by multigated radionuclide ejection fractions. When the results were stratified using a baseline ejection fraction, a mild depression was observed with therapy.

Pharmacokinetics

Propafenone is probably extensively metabolized, most likely by first-pass hepatic metabolism. The metabolic pathway has not been completely elucidated. Comparison of cumulative urinary excretion over 24 hours shows that 1.3% (70 mg) of the intravenous and 0.65% (600 mg) of the oral drug was excreted in the urine unchanged. The plasma protein binding is about 97%. The half-life is 2.5 hours, with a range of 1.2–4.2 hours. Connolly et al.[101] reported a great intersubject variability in the elimination half-life, 2.4–11.8 hours.

In a study of 21 patients with stable ventricular arrhythmias Blanke et al.[102] investigated the correlation between antiarrhythmic effectiveness and propafenone plasma concentration. On the third day, the mean propafenone plasma concentration of the 9 patients free of arrhythmia was 780 ng/ml, whereas in patients with persistent arrhythmias, it was 350 ng/ml. Pronounced individual variations were found for frequency of extrasystoles and plasma concentration. Wiebringhaus et al.[103] studied 43 patients with different cardiac arrhythmias during long-term oral therapy with propafenone for 1–34 months (average, 13.4 months). Plasma concentrations were repeatedly determined between the third and fourth hours after the last dose. The daily dose ranged from 450–1200 mg and the plasma concentrations from 500–3000 ng/ml. There was no strict correlation between plasma levels and the dose ingested, therapeutic success, and side effects. There was some correlation between plasma levels and widening of the QRS complex, however. Connolly et al.[101] reported that the plasma propafenone concentration which caused over 90% suppression of ventricular ectopic beats ranged from 64–1044 ng/ml (mean, 588 ng/ml).

Various formulations in capsules and sugar-coated tablets containing 300 mg of propafenone were available until the end of 1975. Film-coated tablets of 300 mg (Rytmonorm) and 150 mg (Rytmonorm 150) were developed in 1976. The dosage is 150–300 mg, three times daily.

Efficacy

POTENTIALLY LETHAL VENTRICULAR ARRHYTHMIAS. In a double-blind, crossover trial, in which propafenone was compared against a placebo, DeSoyza et al.[104] reported propafenone to be effective in 25 out of 30 (83%) patients. Ventricular tachycardia, which was present in 29 patients at baseline, was abolished in all patients at the maximum propafenone dosage of 900 mg/day.

In a double-blind, crossover, placebo-controlled study, Salerno et al.[105] used Holter recordings to evaluate the effectiveness of propafenone for the treatment of PVCs in 12 patients. The effectiveness of propafenone was confirmed: 80% suppression of total PVCs in 7 of 12 patients and almost complete suppression of ventricular tachycardia.

CLINICAL TRIALS AGAINST OTHER ANTIARRHYTHMIC AGENTS. In patients with PVCs on Holter monitoring before and after administration of propafenone (900 mg/day) and quinidine (800 mg/day), propafenone completely controlled the arrhythmia in 8 patients, quinidine in only 3.[106]

Naccarella et al.[107] compared the efficacy of propafenone (300 mg, three times daily for 5 days) with disopyramide (200 mg, three times daily for 5 days) using 24-hour Holter monitoring in 12 patients with symptomatic PVCs. The results indicated that both drugs significantly reduced PVCs (a 70%–80% reduction) in 8 of 12 patients receiving propafenone and 6 of 12 receiving disopyramide.

LETHAL VENTRICULAR ARRHYTHMIAS. Podrid and Lown[108] studied the efficacy of propafenone in 30 patients with sustained hemodynamically unstable ventricular arrhythmia. Of the 22 patients who underwent acute testing and received a single dose of 450 mg of propafenone, 11 had suppression of arrhythmia, thus meeting the criteria for drug efficacy. All 30 patients entered a short maintenance period of 72–96 hours (150–300 mg, three times daily), and 17 (57%) had a reduction of PVCs from 678–49 ($P < .01$), a reduction of couplets from 88–0.2/hr ($P > .01$), and a complete abolishment of ventricular tachycardia.

Programmed electrical stimulation studies were performed both before and after intravenous (2 mg/kg, over 10 minutes, followed by up to 2 mg/min) or oral (900 mg/day) administration of propafenone.[109,110] The ventricular tachycardia cycle length increased significantly in both studies. After oral evaluation, 4 of 8 patients were discharged on propafenone therapy and had no symptomatic tachycardia or side effects with a mean follow-up period of 4 months. Lower intravenous doses (1 mg/kg) were less effective; however, 3 of 11 patients treated with high intravenous doses of propafenone had inducibility of sustained ventricular tachycardia suppressed. Both groups of investigators concluded that propafenone is a promising drug for treating patients with ventricular tachycardia. Connolly et al.[111] performed electrophysiologic studies in 16 patients with ventricular tachycardia or nonfatal cardiac arrest. All patients had baseline inducible sustained ventricular tachycardia. During oral propafenone therapy (150–300 mg, three times daily), ventricular tachycardia was not inducible in one patient, was unsustained in one, and was harder to induce in two patients. Two of five patients treated with oral propafenone were arrhythmia-free during a follow-up period of 1–8 months.

In an electrophysiologic study of 14 patients with both clinical and induced sustained ventricular tachycardia by Doherty et al.,[112] 12 of the 14 patients failed to respond to conventional antiarrhythmic drug therapy. Ventricular tachycardia remained inducible or occurred spontaneously in 13 of 14 patients after propafenone administration. The ventricular tachyardia cycle length did not significantly change after drug therapy.

Adverse Side Effects

Side effects include restlessness, disturbed sleep, lack of concentration, syncope, myoclonus, psychosis, convulsion, diarrhea, epigastric pain, urticaria, and alopecia. The prevalence varies considerably in up to 25% of cases. Rare cases of cholestatic hepatitis, agranulocytosis and oligospermia reversible impotence have been reported. In Europe, two cases of cholestatic hepatitis have been related to propafenone treatment.[113] Experience with long-term treatment has shown that extracardiac side effects may still occur after a considerable time.[114]

Drug Interactions

Belz et al.[115] indicated that propafenone (150 mg, every 8 hours) increased plasma digoxin concentrations 37% during coadministration for 2 weeks. In another study, propafenone increased serum digoxin levels in 5 of 5 patients (with a mean increase of 83%).[105] No patients had evidence of digitalis toxicity during this study, however.

A case report by Korst, Brandes, and Littman[116] documents a possible interaction between coumadin and propafenone. Because of the high level of protein binding of propafenone (97%), caution should be observed when administering this drug with oral anticoagulants.

Summary

Propafenone is a new investigational antiarrhythmic drug available for oral and intravenous administration. Propafenone is extensively metabolized, although the metabolic pathways have not been completely elucidated. It is effective in the treatment of ventricular arrhythmias and its tolerance is under study.

Indecainide

History

Indecainide is a new investigational antiarrhythmic agent and its chemical name is 9-[3-(methylethyl) amino]prophyl]-9H-fluorene-9-carboxamide hydrochloride.

Mechanism of Action

In humans, indecainide prolongs cardiac impulse conduction expressed on the surface ECG as lengthening of the PR and QRS intervals.[117] There were maximum prolongations of the PR and QT intervals of 30 and 10 msec, respectively, with return to control values 45–50 minutes after the end of the infusion.

In a study of 10 patients treated with oral indecainide (50–100 mg, every 8 hours), Siddoway et al.[118] noted that the PR interval increased 0.4 ± 0.02 sec in responders ($P < .5$) and only 0.1 sec in nonresponders. Krejci et al.[119] reported a 25% increase in the PR interval, and an 18% increase in the QRS interval; the QT interval nonsignificantly decreased by 1%.

Hemodynamics

Blood pressures, the pulse rate, systolic time intervals, stroke volumes, the cardiac output, and the cardiac index were measured by noninvasive techniques every 5 minutes before, during, and after the infusion of the drug or placebo in 5 patients. Increasing doses were associated with an increase in the diastolic and mean pulmonary pressure, preejection period, and heart rate, and a decrease occurred in the stroke volume, cardiac output, and cardiac index.

Krejci et al.[119] evaluated the effects of indecainide in a short-term, oral dose–ranging, single-blind, efficacy trial in 7 patients with ventricular ectopic depolarizations. The drug produced no significant change in heart rate, systolic time intervals, or any ECG measurements. The negative inotropic effects of the drug are not clearly understood. Caution should be exercised when administering indecainide to patients with compromised cardiac function, or when administered concomitantly with other cardiac depressants.

Pharmacokinetics

In one study, intravenous administration of ^{14}C-radiolabeled indecainide in four normal volunteers resulted in a plasma half-life of 5.63 ± 1.19 hours (range, 4.8–7.9). Eighty-four percent of the drug was excreted in the urine and 11% in the feces.

Oral radiolabeled indecainide given to five subjects (doses of 0.56–0.73 mg/kg) resulted in a plasma half-life of 11.59 ± 5.78 hours (range, 6–12). Eighty-one percent of the radioactivity was excreted in the urine and 17% in the feces. It is thus possible that 17% of the orally administered drug undergoes first-pass metabolism by the liver. Approximately 87% of the oral dose is absorbed through the intestinal tract. Morganroth et al.[117] reported that the metabolite desisopropyl indecainide represented 10% of the active compound. In one study of oral indecainide in five subjects, the maximum plasma concentrations ranged from 152–315 ng/ml (mean, 217.4 ± 72.9) and was reached in 1.9 ± 0.9 hours (range, 0.5–2.5). Krejci et al.[119] reported that indecainide plasma levels in an optimum dose, were 233–658 ng/ml (mean, 413).

Indecainide may be administered orally and intravenously. It is provided for clinical trials as white, opaque capsules equivalent to 50, 75, and 100 mg base. An intravenous solution is equivalent to 5 mg of base drug per milliliter (10 ml vials are available). Oral doses of 50–100 mg are given three or four times a day.

Efficacy

POTENTIALLY LETHAL VENTRICULAR ARRHYTHMIAS. In a dose-ranging study, intravenous indecainide (17.5 μg/kg/min for 25 minutes) produced a 100% suppression of the ventricular ectopic activity for a short period of time. When 60 mg were infused at 12.6 mg/kg/min, PVCs were completely suppressed for 10–11 hours.

Morganroth et al.[117] reported a greater than 70% reduction in PVCs in 93% of the patients and a greater than 90% reduction in 85% of the patients. In another dose-ranging study, all patients achieved at least an 80% reduction. In a study by Siddoway et al.,[118] 8 of 10 patients had satisfactory activity at a mean dosage of 66 ± 19 mg every 8 hours. Krejci et al.,[119] in a short-term, oral dose–ranging, single-blind trial, studied the efficacy of indecainide in 7 patients. Four of them had ventricular tachycardia defined as greater than or equal to 3 repetitive PVCs. The average suppression of ventricular tachycardia was 94.5% for 50 mg, 99.7% for 75 mg, and 100% for 100 mg, three times daily.

In a dose-ranging, single-blind, placebo study, Morganroth et al.[117] administered oral indecainide to 14 patients with nonsustained ventricular tachycardia and frequent PVCs. Indecainide eliminated ventricular tachycardia in 12 patients (86%).

LETHAL VENTRICULAR ARRHYTHMIAS. Electrophysiologic tests in patients with lethal ventricular arrhythmias is limited at present, but one study[120] demonstrated that the initial ventricular tachycardia was eliminated in only 1 of 10 patients, although in most patients the rate of the ventricular tachycardia was slower.

Adverse Side Effects

Siddoway et al.[118] reported side effects in 3 of 10 patients, which consisted of liver transaminase elevation (1 patient), dizziness (2 patients), and a decrease in white blood count from 4880 ± 283 to 3250 ± 212 (2 patients).

Krejci et al.[119] noted side effects in 4 of 7 patients, but none of them required cessation of the drug. Three patients experienced dizziness, 1 patient developed asymptomatic postural hypotension, 1 patient developed right bundle-branch block, and another had blurred vision. In the study by Morganroth et al.[117] 2 of 14 patients reported side effects (blurred vision and paresthesia). Other adverse effects reported include headache, nausea, vomiting, a "funny taste," and drowsiness.

Summary

Indecainide is a promising new antiarrhythmic agent. It appears to be efficacious in eliminating PVCs and nonsustained ventricular tachycardia. It also appears to be well tolerated with few side effects to date. Further investigation of this agent is warranted.

UNCLASSIFIED CLASS I AGENTS

Cibenzoline

History

Cibenzoline is an imidazoline derivative 2-(2,2-diphenylcyclopropyl)-4,5-dihydro-1H-imidazole that is structurally unrelated to other known antiarrhythmic agents.

Mechanism of Action

The effects of cibenzoline on cardiac conduction are primarily of the class I type, exemplified by quinidine and disopyramide. It decreases membrane responsiveness, the amplitude of action potential, and the maximum rate of depolarization by reducing the fast inward sodium current in the myocardium.[121] Cibenzoline also has some class III activity (prolongation of the action potential duration) and class IV activity (calcium antagonism). In one study, the effect of different doses of cibenzoline (1 and 1.25 mg/kg, intravenously) was compared in several conduction parameters. There was no apparent dose-effect relationship, except for the slowing of His-Purkinje conduction, which appears to increase with increased cibenzoline dose.[122]

Kushner et al.[123] studied the electrophysiologic effects of oral cibenzoline in five male patients with chronic stable ventricular arrhythmias in a placebo-controlled ascending dose study. Cibenzoline caused a significant increase in AH and HV intervals, a nonstatistically significant increase in QRS duration, and essentially no changes in QT and QTc intervals.

Browne et al.[124] studied 26 patients with ventricular tachycardia or PVCs treated with cibenzoline. The PR interval and QRS duration significantly increased ($P < .001$), and the QT interval did not change. The drug did not affect electrophysiologic properties of the atrium or atrioventricular node. Cibenzoline significantly prolonged the ventricular effective and functional refractory periods.

Hemodynamics

At effective antiarrhythmic plasma concentrations (250–350 ng/ml), cibenzoline was found to produce a 15% decrease in positive peak left ventricular dp/dt and a 10% reduction in cardiac output, without any significant change in afterload.[122] When compared to control values, cibenzoline produced no significant change in cardiac contractility (as measured by the cirumferential fiber shortening rate, systolic thickening rate, and ejection fraction).

In the study by Browne et al.[124] no patients had worsening or new onset of clinical signs or symptoms of congestive heart failure during cibenzoline therapy. The mean ejection fraction for the group of 12 patients who had multigated blood pool scans did not change significantly. The dosages used were 65–97.5 mg, every 8 hours. The extent to which cibenzoline exerts a negative inotropic effect has not been clearly defined.

Pharmacokinetics

In normal subjects treated with intravenous cibenzoline, the plasma concentration declined biphasically with an initial rapid decline followed by a log-linear elimination phase with a half-life of about 5 hours. Approximatley 60% of the dose was excreted intact in the urine. After oral administration, 55% of the dose was excreted intact in the urine, and the elimination half-life of 4 hours was similar to that observed after intravenous administration. Oral bioavailability of cibenzoline was complete, and approximately 60% of plasma cibenzoline was found to be protein bound.[125]

In 12 patients with renal failure (not requiring dialysis) the elimination half-life increased approximatley twofold, whereas the total plasma clearance decreased approximately threefold as compared with normal subjects. In patients with decreased renal function, the elimination rate of cibenzoline is decreased, and this may result in plasma concentration two to three times higher than in patients with normal renal function. The dosage therefore should be reduced in patients with impaired renal function. In contrast to cibenzoline, the metabolite does not appear to be active.[126]

In a study of 20 patients, oral cibenzoline administered in an increasing dose, resulted in plasma levels that were a linear function of the administered dose. For a dose of 1 mg/kg, serum levels were about 500 ng/ml. A therapeutic effect was achieved in 90% of the patients with a dose greater than or equal to 2 mg/kg/day, and the mean therapeutic dose was 3.2 mg/kg/day. In the other 248 patients studied by European investigators and treated with oral cibenzoline, the dosages ranged from 1–5 65 mg capsules a day.

Brazzell et al.[127] studied the relationship between plasma concentrations of cibenzoline and its antiarrhythmic effect in 25 patients treated with the drug orally. The plasma concentration, corresponding to a 90% reduction in PVC frequency ranged from 215–405 ng/ml. The authors suggested that the antiarrhythmic effect of cibenzoline is proportional to its plasma concentration.

Two controlled trials studied the effect of oral cibenzoline (65 mg, four times daily) in the treatment of PVCs. One was a double-blind, crossover comparison of cibenzoline to a placebo in 8 patients, and the other was a three-way, single-blind, crossover trial in 12 patients, also comparing cibenzoline to a placebo. Overall, cibenzoline therapy resulted in a greater than 80% reduction in PVCs in approximately 75% of the patients.

Kushner et al.,[123] in a placebo-controlled, ascending dose study with oral cibenzoline, reported a greater than 85% reduction in PVCs in 3 of 5 male patients studied, including 2 in whom only relatively low serum concentrations have been achieved.

Browne et al.[124] tested the effect of oral cibenzoline in 26 patients who had symptomatic ventricular tachycardia (24 patients) or PVCs (2 patients). The drug was given to maximum doses of 65–97.5 mg every 8 hours. Cibenzoline prevented spontaneous episodes of ventricular tachycardia in 8 of 16 patients (50%) with ventricular tachycardia during a 72-hour control ECG recording. Furthermore, 7 of 22 patients (32%) had a greater than 83% reduction in PVCs compared with the control. Kostis et al.[128] reported a more than 75% suppression of PVCs in 13 of 21 patients (62%) treated with cibenzoline (130 mg, twice daily). Six additional patients responded to 160 mg twice daily during an open-label titration phase. Ventricular tachycardia was totally suppressed in 9 of 10 patients (90%) and markedly diminished in the 1 remaining patient. In a double-blind, placebo-controlled, crossover phase in 16 patients, cibenzoline significantly reduced the number of PVCs ($P = .02$), ventricular tachycardia ($P = .01$), and ventricular pairs ($P = .01$).

LETHAL VENTRICULAR ARRHYTHMIAS. In the study by Browne et al.,[124] 9 of 10 patients who underwent electrophysiologic testing had ventricular tachycardia induced during the control period. During maximum oral cibenzoline therapy ventricular tachycardia was still induced in 7 patients. The drug prevented induction of tachycardia in 2 patients, and 1 had no arrhythmia induced at baseline or while receiving cibenzoline therapy.

Adverse Effects

The tolerance to oral cibenzoline is rated as good to excellent in the majority of cases. Gastrointestinal effects are the most frequent, occuring in 1%–4% of the patients and consisting of epigastric pain (3.7%), nausea (2.2%), epigastric burning, vomiting, bitter taste, diarrhea, and lingual mycosis (0.4% each). Cardiac toxicity is always a potential problem and consists of heart blocks, conduction problems, and chest pain. Other adverse effects are malaise (1.5%), weakness, headache, and vertigo (0.7% each). Parenteral cibenzoline has been reported to produce hypotension (4.4%), hypertension (0.7%), nausea and vomiting (0.7%), and general malaise (1.5%). A total of 8 deaths were reported in patients receiving oral cibenzoline and in a patient treated intravenously. In only 2 patients was the death possibly related to cibenzoline therapy.

Summary

Cibenzoline is a new antiarrhythmic agent with a unique structure. Clinical studies in Europe showed that oral cibenzoline was as effective as disopyramide in suppressing chronic PVCs. Studies done in the United Stated showed the drug to be reasonably effective in patients with symptomatic PVCs or nonsustained ventricular tachycardia, but ineffective in the few patients evaluated with sustained ventricular tachycardia or ventricular fibrillation. It is generally well tolerated.

Moricizine

History

Moricizine hydrochloride (as Ethmozine) is a phenothiazine derivative with marked antiarrhythmic properties and was developed in the Soviet Union in 1964.[129] The drug is approved for clinical use in the Soviet Union, but is currently under development in the United States. The drug's chemical name is 10-(3-morpholinopropionyl)phenothiazine-2-carbamic acid ethyl ester hydrochloride.

Mechanism of Action

Several mechanisms of antiarrhythmic action have been suggested by the drug's electrophysiologic effects.[130,131] Morcizine significantly decreases the maximum rate of depolarization. Furthermore, this agent prolongs the effective refractory period. Fox et al.[132] noted that moricizine, in canine studies, increased the fibrillation threshold and effectively decreased ventricular premature depolarizations after coronary occlusion. Morganroth et al.[133] did not note significant electrophysiologic changes in 6 patients treated with oral moricizine (5–10 mg/kg). Minimum effects were observed on sinus node recovery time and atrioventricular conduction. Mann et al.[134] observed a prolongation in these parameters, however.

Hemodynamics

Podrid and Lown[135] reported that ethmozine had no significant hemodynamic effects during acute drug testing or maintenance oral therapy. In another study[136] the increase in resting heart and systolic blood pressure was not clinically relevant, nor was the diastolic blood pressure statistically changed. The heart rate and blood pressure at rest and during exercise were unchanged with moricizine compared with the placebo.[137] During diagnostic cardiac catheterizations, hemodynamic evaluations in 6 patients revealed nonclinically significant changes in right atrial, right ventricular, pulmonary artery, pressures. Heart rate and cardiac output decreased by approximately 30% in 3 patients and by 13% in 1 patient. The relationship of the decrease in cardiac output to moricizine administration is unclear.

More invasive hemodynamic studies are needed to thoroughly evaluate the effects of moricizine therapy on hemodynamic parameters.

Pharmacokinetics

Moricizine is well absorbed by the gastrointestinal tract. The drug's major route of elimination is by metabolism, and biotransformation is believed to occur in the liver.[138] After oral administration, the peak moricizine concentration is noted within 1–1½ hours, and the elimination half-life is 2–5 hours.[139] In cardiac patients and in patients with renal insufficiency, the mean elimination half-life was found to be significantly prolonged to 10 and 47 hours, respectively.[140]

To date, no active metabolites of moricizine have been described.

Plasma Level and Dosage

Pratt et al.[136] reported a mean plasma moricizine level of 0.42 ± 0.28 μg/ml at a mean daily dose of 10.1 ± 2.6 mg/kg. There was a poor correlation between daily moricizine dose and plasma level and between plasma level and reduction of ventricular extrasystoles, a fact consistent with later reported data by the same group of investigators.[141] Other investigators[138,142] have noted a delayed onset of antiarrhythmic effect despite an effective plasma concentration. Danilo et al.[143] noted a prompt onset of antiarrhythmic drug effect. Trials performed in the United States have shown that moricizine should be administered at 10–15 mg/kg for adequate ventricular extrasystole suppression. Moricizine is only available orally. The intravenous form has not yet been studied in humans.

Efficacy

POTENTIALLY LETHAL VENTRICULAR ARRHYTHMIAS. Morganroth et al.[138] studied the efficacy of moricizine in 17 patients using a single-blind, placebo-controlled protocol; 10 of 14 patients (71%) had a greater than 70% reduction in the maximum hourly PVC frequency, compared to the control. Podrid et al.[142] studied 37 patients with chronic symptomatic PVCs treated with moricizine. A placebo was given in a single-blind fashion only to responders. Only 2 of 11 patients (2%) who received 225 mg/day had a significant reduction in arrhythmia, and 14 of 26 patients (54%) who received 600 mg/day responded. Singh et al.,[144] using dosages of

10 mg/kg/day, evaluted the efficacy of moricizine in 20 patients with chronic PVCs. Moricizine was effective in reducing the ventricular arrhythmia by 59%. Kennedy et al.[145] found that moricizine (600 mg/day) was effective in 19 of 21 patients in producing a 50% suppression in PVCs, a 100% reduction in couplets, and a 50% reduction in ventricular tachycardia recurrence. Using a higher moricizine dose, Podrid and Lown[135] noted that in 32 of 58 patients (56%), the drug was effective in preventing ventricular tachycardia recurrence. In 39 patients studied by Pratt et al.[136] moricizine given at a mean total daily dose of 830 ± 318 mg resulted in an 80% reduction in PVCs, a 95% suppression in couplets, and a 99% reduction in total runs of ventricular tachycardia.

The same group of investigators[141] conducted a placebo-controlled, double-blind, longitudinal, crossover comparison study of 27 patients and reported that moricizine was superior to disopyramide in suppressing PVCs and in the total abolition of ventricular pairs. The two antiarrhythmics were equally effective in suppressing nonsustained runs of ventricular tachycardia. In a study of 24 patients with frequent PVCs, moricizine was found to have an equivalent antiarrhythmic efficacy to quinidine but with less adverse reactions.[146]

LETHAL VENTRICULAR ARRHYTHMIAS. Mann et al.[134] failed to find moricizine effective in preventing ventricular tachycardia induction in the electrophysiology laboratory in patients with chronic recurrent ventricular tachycardia. The drug lengthened the cycle length of the ventricular tachycardia and decreased the frequency of PVCs.

Adverse Effects

In general, side effects occur in less than 10% of patients.[133,135,144] Central nervous system adverse effects are the ones most frequently seen and are the most frequent cause for discontinuation of therapy. Moricizine may also cause headaches, lightheadedness, paresthesia, dizziness, vertigo, and confusion. Visual disturbances also have been reported. Gastrointestinal side effects include nausea, epigastric discomfort, vomiting, and diarrhea. The carcinogenic potential in humans is unknown, but moricizine given to rats in a dose 6.5 times normal caused a possible increase hepatic carcinoma incidence.

Summary

Moricizine is a promising new antiarrhythmic agent under investigation in the United States. The drug has nervous system effects, and the oral preparation is effective in suppressing PVCs and ventricular tachycardia. Its potential in controlling life-threatening arrhythmias appears promising, but further studies are necessary. Moricizine is well tolerated, perhaps more so than other antiarrhythmic agents studied to date.

Pirmenol

History

Pirmenol hydrochloride is a pyridinemethanol derivative that is currently undergoing clinical investigations. Its chemical name is *cis*-(±-α-[3-2(,6-dimethyl-1-piperidinyl]-α-phenyl-1-pyridinemethanol monohydrochloride.

Mechanism of Action

Electrophysiologic studies in isolated canine Purkinje fibers have shown that pirmenol, like lidocaine, shortens the action potential duration measured to 50% repolarization, decreases the action potential amplitude and upstroke velocity, and at the same time prolongs the effective refractory period. Like procainamide, it significantly depressed membrane responsiveness and slowed conduction.[147]

In contrast to most antiarrhythmics, which show decreased efficacy at low potassium concentrations and increased toxicity at high concentrations, pirmenol has a constant effect over a wide range of potassium concentrations. This agent's activity therefore should be easier to control than other antiarrhythmic drugs. Like several other antiarrhythmic agents, pirmenol suppresses the automaticity of fibers having the fast and the slow response.

Pirmenol was shown by Steffe et al.[148] to increase the ventricular fibrillation threshold of normal and ischemic myocardium in barbiturate-anesthetized dogs. The administration of the drug did not interfere with cardioversion.

Animal studies[148] have shown that pirmenol at high doses causes a modest increase in heart rate and a decrease in the AH interval, probably due to the anticholinergic effect. Also, it slows infranodal and intraventricular conduction with an increased HV interval and QRS duration. In most clinical studies, administration of pirmenol has not been associated with significant changes in the resting heart rate or PR interval. QRS duration has been only slightly decreased, approximately 10%.

Hemodynamics

Pirmenol has a direct negative inotropic effect that appears to be less than other antiarrhythmic agents.[148] The drug does not appear to affect vascular smooth muscle. In addition, there is no evidence that the drug has an alpha- or beta-blocking action. Phillips et al.[149] studied the hemodynamic effect of pirmenol infusions in patients with normal left ventricular function. There was a slight decrease in the ejection fraction and stroke work index, and the left ventricular end-diastolic pressure rose. The effect of pirmenol in patients with impaired cardiac functions awaits further evaluation. Significant increases in diastolic blood pressure but not in systolic pressure have been noted in human studies of oral and intravenous pirmenol.[150] Anderson, Lutz, and Nappi[151] demonstrated that during 2 weeks of chronic oral pirmenol therapy, echocardiographic ejection fractions were not decreased in 12 patients.

Pharmacokinetics

Pirmenol can be administered intramuscularly, intravenously, and orally. The disappearance of this agent from plasma after an intravenous bolus has been described by two-compartment pharmacokinetics, with an initial rapid fall in plasma concentration and a half-life of 10 minutes. This reflects plasma-to-tissue redistribution. After oral administration, absorption is rapid and nearly complete, with peak levels obtained 30 minutes after administration. The bioavailability is about 85%. Pirmenol is 86% bound to plasma proteins and has an elimination half-life of about 8 hours (range, 4–17 hours). The metabolism of pirmenol is not fully understood, but probably consists of both renal and nonrenal mechanisms. About

30%–50% of total drug clearance is renal.[152,153] The nonrenal clearance presumably occurs by hepatic metabolism and fecal elimination. After oral administration, some patients had enterohepatic recycling.

Hamill et al.[152,154] suggested that 1 μg/ml was the minimum therapeutic concentration of pirmenol based on arrhythmia recurrence after short-term infusion. Reiter et al.[150] demonstrated that a stable therapeutic plasma concentration of pirmenol can be rapidly achieved and maintained with a three-stage infusion regimen. The first stage consists of a priming bolus of 50 mg over 2 minutes, a second stage of a rapid loading infusion of 2.5 mg/min for 1 hour, followed by the third stage, consisting of a maintenance infusion of 0.25 mg/min. With this regimen, a stable plasma pirmenol level of 0.9–2.75 μg/ml was effectively and rapidly achieved and maintained.

The long-term therapeutic efficacy of oral pirmenol has not been adequately evaluated. In one study,[155] the mean therapeutic dosage was approximatley 400 mg/day.

Efficacy

Only a handful of studies have examined the efficacy of pirmenol in suppressing PVCs in humans. In these reports, after single intravenous,[152,156] single oral,[154] and intravenous infusion[150], plasma drug levels below 0.7 μg/ml appear to have no antiarrhythmic activity. In contrast, with pirmenol plasma concentrations of 1 μg/ml or a greater than 90% reduction of PVCs was observed in 60%–80% of the patients. Other antiarrhythmics were previously ineffective in many of these patients.[156]

Anderson et al.[156] compared pirmenol to lidocaine in 8 patients. In an intravenous dose of 150 mg given over 30 minutes, pirmenol was effective in suppressing chronic stable PVCs in more patients than 250 mg of lidocaine given over 30 minutes. Although 88% of patients responded to pirmenol, only 25% responded to lidocaine.

Love et al.[155] evaluated the acute and chronic therapeutic efficacy of oral pirmenol and reported that this agent has been effective in suppressing PVCs for up to 9 months. Anderson, Lutz, and Nappi[151] demonstrated that oral pirmenol was effective in essentially eliminating repetitive episodes of PVCs in a 2-week study. Studies now in progress are evaluating the effect of pirmenol in the prevention of lethal ventricular arrhythmias.

Adverse Effects

During long-term oral administration, pirmenol has been associated with a metallic or bitter taste in approximately 15% of the patients. Probably secondary to an anticholinergic effect, this agent also frequently produces constipation and dry mouth. These side effects have not been intolerable, however.

In the study by Anderson et al.[156] comparing pirmenol to lidocaine, the latter drug produced more frequent side effects. One patient experienced flushing, anxiety, tingling, and sinus tachycardia, probably resulting from an idiosyncratic reaction. A patient who experienced mild transient chest discomfort had no ECG changes and a normal coronary angiogram.

Reiter et al.[150] observed no significant toxicity during 142 hours of intravenous pirmenol infusion (12 infusions in 8 subjects, for up to 48 hours). There were no laboratory abnormalities or changes in hematologic, hepatic, or renal parameters associated with pirmenol therapy.

Summary

Pirmenol appears to have promising characteristics. Its therapeutic spectrum is probably comparable to type I agents. Early human studies reported no serious toxicity, and the drug appears to be safe and well tolerated. Oral and intravenous pirmenol are safely and easily administered. Plasma levels appear to correlate well with antiarrhythmic efficacy. Although preliminary data are encouraging, further trials are needed to further explore pirmenol as an antiarrhythmic agent.

CLASS III ANTIARRHYTHMIC AGENTS

Amiodarone

History

Amiodarone hydrochloride (Cordarone) 2-butyl-3-[3,5-diiodo-4-β-diethylamino-ethoxy)-benzoyl]benzofuran hydrochloride was developed in 1962. Initial investigation focused on its use as an antianginal agent because of its marked effect on vascular smooth muscle. Vastesaeger, Gillot, and Rasson[157] first confirmed the clinical efficacy of amiodarone in this role in 1967. Although moderately effective in the treatment of angina, subsequent investigations in Europe, South America, and more recently in the United States revealed that amiodarone possesses impressive antiarrhythmic activities.

Mechanism of Action

Singh and Vaughan Williams[158] reported in 1970 that the drug's major electrophysiologic effect was a homogeneous prolongation of the action potential duration in atrial and ventricular muscle. They found no significant alteration of the resting membrane potential or height of the action potential, and a minimum delay in the maximum rate of diastolic depolarization (phase 0). Graupiel and Lenfant[159] found that amiodarone's most significant electrophysiologic effect on sinus node function in an isolated rabbit preparation was a prolonged action potential duration. The drug's adrenergic blocking action probably also contributes to sinus slowing. Local anesthetic properties have not been reported. Amiodarone, together with bretylium and sotalol, have been placed in class III of Vaughan Williams' antiarrhythmic drug classification (a prolonged action potential duration without significant change in the slope of phase 0 depolarization or resting membrane potential and without competitive adrenergic blockade or local anesthetic properties). The durg causes an increase in atrial, atrioventricular nodal, and ventricular effective refractory periods. In accessory pathway tissue (usually composed of atrial or ventricular musclelike tissue) Wellens et al.[160] found a prolonged antegrade effective refractory periods in 15 of 15 patients studied and lengthening of retrograde effective refractory periods in 8 patients after 14 days of oral amiodarone therapy.

A "pure" class III drug will not directly alter the conduction time in cardiac tissue. After oral amiodarone administration the AH interval increases because of prolongation of atrial effective refractory periods, lengthening of the relative refractory period of the atrioventricular node in response to a series of action potentials,[162] and most significantly to amiodarone's adrenergic blocking action on atrioventricular nodal tissue. Slight increases in the HV and QRS intervals have been reported. Nademanee et al.[161] have suggested that prolongation of intraventricular conduction does not occur in the absence of preexisting conduction disease or concomitant therapy with other cardioactive drugs or both.

Hemodynamics

Amiodarone is a direct vascular smooth muscle relaxant[163] that led, in part, to its initial use as an antianginal agent. In addition, it produces noncompetitive alpha- and beta-adrenergic receptor inhibition.[163] Unlike the prototype beta-adrenergic blocker propranolol, amiodarone reduces cardiac chronotropic and inotropic responses to glucagon.

Amiodarone's negative inotropic effects do not become clinically manifested at intravenous doses less than 10 mg/kg. Administration of the drug in doses up to 5 mg/kg intravenously to patients with severely depressed LVEF did not result in significant hemodynamic deterioration.[164] Similarly, with long-term oral use (200–600 mg/day) no clinically apparent deterioration was reported in patients with significant underlying left ventricular dysfunction.[165,166] The infrequent exacerbation of congestive heart failure noted in these reports may be related to reduction in heart rate rather than a negative inotropic effect.

Pharmacokinetics

The pharmacokinetics of amiodarone have not been completely elucidated despite extensive investigation.

Recent development of a specific amiodarone assay employing high-performance liquid chromatography has permitted more exact determination of pharmacokinetic parameters. In humans after a single oral dose of the drug (200–1800 mg) absorption is slow, incomplete, and highly variable.[167] Studies of the bioavailability approximations in humans showed that the drug's mean absorption fraction (the percentage reaching the general circulation) was approximately 40%–50%. In each study there was a marked interpatient variability (22%–86%), however.

With long-term oral administration (200–800 mg/day) a marked cumulative effect has been noted. Andreasen et al.[168] found that a dose of 200 mg given daily resulted in approximately a twofold to threefold increase in serum through concentration of amiodarone over 30 days. Other investigators[168,169] also reported a remarkably large steady state half-life, although significant interpatient variability was again noted (13–60 days). The clinical observation that antiarrhythmic activity was present as long as 45 days after cessation of amiodarone therapy is consistent with this prolonged elimination half-life.[170] Amiodarone's protein binding is unknown and its exact metabolism is not clear. Andreasen et al.[168] found no unchanged amiodarone in the urine. Shortly after intravenous administration, measurements of urinary excretion of iodine suggest minimum urinary excretion after hepatic biotransformation. *N*-desethylamiodarone is the only metabolite of amiodarone to date, and its pharmacokinetic and pharmacologic properties are unknown.[167]

Plasma Level and Dosage

The serum level of amiodarone may be an insensitive measure of its tissue concentration, and therefore of its direct effect because of its significant cumulative effect and prolonged elimination half-life. Haffajee et al.[166] showed that in patients with supraventricular and ventricular tachyarrhythmias who responded to amiodarone, effective therapeutic control was maintained when apparent steady state serum drug levels were greater than 1 mg/L, and the arrhythmia recurred whenever the serum concentration fell below this level. In those patients with similar arrhythmias in whom therapeutic control was never achieved, serum levels were often greater than 1 mg/L. Tissue drug concentrations were not obtained in most of those subjects. It is apparent that clinical response cannot be predicted from serum levels alone. In humans amiodarone blocks the peripheral conversion of T_4 and T_3, resulting in an increase in reverse T_3 (rT_3). This increase appears to correlate with the drug's antiarrhythmic action and some of its toxic effects. It therefore has been suggested that the serum rT_3 level may be regarded as an indirect "internal assay" and that serial measurements could be useful in adjusting therapy.[167]

It appears that a loading dose of 1–2 g/day orally for 2 weeks is necessary. In emergency situations the drug should be given as a 5–10 mg/kg bolus, followed by a 10 mg/kg/day continuous infusion for 3–5 days. Intravenous therapy probably should be supplemented by concurrent oral administration of at least 600 mg/day for maximum effectiveness. After stabilization, the oral dosage often can be reduced (400–600 mg/day) to minimize dose-related toxicity. An occasional patient may require higher doses.

Oral admiodarone (200–600 mg/day) can be effective in a relatively high percentage of patients with supraventricular tachyarrhythmias in whom previous therapy with conventional antiarrhythmic drugs has been unsuccessful. It appears to be especially useful in patients with refractory tachyarrhythmias associated with the Wolff-Parkinson-White syndrome.

Efficacy

VENTRICULAR TACHYARRHYTHMIAS. At present, the antiarrhythmic efficacy of amiodarone is directed toward the treatment of lethal ventricular arrhythmias. Recent studies have shown that high loading dosages (up to 2000 mg/day), usually 1000 mg/day, have been administered to shorten the "latent" period before full therapeutic effectiveness.[165,171] Furthermore, it has been suggested that higher daily maintenance dosages (400–1200 mg/day) are sometimes required to control the arrhythmia. Rosenbaum et al.[172] studied patients with recurrent ventricular tachycardia who were treated with 300–600 mg/day of amiodarone (25 patients also received other antiarrhythmic medication simultaneously). A complete response occurred in 34 (78%), and a partial response occurred in 5 (11%). In 8 of the 44 cases, ventricular tachycardia was related to a postmyocardial infarction ventricular aneurysm, and amiodarone therapy resulted in a complete response in 6 (78%). No significant side effects occurred, except for 2 patients requiring discontinuation of the drug for severe nausea and erythema nodosum.

Podrid and Lown[173] studied 41 patients and found oral amiodarone therapy effective in treating recurrent symptomatic sustained ventricular tachycardia. These patients had previously failed to respond to treatment with an average of six antiarrhythmic drugs. The etiologic basis for the ventricular tachycardia was not specified but presumably was secondary to coronary artery disease in most of the patients. The overall success rate was 68% after an average of 12 months of treatment using a 1-week loading regimen of 600 mg daily, followed thereafter by 200 mg/day. In the initial treatment group of 22 patients who had significant hemodynamic impairment associated with ventricular tachycardia, the annual sudden death mortality was 18%. Death occurred in the first 12 months but was not classified as sudden in another 18% of the patients. No serious toxic effects were reported, and none of the nonsudden deaths were clearly related to amiodarone therapy.

Nadamanee et al.[174] used serial 24-hour Holter monitor recordings to assess the effectiveness of amiodarone therapy in 21 patients with recurrent life-threatening ventricular tachycardia. The patients did not receive a loading dose. Oral treatment was begun at 600 mg and subsequently increased up to 1200 mg/day at 3-week intervals, based on therapeutic response as judged by Holter monitoring. Of the 21 patients in whom amiodarone therapy was initiated, 16 had Holter recording before the initiation of therapy. Of these, 1 died suddenly 4 days after beginning treatment at 600 mg/day. In the 15 remaining patients, 11 had almost total suppression of PVCs (>98% decrease in frequency) with amiodarone. Three patients had 90%–95% PVC suppression. In 19 of the surviving 20 patients (including the 5 without previous 24-hour ECG recordings) total abolition of repetitive PVCs could be achieved. After a mean of 12 months of therapy only one patient died suddenly.

Heger et al.[165] studied 45 patients with refractory recurrent ventricular tachycardia (29 patients) or ventricular fibrillation (16 patients) treated with larger doses of amiodarone administered as a loading dosage of 800 mg/day for a minimum of 6–8 weeks. The maintenance dosage was adjusted on the basis of clinical responses. In 2 patients the daily dosage had to be increased to 1800–2000 mg for adequate control; however, in both patients the dose was subsequently decreased because of reversible drug-induced neurotoxicity. Overall, treatment was successful in 30 of 45 patients (67%). Of these, 17 (38%) were controlled by amiodarone alone, whereas the others (29%) required additional antiarrhythmic treatment. Therapy was successful; 21 of 29 patients (71%) had recurrent ventricular tachycardia and 9 of 16 (56%) had recurrent ventricular fibrillation. In 9 patients amiodarone was discontinued because of inadequate arrhythmia control. Seven of these had recurrent ventricular tachycardia or fibrillation during the initial loading period. Therapy was postponed in 2 patients because they developed pulmonary fibrosis, presumed secondary to amiodarone. Five patients died while receiving amiodarone therapy, and in 2 of these patients death was due to recurrent arrhythmia. One patient died as a result of pulmonary insufficiency secondary to probable drug-related pulmonary fibrosis. In 2 other patients death occurred in the setting of progressive congestive heart failure believed to be unrelated to amiodarone. Two surviving amiodarone patients required placement of a permanent atrial pacemaker for significant sinus bradycardia.

In conclusion, this study again demonstrates that higher drug doses are often necessary for adequate therapeutic control of recurrent sustained ventricular tachycardia. The fact that 7 patients experienced recurrent arrhythmia during loading with a moderate daily dosage (800 mg) emphasizes that a higher initial dosage may sometimes be required to accelerate the onset of maximum efficacy. This investigation also demonstrated that a higher amiodarone dosage can be associated with more significant toxicity than previously reported, however.

Waxman et al.[175] confirmed these findings in a study of 51 patients in whom amiodarone was administered initially at a dosage of 1400 mg/day for 7–35 days, adjusting the loading period on the basis of clinical response. The subsequent dosage (400–800 mg) was determined either by the rapidity of response to the loading regimen or by the results of electrophysiologic study. The effect of amiodarone therapy was evaluated by clinical effect and electrophysiologic study. Five patients were eliminated early from the study for reasons not related to amiodarone therapy. After a mean follow-up of 8.6 months, amiodarone therapy prevented arrhythmia recurrence in 23 of 46 patients (50%), and therapy was judged partially effective in 13 (38%). In this group amiodarone alone failed to prevent spontaneous recurrences in 10 patients, and a type IA agent was added for control. In 3 patients spontaneous ventricular tachycardia did not occur, but a hemodynamically compromising arrhythmia was induced during electrophysiologic study with amiodarone alone. The addition of a type IA agent in these patients slowed the rate of induced arrhythmia, and combined therapy was continued long term. Amiodarone, alone or in combination, was ineffective in 10 of the 46 patients (22%).

In the study by Nadamanee et al.,[176] 22 patients underwent electrophysiologic testing and 24-hour ECG recordings before the initiation of treatment and after stabilization of therapy. Before antiarrhythmic therapy all 22 had inducible ventricular tachycardia and after amiodarone alone, 9 patients remained inducible, although the cycle length of the induced ventricular tachycardia was usually significantly prolonged. The long-term clinical outcome was not different between the inducible and noninducible group. All had excellent arrhythmia control, and there was generally a greater than 90% reduction in PVC frequency on serial Holter recordings.

Other investigators have reported similar findings. Horowitz et al.[177] evaluated 69 patients with programmed electrical stimulation after a standardized amiodarone loading regimen. In 22 patients no arrhythmia could be induced during amiodarone (or combination) therapy, and there were no recurrent episodes of sustained ventricular tachycardia or ventricular fibrillation. In the 47 patients in whom ventricular tachyarrhythmias remained inducible, 15 (32%) had recurrences during a similar follow-up period. In addition, the severity of the recurrent episodes (ventricular tachycardia characteristics and hemodynamic sequelae) were accurately predicted by programmed stimulation.

In many patients follow-up electrophysiologic studies may be a useful prognostic tool and may also aid in selecting additional antiarrhythmic agents, which, when used in combination with amiodarone, can produce an effective clinical response. Although the predictive accuracy of programmed stimulation with amiodarone therapy may be somewhat lower than that with other antiarrhythmic agents, this technique does appear to be of significant value during amiodarone therapy. In conclusion, amiodarone can be highly effective in the treatment of refractory ventricular tachyarrhythmias if the appropriate dosage (intravenous, oral, or both) is employed.

Although there are rare reports[178] of amiodarone administration for PVC suppression in patients without a history of life-threatening ventricular arrhythmias, the relatively frequent occurrence of adverse reactions will most likely restrict its application to those with recurrent ventricular tachycardia or fibrillation.

Adverse Effects

Amiodarone produced few and relatively mild side effects when initially used in a low dose. Since its clinical exposure has broadened, particularly with the use of a larger dosage and with longer follow-up periods, it has become apparent that drug-related toxicity is fairly common and sometimes severe. Most of the observed toxic effects are probably reversible and appear to be related to the dose and duration of treatment. Although it is difficult to correlate serum amiodarone levels with clinical effect, it has been suggested recently that toxic reactions appear more frequently at steady state levels greater than 2.5 mg/L.[166,179]

CARDIAC EFFECTS. Most patients receiving the drug developed a sinus bradycardia; however, less than 5% required a pacemaker for severe sinus slowing or sinus arrest.[165,175,176] Development of high-degree atrioventricular block is also uncommon. The QTc interval lengthens in virtually all patients receiving amiodarone as a manifestation of prolongation of the ventricular muscle action potential duration. Torsades de pointes or a more malignant ventricular tachycardia occurs only rarely.[180] Exacerbation of congestive heart failure is also apparently unusual despite the drug's negative inotropic property. The occurrence of progressive congestive heart failure in patients receiving amiodarone is most likely the result of the drug's negative chronotropic effects and might be resolved by pacemaker placement.

THYROID EFFECTS. The amiodarone molecule is structurally similar to thyroxine. A 200 mg tablet contains approximately 75 mg of organic iodine. It is therefore not surprising that abnormal thyroid function abnormalities have been noted in patients receiving the drug. There are several mechanisms by which amiodarone can affect thyroid function. Clinically manifested thyroid dysfunction occurs infrequently. Thyrotoxicosis resembling Graves' disease can occur in patients without prior evidence of thyroid dysfunction. In patients with nodular goiter the large iodine load associated with amiodarone therapy can induce hyperthyroidism but can also result in hypothyroidism, possibly secondary to inhibition of thyroglobulin proteolysis.[181] It is probably not necessary to alter amiodarone therapy in patients who only have abnormalities in thyroid function tests. In patients who develop clinically overt thyroid dysfunction, the amiodarone dosage should be decreased (in conjunction with the institution of thyroid-specific therapy), but complete discontinuation may not always be necessary.

PULMONARY EFFECTS. Pulmonary toxicity is one of the most severe adverse effects of amiodarone therapy. It was not recognized as a complication until the 1980 report of Rotmensch et al.[182] Since then this complication has been described in most studies evaluating amiodarone for the treatment of ventricular tachyarrhythmias.[183,184] The reported incidence varies from approximately 0.5%–10% of the patients treated. The clinical findings consist of increasing dyspnea, hypoxemia, and hypocapnia; an elevated erythrocyte sedimentation rate; leukocytosis without eosinophilia; and a restrictive pattern on pulmonary function testing.[183] Radiographic findings include diffuse interstitial and patchy alveolar infiltrates predominantly involving the upper lobes. Histologically, there is nonspecific interstitial or alveolar fibrosis with hyperplasia of type II pneumocytes, and foamy macrophages are seen in alveolar spaces.

Clinical symptoms and radiographic changes appear reversible after amiodarone therapy is discontinued, although radiographic resolution often takes longer than 2 months.[183] Corticosteroids have been used for treatment, in addition to discontinuation of amiodarone; however, an immunologic basis for pulmonary toxicity has not been established. It has been suggested that this adverse effect may, in part, be dose related, is cumulative in nature, and only certain patients may be susceptible. Most patients receiving amiodarone for extended periods will have abnormal pulmonary function tests (a decreased total lung capacity and decreased diffusing capacity), but clinically overt pulmonary fibrosis is uncommon.

OPHTHALMOLOGIC EFFECTS. The development of microdeposits in the corneal epithelium was one of the first reported side effects of amiodarone therapy. Amiodarone, like other iodinated compounds, is excreted through the lacrimal gland and deposited directly on the cornea. These deposits can be detected by slit-lamp examination in virtually all patients receiving the drug even for as short a period as a few days.[184] Amiodarone keratopathy is progressive and is believed to be related to the dosage and duration of treatment.[185] Treatment with methylcellulose eyedrops and reduction of the amiodarone dose may limit the extent of opacification. Complete regression probably requires that the drug be discontinued; however, since the majority of patients are asymptomatic or only minimally symptomatic, this is usually not necessary.

DERMATOLOGIC EFFECTS. Cutaneous photosensitivity without hyperpigmentation has been reported in approximately 1%–10% of patients treated with amiodarone. A blue-gray discoloration of sun-exposed areas is a rare adverse effect. It can appear in patients receiving long-term therapy and generally more than 600 mg/day of amiodarone. Biopsy of affected skin reveals that the pigmentation is most likely due to increased lipofusion deposits in dermal cells.[186] This appears to be a more reversible effect with discontinuation of the drug, but regression may be slow, with discoloration persisting for more than 1 year.

Gastrointestinal Effects

Anorexia, nausea, and constipation are frequent adverse effects with amiodarone administration. Constipation is particularly common during the initial loading period of oral therapy. Approximately 15%–20% of patients have asymptomatic and frequently transient elevation of hepatic aminotransferase levels with return to normal during continued treatment. Clinically overt hepatitis associated with amiodarone has been reported,[165] and data obtained from biopsy in both symptomatic and asymptomatic patients are nonspecific.

NEUROLOGIC EFFECTS. Neurotoxicity associated with amiodarone use appears in several forms. A peripheral neuropathy has been reported, but it appears to regress completely with a decrease or withdrawal of amiodarone.

Drug Interactions

A number of investigators[173] have reported an increase in prothrombin time when amiodarone was added to stable warfarin regimens. The mechanism of this apparent interaction (altered protein binding or inhibition of metabolism) is unknown.

Mosey et al.[187] reported on interaction with digoxin resulting in significant increases in plasma digoxin levels 1 week after initiation of amiodarone therapy. The mechanism for this is not apparent. Saal et al.[188] reported clinically relevant increases in serum quinidine and serum procainamide levels when these agents are administered concomitantly with amiodarone.

Summary

Amiodarone is a class III antiarrhythmic agent that appears to be highly effective in the treatment of various supraventricular and ventricular tachyarrhythmias. It has an extremely long elimination half-life, which permits a once daily dosage schedule, thus increasing patient compliance. Its use is associated with relatively frequent and sometimes severe toxic effects that will probably limit its clinical use in patients with refractory life-threatening lethal ventricular arrhythmias.

Sotalol

History

Sotalol (Sotacor) is a beta-adrenergic blocking agent developed in 1960. This agent is unique in that it combines class II (beta-adrenergic blockers) with class III (similar to amiodarone) antiarrhythmic effects. Its chemical name is 4′-[1-hydroxy-2-(isopyropylamino)ethyl]methanesulfonanilide hydrochloride.

Mechanism of Action

Ward, Camm, and Spurrel[189] administered intravenous sotalol (0.4 mg/kg) to 10 patients and studied the acute electrophysiologic effects. The drug produced a significant increase in the basic sinus cycle length, sinus node recovery time, atrial-His conduction interval, and the effective and functional refractory period of the atrioventricular node. These effects were consistent with beta-adrenergic blockade and not class III antiarrhythmic effect. In a study of 24 patients (13 with the Wolff-Parkinson-White syndrome), Nathan et al.[190] found that sotalol prolonged the atrial, ventricular, and atrioventricular nodal effective and functional refractory periods. An increase of the accessory pathway antegrade and retrograde effective refractory periods was noted in the 13 patients with ventricular preexcitation.

Edvardsson et al.[191] reported that the acute administration of intravenous sotalol (40–100 mg) in humans consistently increased the left ventricular repolarization time, confirming the existence of a class III mode of action.

Echt et al.[192] compared the effect of intravenous sotalol (0.3 or 0.6 mg/kg, in 9 patients) and intravenous propranolol (0.15 or 0.2 mg/kg, in 8 patients) in 17 patients in a double-blind, randomized study. Sotalol, but not propranolol, prolonged atrial and ventricular effective refractory periods, lengthened the action potential duration and the QT interval.

Hemodynamics

Dexter et al.[193] reported that intravenous injection of sotalol (0.6 mg/kg) in patients with heart failure produced a reduction in cardiac output proportional to the degree of bradycardia. There was no change in stroke volume, mean arterial blood pressure, or pulmonary vascular pressures. In contrast, in normotensive subjects, an intravenous injection of sotalol (10–40 mg) did not reduce cardiac output, although it blocked the response to isoproterenol.[194]

Lawrie et al.[195] studied the hemodynamic effects of sotalol in two groups of cardiac patients. In the first group, intravenous sotalol (0.2 mg/kg) resulted in a significant reduction in the cardiac output and heart rate and the stroke volume was not changed. In the second group, the effects of intravenous sotalol on cardiac function were measured. The drug did not significantly raise the left ventricular end-diastolic pressure, but it significantly decreased the left ventricular dp/dt. These results indicate that sotalol has both a negative chronotropic and a modest negative inotropic effect.

Pharmacokinetics

It was reported by Schnelle, Klein, and Schinz[196] that after intravenous injection in healthy subjects, sotalol followed a two-compartment distribution pattern, with a first order-process of distribution and elimination. The elimination half-life was 6–8 hours. Sotalol was mainly excreted by the kidney and no metabolites were found. Oral sotalol is rapidly absorbed and produces peak blood levels in 2–3 hours.

Tjandramaga et al.[197] reported that in patients with impaired renal function sotalol could be removed by hemodialysis. Off dialysis the plasma half-life was about 42 hours, and during hemodialysis it was about 7 hours.

Plasma Level and Dosage

Shanks et al.[198] administered oral sotalol to healthy subjects and found that the plasma concentration 2 hours after administration of 400 and 800 mg doses showed a fourfold variation. The peak plasma level occurred 2–3 hours after administration and declined slowly, with a measurable amount present after 24 hours.

Brown et al.[199] reported that the plasma levels of sotalol measured 2 hours after the oral administration of 25–800 mg never showed more than a sixfold variation between different subjects. Peak plasma levels were produced in 2–3 hours. After administration of 100 mg intravenously, sotalol plasma levels ranged from 3.7–4.75 μg/ml (average, 4.2 μg/ml).[200] The usual dose is 160–320 mg, twice daily.

Efficacy

POTENTIALLY LETHAL VENTRICULAR ARRHYTHMIAS. According to Latour et al.,[201] intravenous sotalol (20–60 mg) was effective in 9 out of 11 patients with ventricular arrhythmias, particularly in lidocaine-resistant patients.

Simon and Berman[202] studied 38 patients with atrial and ventricular arrhythmias, 5 of whom had PVCs. Oral sotalol (40–240 mg/day) controlled the ventricular arrhythmias in 4 (80%) of 5 patients; 1 patient did not improve.

Myburgh et al.[203] compared the antiarrhythmic efficacy of sotalol with that of nadolol in 22 patients with stable chronic ventricular arrhythmias after myocardial infarction. The study was a single-blind, crossover format, with placebo periods before active drug administration and during the crossover periods. Both oral sotalol (160 and 320 mg) and oral nadolol (80 and 160 mg) significantly suppressed PVCs ($P < .001$).

LETHAL VENTRICULAR ARRHYTHMIAS. Senges et al.[204] assessed the efficacy of sotalol in 18 patients with sustained ventricular tachycardia who underwent electrophysiologic testing. In each patient, the arrhythmia could be induced by programmed stimulation during control studies. Sotalol prevented induction of sustained ventricular tachycardia in 12 of the 18 patients (67%). Furthermore, 9 patients were given long-term oral therapy with sotalol and 4 patients were given another effective agent. Complete (12 patients) or partial (1 patient) long-term prophylaxis against ventricular tachycardia was demonstrated over a mean follow-up period of 16 months (Range, 8–24). Sotalol therefore can provide effective prophylaxis against sustained ventricular tachycardia.

Adverse Effects

Arnold[205] reported the clinical safety of sotalol (20–160 mg/day) in 49 male subjects in a double-blind study. Generally, sotalol was well tolerated. Gastrointestinal complaints (upset stomach, stomachache, nausea, and diarrhea) were reported by 6 subjects; however, these complaints were not attributed to sotalol therapy. One patient developed peroneal nerve palsy while receiving sotalol. The palsy cleared on withdrawal of the drug. The same investigator conducted a trial to determine the safety of a maximum dosage of 1.28 g/day of sotalol in 12 male "normal" subjects. Throughout the study there were no complaints or physical findings attributable to the administration of sotalol.[205] These two studies indicate that the administration of sotalol was well tolerated.

Neuvonen et al.[206] described the findings in 6 patients admitted to the hospital 0.5–4.5 hours after the ingestion of an overdose of 2.4–8 g of sotalol. All patients developed bradycardia and hypotension. Severe ventricular tachyarrhythmias occurred in 5 of the 6 patients. Polymorphous ventricular tachycardia was observed in 12 of 13 patients who developed syncope and a prolonged Qtc interval while taking therapeutic doses of sotalol. Serum potassium concentrations were reduced in 8 of 12 patients taking a diuretic and sotalol combined.[207] Even in low doses sotalol may be hazardous in the presence of hypokalemia. Isolated cases of torsade de pointes[208] and retroperitoneal fibrosis[209] associated with sotalol therapy have been reported. High doses of sotalol in patients with marked left ventricular dysfunction should be given with caution, with particular attention given to changes in repolarization on the surface ECG (QT interval).

Summary

Sotalol exerts classes II and III antiarrhythmic effects. In contrast to amiodarone, sotalol produces an immediate antiarrhythmic effect. It is characterized by having only a minimum direct myocardial depressant activity. Because it is minimally metabolized and appears to be well tolerated, sotalol may prove to be a unique and effective antiarrhythmic drug for control of ventricular arrhythmias.

REFERENCES

1. Panidis I, Morganroth J: Holter monitoring during cardiac sudden death: Clues to its etiology and prevention. J Am Coll Cardiol 2:798, 1983
2. The Multicenter Post-Infarction Research Group: Risk stratification and survival after myocardial infarction. N Engl J Med 309:331, 1983
3. Morganroth J: Premature ventricular complexes: Diagnosis and indications for therapy. JAMA 252:673, 1984
4. Kostis JB, McCrone K, Moreya AE, et al: Premature ventricular complexes in the absence of identifiable heart disease. Circulation 63:1351, 1981
5. Moore EN, Feldman SH, Horowitz LN, et al: Electrophysiologic properties of a new antiarrhythmic drug tocainide. Am J Cardiol 41:703, 1978
6. Griffin J, Schnittger F, Peters PJ, et al: Effects of tocainide on ventricular fibrillation threshold. Circulation 56:158, 1977
7. Horowitz LN, Josephson ME, Farshidi A: Human electropharmacology of tocainide, a lignocaine congener. Am J Cardiol 42:276, 1978
8. Anderson JL, Mason JW, Winkle RA, et al: Clinical electrophysiologic effects of tocainide. Circulation 57:685, 1978
9. Ryan WF, & Karliner JS: Effects of tocainide on left ventricular performance at rest and during acute alterations in heart rate and systemic arterial pressure. Br Heart J 41:175, 1979
10. Graffner C, Conradson T, Horvendahl S, et al: Tocainide kinetics after intravenous and oral administration in healthy subjects and in patients with acute myocardial infarction. Clin Pharmacol Ther 27:64, 1980
11. Winkle RA, Meffin PJ, Fitzgerald JW, et al: Clinical efficacy and pharmacokinetics of a new orally effective antiarrhythmic, tocainide. Circulation 54:884, 1976
12. Ronfeld PA, Wolshin EM, & Block AJ: Tocainide and metabolites: Human pharmacokinetics and animal pharmacology. Clin Pharmacol Ther 27:282, 1980
13. Woosley RL, McDevitt DG, Nies AS, et al: Suppression of ventricular ectopic depolarizations by tocainide. Circulation 56:980, 1977
14. Maloney JD, Nissen RG, & McColgan JM: Open clinical studies at a

referral centre: Chronic maintenance tocainide therapy in patients with recurrent sustained ventricular tachycardia refractory to conventional antiarrhythmic agents. Am Heart J 100: 1023, 1980
15. LeWinter MM, Engler RL, & Karliner JS: Tocainide therapy for treatment of ventricular arrhythmias: Assessment with ambulatory electrocardiographic monitoring and treadmill exercise. Am J Cardiol 45:1045, 1980
16. Campbell RWF, Bryson LG, Bailey BJ, et al: Oral tocainide in suspected acute myocardial infarction. Circulation 60(suppl 3):70, 1979
17. Roden DM, Reele SB, Hisgens SB, et al: Tocainide therapy for refractory reventricular arrhythmias. Am Heart J 100:15, 1980
18. Winkel RA, Mason JW, & Harrison DC: Tocainide for drug-resistant ventricular arrhythmias: Efficacy, side effects, and lidocaine responsiveness for predicting tocainide success. Am Heart J 100:1031, 1980
19. Morganroth J, Price B, Dreifus LS: Comparative efficacy and tolerance of quinidine vs low dose tocainide. Clin Res 30:207A, 1982
20. Velebit V, Podrid P, Lown B, et al: Agravation and provocation of ventricular arrhythmias by antiarrhythmic drugs. Circulation 65:886, 1982
21. Engler RL, LeWinter M: Tocainide induced ventricular fibrillation. Am Heart J 101:494, 1981
22. Singh BN, Vaughn Williams EM: Electrophysiological and other effects on cardiac function of koll73. Br Heart J 35:558, 1973
23. Roos, JC, Paalman ACA, Dunning AJ: Electrophysiologic effects of mexiletine in man. Br Heart J 38:1262, 1976
24. Saunamaki KI: Hemodynamic effects of a new antiarrhythmic agent, mexiletine (koll73) in ischemic heart disease. Cardiovasc Res 9:788, 1975
25. Campbell NPS, Zaidi SA, Adgey AAJ, et al: Observations on hemodynamic effects of mexiletine. Br Heart J 41:182, 1979
26. Prescott LF, Clements JA, Pottage A: Absorption, distribution and elimination of mexiletine. Postgrad Med J 53(suppl 1):50, 1977
27. Baudinet G, Henrard L, Quinaux N, et al: Pharmacokinetics of mexiletine in renal insufficiency. Acta Cardiol 25(suppl):55, 1980
28. Campbell NPS, Chatarvedi NC, Kelly JG, et al: Mexiletine (koll73) in the management of ventricular dysrhythmias. Lancet 2:404, 1973
29. Middleton D: Baseline pharmacology, electrophysiology and pharmacokinetics of mexiletine. Acta Cardiol 25(supp):45–53, 1980
30. Pottage A: Oral dosage schedules for mexiletine. Postgrad Med J 53(suppl 1):155, 1977
31. Campbell RWF, Talbot RG, Doller MA, et al: Comparison of procainamide and mexiletine in the prevention of arrhythmias after acute myocardial infarction. Lancet 1:1252, 1975
32. Achuff SC, Campbell RWF, Pottage A, et al: Mexiletine in the prevention of ventricular arrhythmias in acute myocardial infarction. Postgrad Med J 53(suppl 1):163, 1977
33. Campbell NPS, Pantridge JR, Adgey AAJ: Long-term oral antiarrhythmic therapy with mexiletine. Br Heart J 40:796, 801, 1978
34. Mehta J, Conti CR: Mexiletine, a new antiarrhythmic agent for treatment of premature ventricular complexes. Am J Cardiol 49:455, 1982
35. Abinader EG, Cooper M: Mexiletine: Used in control of chronic drug-resistant ventricular arrhythmia. JAMA 242:337, 1979
36. Podrid PJ, Lown B: Mexiletine for ventricular arrhythmias. Am J Cardiol 47:895, 1981
37. DiMarco JP, Garon H, Ruskin JN: Mexiletine for refractory ventricular arrhythmias: Results using serial electrophysiologic testing. Am J Cardiol 47:131, 1981

38. Duff HJ, Roden D, Primm RK, et al: Mexiletine in treatment of resistant ventricular arrhythmias: Enhancement of efficacy and reduction of dose-related side effects by combination with quinidine. Circulation 67:1124, 1983
39. Palileo EV, Welch W, Hoff J, et al: Lack of effectiveness of oral mexiletine in patients with drug-refractory paroxysmal sustained ventricular tachycardia. Am J Cardiol 50:1075, 1982
40. Waspe LE, Waxman HL, Buxton AE, et al: Mexiletine for control of drug-resistant ventricular tachycardia: Clinical and electrophysiologic results in 44 patients. Am J Cardiol 51:1175, 1983
41. Talbot RG, Clark RA, Nimmo J, et al: Treatment of ventricular arrhythmias with mexiletine (koll73). Lancet 2:399, 1973
42. Vik-Mo H, Ohm O, Lund-Johansen P: Electrophysiologic effects of flecainide acetate in patients with sinus node dysfunction. Am J Cardiol 50:1090, 1982
43. Hellestrand KJ, Bexton RS, Nathan AW, et al: Acute electrophysiologic effects of flecainide acetate on cardiac conduction and refractoriness in man. Br Heart J 48:140, 1982
44. Legrand V, Vandormael M, Co-Lignon P, et al: Hemodynamic effects of a new antiarrhythmic agent, flecainide (R-818), in coronary heart disease. Am J Cardiol 51:422–26, 1983
45. Conard GJ, Carlson GL, Frost JW, et al: Human palsma pharmacokinetics of flecainide acetate (R-818); A new antiarrhythmic following single oral and intravenous doses (abstract). Clin Pharmacol Ther 25:218, 1979
46. Hodges M, Haughland M, Granrud G, et al: Suppression of ventricular ectopic depolarizations by flecainide acetate, a new antiarrhythmic agent. Circulation 65:879, 1982
47. Anderson JL, Stuart JR, Perry B, et al: Oral flecainide acetate for the elimination of ventricular arrhythmias. N Engl J Med 305:473, 1981
48. Duff HJ, Roden DM, Maffucci RJ, et al: Suppression of resistant ventricular arrhythmias by twice daily dosing with flecainide. Am J Cardiol 48:1133, 1981
49. The Flecainide-Quinidine Research Group: Flecainide versus quinidine for treatment of chronic ventricular arrhythmias: A multicenter clinical trial. Circulation 67:1117, 1983
50. Anderson JL, Lutz JR, Allison SB: Electrophysiologic and antiarrhythmic effects of oral flecainide in patients with inducible ventricular tachycardia. J. Am. Coll. Cardiol 2:105, 1983
51. Morganroth J, Horowitz LN: Flecainide: Its proarrhythmic effect and expected changes on the surface electrocardiogram. Am J Cardiol 53:898, 1984
52. DiBianco R, Fletcher RD, Cohen AI, et al: Treatment of frequent ventricular arrhythmia with encainide: Assessment using serial ambulatory electrocardiograms, intracardiac electrophysiologic studies, treadmill exercise tests, and radionuclide cineangiographic studies. Circulation 65:1134, 1982
53. Sami M, Mason JW, Peters F, et al: Clinical electrophysiologic effects of encainide, a newly developed antiarrhythmic agent. Am J Cardiol 44:526, 1979
54. Jackman WM, Zipes DP, Naccarelli GV, et al: Electrophysiology of oral encainide. Am J Cardiol 49:1270, 1982
55. Prystowsky EN, Klein GJ, Rinkenberger RL, et al: Clinical efficacy and electrophysiologic effects of encainide in patients with Wolff-Parkinson-White syndrome. Circulation 68:385, 1983
56. Roden DM, Duff HJ, Priman RK, et al: Control of ventricular preexcitation and associated arrhythmias by encainide. Am Heart J 102:794, 1981
57. Roden DM, Reele SB, Higgins SB, et

al: Total suppression of ventricular arrhythmias by encainide: Pharmacokinetic and electrocardiographic characteristics. N Engl J Med 302:877, 1980
58. Sami MH, Derbekyan VA, Lisbona R: Hemodynamic effects of encainide patients with ventricular arrhythmia and poor ventricular function. Am J Cardiol 52:507, 1983
59. Winkle RA, Peters F, Kates RE, et al: Clinical pharmacology and antiarrhythmic efficacy of encainide in patients with chronic ventricular arrhythmias. Circulation 64:290, 1981
60. Wang T, Roden DM, Wolfenden HT, et al: Pharmacokinetics of encainide and its metabolites in man (abstract). Clin Pharmacol Ther 31:278, 1982
61. Roden DM, Duff HJ, Altenberg D, et al: Antiarrhythmic activity of the O-demethyl metabolite of encainide. J Pharmacol Exp Ther 221:552, 1982
62. Elharrar V, Zipes DP: Effects of encainide and metabolites (MJ14030) and (MJ9444) on canine cardiac Purkinje and ventricular fibers. J Pharmacol Exp Ther 220:440, 1982
63. Kates RE, Harrison DC, Winkle RA: Metabolite cumulation during long-term oral encainide administration. Clin Pharmacol Ther 31:427, 1982
64. Winkle RA, Peters F, Kates RE, et al: Possible contribution of encainide metabolites to the long-term antiarrhythmic efficacy on encainide. Am J Cardiol 51:1182, 1983
65. Duff HJ, Dawson AK, Roden DM, et al: Electrophysiologic actions of O-demethyl encainide: An active metabolite. Circulation 68(suppl 2): 385, 1983
66. Kate RE, Woosley RL, Harrison DC: Clinical importance of metabolites of antiarrhythmic drugs. Am J Cardiol 53:248, 1984
67. Morganroth J, Hodges M, Ruffy R, et al: The cooperative encainide trial: efficacy, tolerance and dose findings in chronic severe ventricular ectopy (abstract). Am J Cardiol 49:1003, 1982
68. Sami M, Harrison DC, Kruaemer H, et al: Antiarrhythmic efficacy of encainide and quinidine: validation of a model for drug assessment. Am J Cardiol 48:147, 1981
69. Winkle RA, Mason JW, Griffin JC: Malignant ventricular tachyarrhythmias associated with the use of encainide. AM Heart J 102:857, 1981
70. Chesnie B, Podrid P, Lown B, et al: Encainide for refractory ventricular tachyarrhythmia. Am J Cardiol 52:495, 1983
71. Manz M, Steinbeck G, Luderitz B: Electrophysiological effects of lorcainide in sinoatrial disease and in Wolff-Parkinson-White syndrome. Eur Heart J 3:56, 1982
72. Bar FW, Farre J, Ross D, et al: Electrophysiological effects of lorcainide, a new antiarrhythmic drug: Observations in patients with and without pre-excitation. Br Heart J 45:292, 1981
73. Kasper W, Meinertz T, Kersting F, et al: Electrophysiological actions of lorcainide in patients with cardiac disease. J Cardiovasc Pharmacol 1:343, 1979
74. Kasper W, Treese N, Meinertz T, et al: Electrophysiologic effects of lorcainide on the accessory pathway in the Wolff-Parkinson-White syndrome. Am J Cardiol 51:1618, 1983
75. Echt DS, Mitchell LB, Kates RE, et al: Comparison of the electrophysiologic effects of intravenous and oral lorcainide in patients with recurrent ventricular tachycardia. Circulation 68:392, 1983
76. Saksena S, Rothbart ST, Cappello G et al: Clinical and electrophysiologic effects of chronic lorcainide therapy in refractory ventricular tachycardia J Am Coll Cardiol 2:538, 1983
77. Meinertz T, Kasper W, Kersting F et al: Lorcainide II: Plasma concentration-effect relationship. Clin Pharmacol Ther 26:196, 1979
78. Ng CK, Gstottner M, Gneiner R: Intracardiac electrophysiological ef-

fects of lorcainide in man. Eur J Clin Pharmacol 15:241, 1979

79. Myburgh DP, Goldman AP, Schamroth JM: Lorcainide—An antiarrhythmic agent for ventricular arrhythmias. S Afr Med J 57:236, 1980
80. Meinertz T, Kersting F, Kasper W, et al: Haemodynamic effect of a single intravenous dose of lorcainide in patients with heart disease. Eur J Clin Pharmacol 18:461, 1980
81. Shita A, Bernard R, Mostinick R, et al: Haemodynamic reactions after intravenous injection of lorcainide hydrochloride in acute myocardial infarction. Eur J Cardiol 12:237, 1981
82. Jahnchen E, Bechtold H, Kasper W, et al: Lorcainide I: Saturable presystemic elimination. Clin Pharmacol Ther 26:187, 1979
83. Klotz U, Muller-Seydiltz P, Heimburg P: Pharmacokinetics of lorcainide in man: A new antiarrhythmic agent. Clin Pharmacol Ther 3:407, 1978
84. Klotz U, Muller-Seydlitz P, Heimburg P: Lorcainide infusion in the treatment of ventricular premature beats (VBP). Eur J Clin Pharmacol 16:1, 1979
85. Klotz U, Muller-Seydlitz P, Heimburg P: Pharmacokinetics of lorcainide in disease states, in Jahnchen et al (Eds): Prognosis and Pharmacotherapy of Life-Threatening Arrhythmias. Royal Society of Medicine, London, 1981, p 45
86. Somani P: Pharmacokinetics of lorcainide, a new antiarrhythmic drug in patients with cardiac rhythm disorders. Am J Cardiol 48:157, 1981
87. Kates RE, Keefe DL, Winkle RA: Lorcainide disposition kinetics in arrhythmia patients. Clin Pharmacol Ther 33:28, 1983
88. Morganroth J: The efficacy and safety of lorcainide in the treatment of ventricular arrhythmias as assessed by frequent Holter monitoring, in Jahnchen et al (Eds): Prognosis and Pharmacotherapy of Life-Threatening Arrhythmias, Royal Society of Medicine, London, 1981, p 149
89. Meinertz T, Kasper W, Kersting F, et al: Antiarrhythmic effect of lorcainide during chronic treatment. Arzneimittelforsch 30:1593, 1980
90. Kesteloot H, Stroobandt R: Clinical experience with lorcainide (R15889), a new antiarrhythmic drug. Arch Int Pharmacodyn Ther 230:225, 1977
91. Amery WK, Heykants JJP, Xhonneux R, et al: Lorcainide (R15889): a first review. Acta Cardiol 36:207, 1981
92. Sung RJ, Somani P: Discordant antiarrhythmic effects of intravenous lorcainide on ventricular premature beats and ventricular tachycardia. Circulation 64(suppl 4):37, 1981
93. Somberg JC, Willens H, Camilleri W, et al: Effect of lorcainide on suppressing ventricular tachycardia induced by programming stimulation. Circulation 64(suppl 4):37, 1981
94. Lloyd EA, Workman LJ, Commerford PJ, et al: Evaluation of lorcainide, a new antiarrhythmic agent. S Afr Med J 60:929, 1981
95. Chesnie B, Lampert S, Podrid P et al: Lorcainide for refractory ventricular arrhythmia. JACC 1:708, 1983
96. Seipel L, Breithardt G, Both A, et al: Effects of propafenone on the sinus nodes and intracardiac conduction in man (Ger). Drug Dev Eval 1:45, 1977
97. Probst P, Pachinger O: The influence of propafenone on the hemodynamics of the left ventricle and the atrioventricular conduction with special reference to the WPW syndrome (Ger). Z Kardiol 65:212, 1976
98. Bachour G, Hochrein H: Hemodynamic responses to propafenone (Ger). Drug Dev Eval 1:39, 1977
99. Lamounier EN, Martinez Filho EE, Hermann JL, et al: Hemodynamic action of propafenone in patients with atherosclerotic coronary disease (Por). Arq Bras Cardiol 33:73, 1979
100. Baker BJ, DeSoyza N, Boyd CM, et al: Effects of propafenone on left

ventricular function. Circulation 67(suppl 2):267, 1982

101. Connolly SJ, Kates RE, Lebsack CS, et al: Clinical pharmacology of propafenone. Circulation 68:589, 1983
102. Blanke H, Aschbrenner B, Karsch KR, et al: Plasma level, effectiveness and organ distribution of propafenone. Dtsch Med Wochenschr 104:587, 1979
103. Wiebringhaus E, Seipel L, Breithardt G, et al: Long-term results with the new antiarrhythmic drug propafenone with respect to plasma levels (Ger). Z Kardiol 66:625, 1977
104. DeSoyza N, Murphy M, Sakhaii M, et al: The safety and efficacy of propafenone in suppressing ventricular ectopy. Circulation 67(suppl 2):266, 1982
105. Salerno DM, Granrud G, Sharkey P, et al: A controlled trial of propafenone for treatment of frequent and repetitive ventricular premature complexes. Am J Cardiol 53:77, 1984
106. Barros RB, et al: Propafenone: A new chance for the treatment of ventricular arrhythmias. Paper presented at the Third International Congress of Cardiologists, Porto Alegre, Brazil, July 10-16, 1977
107. Naccarella F, Palmieri M, Del Croso G, et al: Comparison of the efficacy of propafenone vs disopyramide for complex premature ventricular contractions. Drug Res 32:547, 1982
108. Podrid PJ, Lown B: Propafenone: A new agent for ventricular arrhythmia. J Am Coll Cardiol 4:117, 1984
109. Shen EN, Sung RJ, Morady F, et al: Electrophysiologic and hemodynamic effects of intravenous propafenone in patients with recurrent ventricular tachycardia. J Am Coll Cardiol 3:1291, 1984
110. Chilson DA, Zipes DP, Heger JJ, et al: Propafenone: Clinical and electrophysiology effects in patients with ventricular tachycardia (abstract). Clin Res 30:706A, 1982
111. Connolly SJ, Kates RE, Lebsack CS, et al: Clinical efficacy and electrophysiology of oral propafenone for ventricular tachycardia. Am J Cardiol 52:1208, 1983
112. Doherty JU, Waxman HL, Kienzle MQ, Cassidydm, Marchlinski FE, Buxton AE, Josephson ME: Limited role of intravenous propafenone hydrochloride in the treatment of sustained ventricular tachycardia: Electrophysiologic effects and results of programmed ventricular stimulation. J Am Coll Cardiol 4:378–381, 1984.
113. Schuff-Werner P, Kaiser D: Cholestatic hepatitis following antiarrhythmic therapy with propafenone (Ger). Dtsch Med Wochenschr 105:137, 1980
114. Fischer G, Seipel L: Clinical experience with oral propafenone (Ger). Drug Dev Eval 1:109, 1977
115. Belz GG, Matthews J, Sci M, et al: Digoxin—antiarrhythmias, pharmacodynamics and pharmacokinetic studies with quinidine, propafenone and verapamil (abstract). Clin Pharmacol Ther 31:202, 1982
116. Korst HA, Brandes JW, Littmann KP: Warning: Propafenone potentiates the effects of oral anticoagulants (Ger). Med Klin 76:349, 1981
117. Morganroth J, Horowitz LN, Mulhern C, et al: Indecainide: A new class IC antiarrhythmic: Pharmacokinetics, efficacy and safety (abstract). Circulation (suppl 68:3):311, 1983
118. Siddoway LA, Bergstrand RH, Primm KR, et al: Antiarrhythmic efficacy, safety and pharmacokinetics of indecainide (abstract). Circulation (suppl 68:3):311, 1983
119. Krejci J, Grandrud G, Salerno D, et al: Indecainide, a dose-ranging efficacy trial for treatment of ventricular ectopic depolarizations (abstract). Circulation (suppl 68:3):311, 1983
120. Horowitz LN, Morganroth J, Webb CR et al: Clinical electrophysiology of indecainide, Circulation 107:II-1769, 1984
121. Miller JS, Vaughan Williams ES: Effects on rabbit nodal atrial, ventricu-

lar, and Purkinje cell potentials of a new antiarrhythmic drug, cibenzoline, which protects against action potential shortening in hypoxia. Br J Pharmacol 75:469, 1982

122. Investigational Drug Brochure: Cibenzoline: Pharmacodynamics. Nutley, NJ, Hoffmann-LaRoche, p 16–21, June, 1982
123. Kushner M, Magiros E, Peters R, et al: The electrophysiologic effects of oral cibenzoline. J Electrocardiol 17:15, 1984
124. Browne KF, Prystowsky EN, Zipes DP, et al: Clinical efficacy and electrophysiologic effects of cibenzoline therapy in patients with ventricular arrhythmias J. Clin Coll Cardiol 3:857–864, 1984
125. Canal M, Flouvat B, Tremelay D, Pharmacokinetics in man of a new antiarrhythmic drug, cibenzoline. Eur J Clin Pharmacol 24:509, 1983
126. Leinweber, FJ, Loh AC, Szuna AJ, et al: Biotransformation of cibenzoline to 2-(2,2-diphenylcycloprophyl)-1H-imidazole. Xenobiotica 13:287, 1983
127. Brazzell RK, Aogaichi K, Heger JJ Jr, et al: Cibenzoline plasma concentration and antiarrhythmic effect. Clin Pharmacol Ther 35:307, 1984
128. Kostis JB, Krieger S, Moreyra A, et al: Cibenzoline for treatment of ventricular arrhythmias: A double-blind placebo-controlled study. J Am Coll Cardiol 4:372, 1984
129. Gritsenko AN, Yermakova ZI, Zhuranlev SV: Synthesis of ethmozine—a new drug having antiarrhythmic action. Chem Pharmacol J 6:17, 1971
130. Arita M, Surawicz B: Electrophysiologic effects of phenothiazines on canine cardiac fibers. J Pharmacol Exp Ther 184:619, 1973
131. Tsuji Y, Nishimura M, Osada M, et al: Membrane action of ethmozine on normoxic and hypoxic canine Purkinje fibers. J Cardiovasc Pharmacol 5:961, 1983
132. Fox S, Hoffman B, Rosen M, et al: Effects of ethmozine and lidocaine on ventricular fibrillation and defibrillation in anesthetized dogs (abstract). Am J Cardiol 45:474, 1980
133. Morganroth J, Michelson EL, Kitchen JG, et al: Ethmozine: Electrophysiologic effects in man (abstract). Circulation 64(suppl 4):263, 1981
134. Mann DE, Luck JC, Pratt CM, et al: Clinical and electrophysiologic effects of ethmozine in man (abstract). Clin Res 29:813A, 1981
135. Podrid PJ, Lown BL: Ethmozine therapy for malignant ventricular arrhythmia (abstract). Am J Cardiol 49:1015, 1982
136. Pratt CM, Yepsen SC, Taylor AA, et al: Ethmozine suppression of single and repetitive ventricular premature depolarizations during therapy: Documentation of efficacy and long-term safety. Am Heart J 106:85, 1983
137. Singh SN, DiBianco R, Gottdiener JS, et al: Effect of moricizine hydrochloride in reducing chronic high frequency ventricular arrhythmia: Results of a prospective controlled trial. Am J Cardiol 53:745, 1984
138. Morganroth J, Pearlman AS, Dunkman WB, et al: Ethmozine: A new antiarrhythmic agent developed in the USSR: Efficacy and tolerance. Am Heart J 98:621, 1979
139. Whitney CC, Weinstein SH, Gaylord JC: High performance liquid chromatographic determination of ethmozine in plasma. J Pharmacol Sci 70:462, 1981
140. Keefe DL, Kates RE, Harrison DC: New antiarrhythmic drugs: Their place in therapy. Drugs 22:363, 1981
141. Pratt CM, Young JB, Francis MJ, et al: Comparative effect of disopyramide and ethmozine in suppressing complex ventricular arrhythmias by use of a double-blind, placebo controlled, longitudinal crossover design. Circulation 69:288, 1984
142. Podrid PJ, Lyakishev A, Lown B, et al: Ethmozine, a new antiarrhythmic drug for suppressing ventricular pre-

mature complexes. Circulation 61:450, 1980

143. Danilo P, Langan WB, Rosen MR, et al: Comparative antiarrhythmic efficacy and tolerance of ethmozine and quinidine (abstract). Circulation 57:103, 1978

144. Singh SN, DiBianco R, Fletcher RD, et al: Ethmozine shown effective in reducing chronic high frequency ventricular arrhythmia: Results of a prospective, controlled trial (abstract). Am J Cardiol 49:1015, 1982

145. Kennedy HL, Pescarmona JE, Jayner, V et al: The efficacy and tolerance of ethmozine for chronic ventricular ectopy. Circulation 57(suppl 2):177, 1978

146. Morganroth J, Orth DW, Michelson EL, et al: Comparative antiarrhythmic efficacy and tolerance of ethmozine and quinidine (abstract). Circulation 57:103, 1978

147. Reder RF, Danilo P, Rosen MR: Effects of pirmenol HC1 on electrophysiologic properties of cardiac Purkinje fibers. Eur J Pharmacol 61:321, 1980

148. Steffe TJ, Mertz TE, Hastings SG, et al: CI-845 (pirmenol hydrochloride): A new orally effective long-acting antiarrhythmic agent. J Pharmacol Exp Ther 214:50, 1980

149. Phillips HR, Stack RS, David DD, et al: Hemodynamic effects of the antiarrhythmic drug, pirmenol. Clin Pharmacol Ther 32:235, 1982

150. Reiter MJ, Hammill SC, Shand DG, et al: Efficacy, safety and pharmacokinetics of a concentration-maintaining regimen of intravenous pirmenol. Am J Cardiol 52:83, 1983

151. Anderson JL, Lutz JR, Nappi JM: A controlled study of multiple dose oral pirmenol for the treatment of ventricular arrhythmias. Circulation 68:273, 1983

152. Hammill SC, Shand DG, Routledge PA, et al: Pirmenol, a new antiarrhythmic agent: Initial study of efficacy, safety and pharmacokinetics. Circulation 65:369, 1982

153. Sanders SW, Nappi JM, Folta RL, et al: Disposition of intravenous pirmenol (abstract). J Clin Pharmacol 23:113, 1983

154. Hammill SC, Shand DG, Harell FE, et al: Pirmenol kinetics and effective oral dose. Clin Pharmacol Ther 32:686, 1982

155. Love J, Haffajee C, Johnson B, et al: Oral pirmenol in effective, acute and chronic therapy for ventricular arrhythmias (abstract). Circulation 68:273, 1983

156. Anderson JL, Lutz JR, Sanders SW, et al: Efficacy of intravenous pirmenol hydrochloride for treatment of ventricular arrhythmias: A controlled comparison with lidocaine (abstract). J Cardiovasc Pharmacol 5:213, 1983

157. Vastesaeger M, Gillot P, Rasson G: Etude clinique d'une nouvelle medication antiangoreuse. Acta Cardiol 22:483, 1967

158. Singh BN, Vaughan Williams EM: The effect of amiodarone, a new antianginal drug on cardiac muscle. Br J Pharmacol 39:657, 1970

159. Graupill N, Lenfant J: The effects of amiodarone on the sinus node of the rabbit heart. Eur J Pharmacol 39:357, 1979

160. Wellens HJJ, Lie KI, Bar FW, et al: Effect of amiodarone in the Wolff-Parkinson-White syndrome. Am J Cardiol 38:189, 1976

161. Nademanee K, Hendrickson J, Kannan R, et al: Antiarrhythmic efficacy and electrophysiologic actions of amiodarone in patients with life-threatening ventricular arrhythmias: Potent suppression of spontaneously occurring tachyarrhythmias vs inconsistent aboliton of induced ventricular tachycardia. Am Heart J 103:950, 1982

162. Finerman WB, Hamer A, Peter T, et al: Electrophysiologic effects of chronic amiodarone therapy in patients with ventricular arrhythmias. Am Heart J 104:987, 1982

163. Charlier R, Deltour G, Baudine A, et al: Pharmacology of amiodarone, an

antianginal drug with a new biological profile. Arzneimittelforsch 18:1408, 1968

164. Horowitz LN, Mattleman SJ, Spielman SR, et al: Intravenous amiodarone loading for ventricular tachycardia. Circulation 66(suppl 2):222, 1982

165. Heger JJ, Prystowsky EN, Jackman WM, et al: Amiodarone—clinical efficacy during long-term therapy for recurrent ventricular tachycardia or ventricular fibrillation. N Engl J Med 305:539, 1981

166. Haffajee CI, Love JC, Canada AT, et al: Clinical pharmacokinetics and efficacy of amiodarone for refractory tachyarrhythmias. Circulation 67:1347, 1983

167. Kannan R, Nadamanee K, Hendrickson J, et al: Amiodarone Kinetics after oral doses. Clin Pharmacol Ther 31:438, 1982

168. Andreasen F, Agerbaek H, Bjerregaard P, et al: Pharmacokinetics of amiodarone after intravenous and oral administration. Eur J Clin Pharmacol 19:923, 1981

169. Canda AT, Lesko LJ, Haffajee CI: Disposition of amiodarone in patients with tachyarrhythmias. Curr Ther Res 30:968, 1981

170. Rosenbaum MB, Chiale PA, Ryba D, et al: Control of tachyarrhythmias associated with Wolff-Parkinson-White syndrome by amiodarone hydrochloride. Am J Cardiol 34:215, 1974

171. Kaski JC, Girotti L, Messuit H, et al: Long-term management of sustained, recurrent, symptomatic ventricular tachycardia with amiodarone. Circulation 64:273, 1981

172. Rosenbaum MB, Chiale PA, Halpern MS, et al: Clinical efficacy of amiodarone as an antiarrhythmic agent. Am J Cardiol 38:934, 1976

173. Podrid PS, Lown B: Amiodarone therapy in symptomatic sustained refractory atrial and ventricular tachyarrhythmias. Am Heart J 101:374, 1981

174. Nadamanee K. Hendrickson J, Cannom DS, et al: Control of refractory life-threatening ventricular tachyarrhythmias by amiodarone. Am Heart J 101:759, 1981

175. Waxman HL, Groh WC, Marchlilnski FE, et al: Amiodarone for control of sustained ventricular tachyarrhythmia: Clinical and electrophysiologic effects in 51 patients. Am J Cardiol 50:1066, 1982

176. Nadamanee K. Singh BN, Hendrickson J, et al: Amiodarone in refractory life-threatening ventricular arrhythmias. Ann Intern Med 98:577, 1983

177. Horowitz LN, Spielman SR, Greenspan AM, et al: Ventricular arrhythmias—Use of electrophysiologic studies. Am Heart J (in press)

178. Toruncha A, Garcia-Baretto D, Gonzalez-Domex A, et al: Oral amiodarone in high risk ventricular arrhythmias. Cor Vasa 24:354, 1982

179. Rotmensch HH, Schoshani S, Spielman S, et al: Relationship between adverse reactions to amiodarone and steady-state serum concentrations. Circulation 68(suppl 3):279, 1983

180. Rinkenberger RL, Prystowsky EN, Jackman WM, et al: Drug conversion of nonsustained ventricular tachycardia to sustained ventricular tachycardia during serial electrophysiologic studies: Identification of drugs that exacerbate tachycardia and potential mechanisms. Am Heart J 103:177, 1982

181. Staubli M, Bischof P, Wimpfheimer C, et al: Amiodarone and the thyroid pathology. Ann Endocrinol 42:446, 1981

182. Rotmensch HH, Liron M, Tupilski M, et al: Possible association of pneumonitis with amiodarone therapy (letter). Am Heart J 100:412, 1980

183. Marchilinski FE, Gansler TS, Waxman HL, et al: Amiodarone pulmonary toxicity. Ann Intern Med 97:839, 1982

184. Sobol SM, Rakita L: Pneumonitis and pulmonary fibrosis associated

with amiodarone treatment: A possible complication of a new antiarrhythmic drug. Circulation 65:819, 1982

185. Kaplan LJ, Cappaert WE: Amiodarone keratopathy: Correlation to dosage and duration. Arch Ophthalmol 100:601, 1982

186. Korting HC, Kolz R, Schmoeckel C, et al: Amiodarone pigmentation: A rare, but typical durg side effect. Hautarzt 32:301, 1981

187. Mosey JO, Jaggarao NS, Grundy EN, et al: Amiodarone increases plasma digoxin concentrations. Br Med J 282:272, 1981

188. Saal AK, Werner JA, Greene HL, et al: Effect of amiodarone on serum quinidine and procainamide levels. Am J Cardiol 53:1264, 1984

189. Ward DE, Camm AJ, Spurrel RAJ: The acute cardiac electrophysiological effects of intravenous sotalol hydrochloride. Clin Cardiol 2:185, 1979

190. Nathan AW, Hellestrand KJ, Bexton RS, et al: Electrophysiologic effects of sotalol—just another beat-blocker? Br Heart J 47:515, 1982

191. Edvardsson N, Hirsch I, Emanuelsson H, et al: Sotalol-induced delayed ventricular repolarization in man. Eur Heart J 1:335, 1980

192. Echt DS, Berte LE, Clusin WT, et al: Prolongation of the human cardiac monophasic action potential by sotalol. Am J Cardiol 50:1082, 1982

193. Dexter L, Brooks H, Banas JS Jr, et al: Effects of sotalol on myocardial function in dogs and in patients with heart failure, in Snart AG (Ed): Advances in Beta-Adrenergic Blocking Therapy—Sotalol, Vol 1. Amsterdam, Excerpta Medica, 1974, p 41

194. Frankl WS, Soloff LA: Sotalol: A new, safe beta-adrenergic receptor blocking agent. AM J Cardiol 22:266, 1968

195. Lawrie TDV, Hutton I, Lorimer AR, et al: Haemodynamic effects of sotalol, in Snart AG (Ed): Advances in Beta-Adrenergic Blocking Therapy—Sotalol, Vol 1. Amsterdam, Excerpta Medica, 1974 p 35

196. Schnelle K, Klein G, Schinz A: Studies on the pharmacokinetics and pharmacodynamics of the beta-blocking adrenergic blocking agent sotalol in normal man. J Clin Pharmacol 19(suppl 2):516, 1979

197. Tjandramaga TB, Verbeeck R, Thomas J, et al: The effect of end-stage renal failure and haemodialysis on the elimination kinetics of sotalol. Fr J Clin Pharmacol 3:259, 1976

198. Shanks RG, Brown HC, Carruthers SG, et al: Clinical pharmacology of sotalol, in Snart AG (Ed): Advances in Beta-Adrenergic Blocking Therapy—Sotalol, Vol 1. Amsterdam, Excerpta Medica, 1974, p 23

199. Brown HC, Carruthers SG, Kelly JG, et al: Observations on the efficacy and pharmacokinetics of sotalol after oral administration. Eur J Clin Pharmacol 9:367, 1976

200. Stroabandt R, Kesteloot H: Efficacy of intravenous sotalol on ventricular arrhythmias occurring during maximal exercise stress testing. Arch Int Pharmacol Ther 264:290, 1983

201. Latour Y, Dumont G, Brosseau A, et al: Effects of sotalol in twenty patients with cardiac arrhythmias. Int J Clin Pharmacol Biopharm 15:275, 1977

202. Simon A, Berman E: Long-term sotalol therapy in patients with arrhythmias. J Clin Pharmacol 19:547, 1979

203. Myburgh DP, Smith R, Diamond TH, et al: A comparison of the efficacy of sotalol and nadolol in the suppression of ventricular ectopic beats. S Afr Med J 63:263, 1983

204. Senges J, Lengfelder W, Jauernig R, et al: Electrophysiologic testing in assessment of therapy with sotalol for sustained ventricular tachycardia. Circulation 69:577, 1984

205. Arnold JD: Sotalol: Clinical safety brochure No. MJ1999, Bristol-Myers Co, Evansville, Indiana March, 1983, p 45

206. Neuvonen PJ, Elonen B, Buorenmaa T, et al: Prolonged QT interval and severe tachyarrhythmias, common

features of sotalol intoxication. Eur J Clin Pharmacol 20:85, 1981

207. McKibbin JK, Pocock WA, Barlow JB, et al: Sotalol, hypokalemia, syncope, and torsades de pointes. Br Heart J 51:157, 1984
208. Kuck KH, Kunze KP, Roewer N, et al: Sotalol-induced torsades de pointes. Am Heart J 10:179, 1984
209. Laakso M, Arvala I, Tervonen S, et al: Retroperitoneal fibrosis associated with sotalol. Br Med J 285:1085, 1982

Peter L. Frommer
Curt Furberg

12

BETA-BLOCKING DRUGS IN THE PREVENTION OF SUDDEN CARDIAC DEATH

The clinical circumstances in which sudden cardiac death sometimes occurs suggest a potential contributory role of the autonomic nervous system. Based on the experience of emergency medical care systems, ventricular fibrillation plays an important role in sudden cardiac death. Experimental studies have shown that interruption of the sympathetic innervation of the heart will substantially decrease the frequency of ventricular arrhythmias and fibrillation in animals.[1-3] In dogs with prior cardiac denervation, experimental myocardial infarction did not result in ventricular fibrillation, although ventricular fibrillation occurred in 60% of the controls that had had the sham operation.[3] These and other findings (Chapter 3) prompted considerable interest in testing the potential effectiveness of beta-adrenergic blocking agents in the prevention of sudden cardiac death in humans.

Blockers of the beta-adrenoreceptors have several features that have been postulated as protective against sudden cardiac death. First, a role for the autonomic nervous system has been thought to exist, and the beta-blockers would interfere with a significant component of the autonomic nervous system's influence on the heart. Second, some beta-blockers have direct intrinsic antiarrhythmic properties through raising the threshold for ventricular fibrillation and suppressing atrial and ventricular premature depolarization. Third, their overall hemodynamic effects result in a decreased workload on the heart and are compatible with a protective effect on the myocardium. More subtle but potentially tangentially relevant effects of beta-blockers include alterations in platelet aggregation, thromboxane formation, myocardial metabolism, and lipolysis.

Some clinical studies to assess the role of beta-blockers in saving lives have focused on patients in the early acute phase of myocardial infarction; others have focused on long-term therapy in survivors of myocardial infarction. The former studies have been directed at immediate in-hospital mortality and minimizing the

SUDDEN CARDIAC DEATH
0-8089-1725-0

amount of ischemic myocardium that is irreversibly damaged, with the potential decrease in long-term mortality from losing less myocardium. This therapy is not directed specifically against sudden cardiac death, but it might be noted that only 2 of the more than 15 clinical trials involving beta-blockers given early during acute myocardial infarction have reported statistically significant beneficial results, and almost half have shown unfavorable trends! One study reported favorable survival results with 10-day follow-up.[4] In the other,[5] therapy was continued for 90 days, so it is a study of both acute intervention and long-term therapy in the early post-acute phase, the period of relatively high mortality for this patient population.

A dozen clinical trials have enrolled patients who have survived the acute phase of myocardial infarction and compared survival in those given long-term beta-blocker therapy with those receiving placebos. Although the underlying hypotheses behind the potential efficacy of beta-blockers in these circumstances tended to rely most heavily on their postulated success in preventing sudden cardiac death, most such trials have focused on all-cause mortality as the primary endpoint. This may be a consequence of the difficulties in defining and establishing sudden cardiac death and the importance of death from any cause.

METHODS

Review Criteria

Included in this review are the findings from randomized controlled clinical trials that report the effect of beta-blocker therapy on all-cause mortality and sudden cardiac death in patients who have recently suffered an acute myocardial infarction.[6-12] Excluded are studies that did not report their sudden death experience,[13,14] studies that enrolled fewer than 100 patients and thus had very low statistical power, and studies that recruited their patients more than 1 month after myocardial infarction.

Study data are presented using the intent-to-treat analysis, that is, all randomized patients are accounted for and in the group to which they had been assigned. Some reports have used other primary analyses, which explains why rates reported here may differ from those published. In the 7 trials meeting the review criteria, intervention was started after the patients became stabilized, usually 1–3 weeks after admission, and was continued for at least 1 year. Selected design features, including the type and dose of beta-blocker tested, time of initiation of treatment, and average length of intervention are given in Table 12-1.

Definition of Sudden Cardiac Death

The primary endpoint in most of the trials was death from any cause. Various definitions of sudden cardiac death were used. In essence, each trial used the onset of premonitory symptoms or new symptoms as the starting point for the measurement of time. Death occurring within 24 hours constituted the definition in three trials.[6,7,9] Deaths occurring within 1 hour and excluding only violent deaths were the time criteria used in a fourth study.[10] A fifth trial reported all

Table 12-1 *Selected Design Features of Long-Term Beta-Blocker Trials*

Trial (Reference No.)	Patients Randomized	Beta-blocker	Daily Dose (mg)	Entry Time* (days)	Mean Follow-up (mos)
Wilhelmsson et al[6]	230	Alprenolol	400	7–21†	24
Ahlmark et al[7]	393	Alprenolol	400	14	24
Multicenter International Study[8]	3053	Practolol	400	13.2	14
Norwegian Multicenter Study[9]	1884	Timolol	20	11.5	17
BHAT[10]	3837	Propranolol	180–240	13.8	25
Hansteen et al[11]	560	Propranolol	160	4–6	12
Julian et al[12]	1456	Sotalol	320	8.3	12

* Entry into study from the time of admission to hospitalization for myocardial infarction.
† From discharge after hospitalization for myocardial infarction.

nonviolent deaths both for the 24-hour and 1-hour definition.[12] Another study divided the cardiac deaths known to have taken place within 24 hours into four time segments: 1 hour or less, 1-2 hours, 2-12 hours, and 12-24 hours.[8] The seventh report applied the following three definitions: witnessed instantaneous death, death witnessed but preceded by chest pain of less than 1 hour duration, and patients found dead but seen alive and free of chest pain less than 12 hours earlier.[11] For three trials[9-11] data on instantaneous death have been reported subsequently.

RESULTS

Antiarrhythmic Effect of Beta-Blockers

Because the overall antiarrhythmic effect of these drugs is reviewed in Chapter 13, the arrhythmia data from the post-myocardial infarction trials are only summarized here. Three of the seven trials obtained 24-hour ambulatory ECG recordings in a subset of participants both on entry into the trial and at a subsequent follow-up visit.[9,10,12] The findings of the three trials are similar. In the subgroup of myocardial infarction survivors who entered the trials with frequent VPBs, fewer patients in the beta-blocker group had this arrhythmia at a follow-up visit than in the placebo group. Some of the patients without frequent VPBs at entry had frequent VPBs at follow-up; this occurred more in patients in the placebo group than in the beta-blocker group. Although few episodes of ventricular tachycardia were recorded at follow-up in all trials, this arrhythmia was less common in patients receiving beta-blockers than placebos.

Effect on All-Cause Mortality and Sudden Cardiac Death

All-cause mortality was lower in the beta-blocker group compared to the control group for all seven long-term trials (Table 12-2). Statistical significance at $P < 0.05$ was reached in three of the trials.[8-10] The relative differences in mortality rates are expressed at risk ratios (intervention group mortality divided by control group mortality), which range from 0.51–0.82.

Study populations, therapy, definitions of sudden death, and periods of follow-up are not identical for the trials. Nevertheless, among the 5728 patients receiving beta-blockers in seven trials, there were 439 deaths, a 7.7% mortality rate; among the 5454 patients receiving placebos, there were 581 deaths, a 10.7% mortality rate. These mortality rates correspond to a risk ratio of 0.72, which indicates an overall reduction in all-cause mortality in these trials of 28% ($P <$ 0.001).

The sudden cardiac death rates were also lower in the beta-blocker group for all seven trials. There is a trend toward a greater overall reduction in sudden cardiac death than in all-cause mortality resulting from beta-blocker treatment (Table 12-2). Among the patients treated with beta-blockers there were 238 sudden cardiac deaths, or a 4.2% rate; among patients receiving a placebo, there were 344 deaths, or a 6.3% rate. These sudden cardiac mortality rates correspond to a risk ratio of 0.67, indicating an overall reduction of 33% in sudden cardiac deaths ($P <$ 0.001). Indeed, if the sudden cardiac deaths are subtracted from all-cause mortality, the remaining death rates—3.5% in the intervention group and 4.4% in the control—represent an intervention/control risk ratio of 0.80 ($P < 0.03$). Thus deaths from all other causes are reduced by 20%, but the sudden cardiac death rate is reduced an average of 33% ($P = 0.1$).

From the data in Table 12-2, it can be calculated that in the five largest trials, the intervention/control risk ratio for nonsudden death ranged from 0.75–1.02. The two smallest trials, which had the most favorable intervention/control risk ratios—0.51 and 0.61 for all-cause mortality and 0.28 and 0.15 for sudden cardiac death—had intervention/control ratios of 1.4 and 2.8 for nonsudden death. It might be argued that this difference is a consequence of the beta-blocker used in those two studies, but more probable explanations include the potential for biased classification of sudden death in an open trial and chance variability associated with small numbers.

Witnessed instantaneous deaths were reported in three trials, at a 2.2% rate (69 deaths) in the 3139 beta-blocker treated patients and at a 4.1% rate (128 deaths) in the 3142 control patients. This represents an intervention/control risk ratio of 0.54 or an average 46% lower rate of instantaneous death in the treated group (P <0.001). For these three trials, the pooled all-cause mortality rates were 8.3% and 12.0%, respectively, corresponding to a relative risk ratio of 0.69 ($P <0.001$). When the instantaneous deaths are removed from the all-cause mortality, the pooled difference in the noninstantaneous deaths becomes 23%, only half of the corresponding difference in instantaneous death ($P <0.05$).

Table 12-2 *Selected Results of Long-Term Beta-Blocker Trials*

Wilhelmsson et al[6]	114	116	6.1	12.1	0.51	≤ 24	2.6	9.5	0.28
Ahlmark et al[7]	69*	93*	7.2	11.8	0.61	≤ 24	1.4	9.7	0.15
Multicentre International Study[8]	1533	1520	6.7	8.4	0.80	≤ 1	2.9‡	4.2‡	0.70
Norwegian Multicenter Study[9]	945	939	10.4	16.2	0.64	≤ 24	7.0	11.7	0.60
BHAT[10]	1916	1921	7.2	9.8	0.74	≤ 1	3.3	4.6	0.72
Hansteen et al[11]	278	282	9.0	13.1	0.69	≤ 1†	4.0	8.2	0.49
Julian et al[12]	873	583	7.3	8.9	0.82	≤ 24	5.5	6.5	0.84
TOTAL	5728	5454	7.7	10.7	0.72		4.2	6.3	0.67

* Incomplete reporting.
† See text for exact definition.
‡ Sudden cardiac death rates underestimated due to missing information.

DISCUSSION

When the data of all randomized clinical trials involving the long-term administration of beta-blockers to survivors of recent myocardial infarction that enrolled over 100 patients and reported sudden cardiac death experience are pooled, a 28% decrease in all-cause mortality is noted in patients treated and followed over an average of 12–25 months when compared to patients receiving a placebo. The varied definitions and the difficulty of ascertaining sudden cardiac death are recognized. When the results of these seven trials involving 11,182 patients are combined, however, and the all-cause mortality is subdivided into sudden cardiac death and all other causes of death, the reductions in mortality become 33% and 20%, respectively. When data from the three trials reporting instantaneous cardiac death are combined, chronic beta-blockade was associated with a 46% lower relative rate of instantaneous death compared to a 23% lower rate of death from all other causes.

From these progressively more favorable effects in going from nonsudden to sudden and then to instantaneous cardiac death rates, it appears that the antiarrhythmic effects of beta-blockers are important in their beneficial effect in this patient population. The reduction in nonsudden deaths, the majority of which were from coronary heart disease, and in the incidence of nonfatal myocardial infarction[15] suggests that other mechanisms play a beneficial role as well.

Efforts will certainly continue to subdivide the population of myocardial infarction survivors into those who have relatively greater or lesser benefits from chronic beta-adrenergic blockade. In the judgment of some, the prognosis of certain patient subgroups may be sufficiently favorable without this prophylactic therapy that the improvement achieved does not outweigh the potential side effects, cost, and inconvenience.[16,17] Others do not share the view that these groups have been adequately separated.[18] There is increasing evidence that those with uncomplicated myocardial infarction and little or no evidence of ventricular irritability have a very favorable prognosis even without beta-blockers. Although beta-blockade seems to reduce risk further even in this patient group, the amount of risk reduction in terms of lives saved for each year of therapy raises questions about the net benefit of treating such patients, even by some of those who had taken a different view earlier.

The length of time after myocardial infarction for which such therapy continues to yield clinical benefit remains undefined. The consensus seems to have been that therapy for at least 2 or 3 years is warranted. For survivors of myocardial infarction, however, the risk of death is greatest in the first few months and decreases substantially after 6 months of survivorship. The benefits of beta-blockade are more prominent in this earlier period. Although some incremental benefit seems to continue, the amount of risk reduction in terms of lives saved for each year of therapy again raises questions about the net benefit of continuing prophylactic beta-blockade routinely beyond 1 year after myocardial infarction, particularly in patients with uncomplicated first infarcts.

A recently reported study with a beta-blocker, oxprenolol, which has both intrinsic sympathomimetic activity and a primary beta-blocking action, failed to show any trend of improved all-cause or cardiac mortality, and recruitment was stopped early.[19] This finding is consistent with the results of a trial of pindolol, which also has mixed beta-blocking and sympathomimetic actions.[20] It would seem plausible that in postinfarction patients, beta-blockers that have mixed actions do not achieve the prophylactic effects of the beta-blockers free of intrinsic sympathomimetic activity. However, practolol, which also has mixed action, reduced all-cause mortality with borderline statistical significance ($p = 0.05$).[8]

Although some details of patient selection and the duration of therapy may undergo refinement, the role of beta-adrenergic blockers in the management of survivors of myocardial infarction is established as a means of decreasing both all-cause and sudden cardiac deaths.

REFERENCES

1. Yodice A: Sympathectomy and experimental occlusion of a coronary artery. Am Heart J 22:545, 1941
2. Harris A, Estandia A, Tillotson R: Ventricular ectopic rhythms and ventricular fibrillation following cardiac sympathectomy and coronary occlusion. Am J Physiol 165:505, 1951
3. Ebert P, Allgood R, Sabiston D: The anti-arrhythmic effects of cardiac denervation. Ann Surg 168:728, 1968
4. Yusuf S, Sleight P, Rossi P, et al: Reduction in infarct size, arrhythmias, and chest pain by early intravenous beta blockade in suspected acute myocardial infarction. Circulation 67 (suppl 1): I-32, 1983
5. Hjalmarson A, Herlitz J, Malek I, et al: Effect on mortality of metoprolol in acute myocardial infarction. Lancet 2:823, 1981
6. Wilhelmsson C, Vedin JA, Wilhelmsen L, et al: Reduction of sudden deaths after myocardial infarction by treatment with alprenolol: Preliminary results. Lancet 2:1157, 1974
7. Ahlmark G, Saetre H: Long-term treatment with beta-blockers after myocardial infarction. Eur J Clin Pharmacol 10:77, 1976
8. Multicentre International Study: Reduction in mortality after myocardial infarction with long-term beta-adrenoreceptor blockade. Supplementary report. Br Med J 2:419, 1977
9. Norwegian Multicenter Study Group: Timolol-induced reduction in mortality and reinfarction in patients surviving acute myocardial infarction. N Engl J Med 304:801, 1981
10. Beta-Blocker Heart Attack Trial Research Group: A randomized trial of propranolol in patients with acute myocardial infarction. I. Mortality results. JAMA 247:1707, 1982
11. Hansteen V, Moinichen E, Lorentsen E, et al: One year's treatment with propranolol after myocardial infarction: Preliminary report of Norwegian multicentre trial. Br Med J 284:155, 1982
12. Julian DG, Prescott RJ, Jackson FS, et al: A controlled trial of sotalol for one year after myocardial infarction. Lancet 1:1142, 1982
13. Baber NS, Wainwright-Evans D, Howitt G, et al: Multicentre postinfarction trial of propranolol in 49 hospitals in the United Kingdom, Italy and Yugoslavia. Br Heart J 44:96, 1980
14. Coronary Prevention Research Group: An early intervention secondary prevention study with oxprenolol following myocardial infarction. Eur Heart J 2:389, 1981
15. Furberg CD, Bell RL: Effect of beta-blocker therapy on recurrent nonfatal myocardial infarction. Circulation 67 (suppl I): I-83, 1983
16. Chamberlain DA: Beta-adrenoceptor antagonists after myocardial infarc-

tion—Where are we now? Br Heart J 49:105, 1983

17. Griggs TR, Wagner GS, Gettes LS: Beta-adrenergic blocking agents after myocardial infarction: An undocumented need in patients at lowest risk. J Am Coll Cardiol 1:1530, 1983
18. Turi ZG, Braunwald E: The use of B-blockers after myocardial infarction. JAMA 249:2512, 1983
19. The European Infarction Study Group: The European Infarction Study: A secondary beta-blocker prevention trial after myocardial infarction. Circulation 68 (suppl III):III-294, 1983
20. Australian and Swedish Pindolol Study Group: The effect of pindolol on the two years' mortality after complicated myocardial infarction. Eur Heart J 4:367, 1983

Lawrence M. Friedman

13

PLATELET-ACTIVE AGENTS IN THE PREVENTION OF SUDDEN CARDIAC DEATH

The evidence concerning the use of platelet-active agents to prevent sudden cardiac death is preliminary and somewhat contradictory. In this chapter, evidence that platelet activity might be associated with sudden death will be briefly presented. In addition, some animal studies that suggest a role for platelet-active agents in preventing sudden death, as well as clinical studies that have employed such drugs will be discussed. Only platelet-active agents, and not the use of anticoagulants, will be addressed.

PATHOPHYSIOLOGIC MECHANISM

Although the common pathway for sudden cardiac death is usually an arrhythmia, a number of factors can predispose to serious arrhythmias.[1] One factor appears to be the acute formation in the coronary circulation of platelet aggregates, which causes myocardial damage.[2] The frequency with which these aggregates occur is not clear, nor is it proven that they lead to sudden death in clinical situations.

Jorgensen et al.[3] infused adenosine diphosphate into coronary arteries of anesthetized pigs. Transitory circulatory collapse was noted, accompanied by ECG ST wave changes indicative of myocardial ischemia. In some cases, ventricular fibrillation and heart block were observed. Platelet counts in the systemic circulation temporarily fell. Tissue studies showed numerous platelet aggregates in the vasculature. These changes were not seen with adenosine monophosphate infusions, nor with adenosine diphosphate infusions in thrombocytopenic pigs.

Haerem[4,5] examined 81 consecutive autopsied patients. Of these, 47 were patients who were classified as having had sudden cardiac death (33 of these were instantaneous deaths), 21 had chronic cardiac disease, but died of other causes, and 13 had no cardiac disease. The presence and magnitude of platelet aggregates were determined in the epicardial arteries. Platelet aggregates were significantly larger and more numerous in sudden death patients than in the 13 patients with no coronary disease. The difference between the sudden death patients and patients with chronic coronary disease was not significant, although a trend was noted. There was no difference between sudden death patients dying instantaneously and those who did not. Similar findings were seen in intramyocardial arteries. Mural platelet microthrombi in the epicardial arteries were also evaluated, and the results, again, were comparable. In some of the sudden death patients, thrombi, emboli, and other major lesions were found in arteries supplying the sinus and atrioventricular nodes. The importance of these lesions is not clear.

The conversion of arachidonic acid to prostaglandin endoperoxides leads to platelet aggregation. Silver et al.[6] found that injections of sodium arachidonate can cause platelet aggregation and death in rabbits within 3 minutes. Platelet thrombi were found in the lung microvasculature. Pretreatment with aspirin, which blocks the conversion of arachidonic acid to the endoperoxides, protected against sudden death.

The endoperoxide-thromboxane A_2 pathway also may be implicated in sudden death.[7] Thromboxane A_2 is both a potent aggregator of platelets and a vasoconstrictor.[6]

Needleman et al.[8] added human platelet-rich plasma plus one of several agonists (thrombin, collagen, or adenosine diphosphate) to rabbit aorta strips. Incubation of the platelets with imidazole, a selective inhibitor of thromboxane synthetase, did not interfere with platelet aggregation, but contraction of the aorta was reduced. There was thus dissociation between the platelet aggregation properties, which may occur in the absence of thromboxane, and the vasoconstrictive property of thromboxane. Imidazole also protects against sudden death in rabbits.[9]

An analog of thromboxane A_2, carbocyclic thromboxane A_2, constricts coronary arteries while inhibiting thromboxane synthesis in platelets.[10] This agent, which does not induce platelet aggregation, causes sudden death in rabbits, presumably as a result of coronary vasospasm.

PREVENTION IN ANIMAL MODELS

Studies employing platelet-active drugs in animals have contributed to our knowledge of platelets and sudden death. Folts, Crowell, and Rowe[11] applied a plastic cylinder to either the circumflex or anterior descending coronary artery in 35 anesthetized dogs. The vessel was narrowed by 60%–80%. In 24 of the dogs, cyclic reductions in blood flow and platelet aggregates were noted. Those dogs receiving aspirin demonstrated a reversal of the blood flow reduction, as opposed to those who did not receive aspirin.

The effect of aspirin on induced coronary occlusions was also studied by Moschos et al.[12] They compared 20 dogs treated with 600 mg of aspirin with 33 untreated dogs. One treated dog died of ventricular fibrillation, as opposed to 13 untreated animals that died, a statistically significant difference. The treated dogs lost less potassium and gained less sodium and water in the myocardium. Plasma-free fatty acid rise was also prevented in the aspirin group. No evidence of microthrombi using microscopic and radioactive labeling techniques was seen in either group of dogs. As noted by the investigators, aspirin thus may have reduced the arrhythmia by its effect on electrolytes, free fatty acids, catecholamines, or through some other mechanism.

Haft et al.[13] infused epinephrine in 30 dogs; 10 were pretreated with aspirin, 10 received dipyridamole, and 10 were not pretreated. The hearts were examined histologically 1 week later. Three dogs in each of the pretreated groups showed evidence of myocardial necrosis, as opposed to all ten of the untreated animals.

Sulfinpyrazone also has been reported to decrease the incidence of ventricular arrhythmias in animals with induced coronary artery occlusions.[14–16] Ectopic beats, ventricular fibrillation, and mortality were all reduced in sulfinpyrazone-treated dogs.[14,15] In cats, sulfinpyrazone pretreatment produced marked decreases in PVBs and episodes of ventricular fibrillation. There was no effect on infarct size.[16] Kelliher et al.[17] found no direct effect of sulfinpyrazone on sympathetic nerve endings in anesthetized cats. They therefore suggested that the drug's ability to reduce arrhythmia and sudden death is probably related to inhibition of prostaglandin synthesis. The effect of sulfinpyrazone on ventricular fibrillation threshold in dogs has also been evaluated.[18] The drug increased the threshold in normal and acutely ischemic hearts and after norepinephrine infusion. The effect was additive to that of practolol and lidocaine.

CLINICAL EXPERIENCE

Aspirin, sulfinpyrazone, and dipyridamole are among the platelet-active agents that have been evaluated in controlled clinical situations. Aspirin has been studied most extensively in patients with myocaridal infarction, and the results are mixed with regard to total mortality.[19,20] Table 13-1 presents results from clinical trials that reported sudden death (defined as cardiac death within 1 hour of the onset of symptoms, although specific criteria differed somewhat). In two of the studies,[21,22] the aspirin-treated groups did better than a placebo control; in two others, the placebo group did better[23,24] (Table 13-1). None of the results are statistically significant. In one of the trials, the Persantine-Aspirin Reinfarction Study,[24] the results were also presented for those patients enrolled less than 6 months from the time of infarction. Despite very favorable trends for total mortality in that subset, sudden death was still more frequent in the aspirin group. A fifth study, which compared aspirin with oral anticoagulants,[25] is also included in Table 13-1. Aspirin was slightly worse than anticoagulant therapy both for total mortality and sudden death, but again, the differences were not significant.

Clinical trials of aspirin in other patient populations have been conducted, including patients with transient cerebral ischemic attacks, shunts for hemodialysis, and prosthetic heart valves. Mortality was generally low in these studies, and sudden death results were unreported. A study of unstable angina patients has shown a 50% reduction in total mortality and nonfatal myocardial infarction due to aspirin, and a 40% reduction in sudden cardiac death.[26] Cairns et al.[27] have confirmed these benefits of aspirin in patients with unstable angina, though they did not report on sudden death. Heikinheimo and Jarvinen[28] studied 430 elderly people. The total mortality was somewhat higher in those patients receiving aspirin (30/209) than in those receiving placebos (22/221), but there was no difference for sudden death (6 versus 7).

Table 13-1 *Clinical Trials of Aspirin in Patients with a Myocardial Infarction*

	Aspirin				Control		
Study (Reference No.)	Daily Dosage (mg)	Number Enrolled	Number of Sudden Deaths	Percentage (%)	Number Enrolled	Number of Sudden Deaths	Percentage (%)
21	972	758	20	2.6	771	25	3.2
22	1500	317	8	2.5	309	12	3.9
23	1000	2267	61	2.7	2257	46	2.0
24	972						
Total		810	45	5.6	406	18	4.4
<6 months		173	10	5.8	95	4	4.2
25*	1500	651	27	4.1	625	23	3.5

* Control was oral anticoagulants

Wilcox et al.[29] randomly allocated 98 patients with acute myocardial infarction to either sulfinpyrazone (200 mg, four times a day) for 10 days or a placebo. Twenty-four hour ambulatory ECGS showed no differences in frequency of ventricular ectopic beats, ventricular tachycardia, or supraventricular arrhythmias. Six patients died during the 10-day treatment period; five received sulfinpyrazone and one received a placebo. In the subsequent 3 weeks, three additional patients who had received sulfinpyrazone died. It is not clear how many of these deaths were considered sudden.

The effect of sulfinpyrazone on mortality also has been evaluated in two large studies of patients recovered from myocardial infarction.[30–32] The Anturane Reinfarction Trial[30,31] enrolled 1629 patients in whom 1 month had elapsed since their infarction. Half were randomized to sulfinpyrazone, 200 mg, four times a day, and half to a placebo. After an average follow-up of 16 months, the sulfinpyrazone group had a statistically nonsignificant difference in total mortality (74 deaths to 89 deaths). Much of this was due to a difference in sudden death (Table 13-2). The difference was even more striking when sudden death within the first 6 months of follow-up are examined. The numbers used in Table 13-2 are from an independent reevaluation of the study data.[31]

The design for the Anturane Reinfarction Italian Study[32] was similar. Sulfinpyrazone (400 mg, twice daily) was administered to 365 patients; 362 patients received a placebo. No difference was noted for either total mortality (29 deaths in the sulfinpyrazone group and 27 in the placebo group) or sudden cardiac death (11 and 9). The reasons for the discrepant results between these two clinical trials are not apparent.

Blakely and Gent[33] compared sulfinpyrazone with a placebo in a geriatric population. The total mortality for all patients was similar in the two groups. Among the patients with atherosclerosis, sulfinpyrazone appeared to reduce the total mortality and death from vascular causes. Sudden death, however, was not reported.

Three major studies of dipyridamole in patients with a myocardial infarction have been conducted. Gent et al.[34] administered 100 mg of dipyridamole four times a day to 51 patients with acute infarctions and placebos to 52 patients. Treatment was continued for 1 month. Of the eight deaths in the dipyridamole group, three were considered to be due to arrhythmias; none of the three placebo group deaths were due to arrhythmias (Table 13-3).

One of the groups in the Persantine-Aspirin Reinfarction Study[25] consisted of patients who received 75 mg of dipyramidamole and 324 mg of aspirin, three times a day. Trends in favor of the combination treatment when compared with placebo were seen for total mortality and sudden death. These trends were more impressive among the patients enrolled within 6 months of their infarction (Table 13-3). A second Persantine–Aspirin Reinfarction Study has recently been completed.[35] There was little difference between dipyridamole plus aspirin and placebo for total mortality, and a nonsignificant trend in favor of treatment for coronary mortality. Sudden cardiac death has not yet been reported.

Dipyridamole has been extensively studied in patients with angina, shunts, and prosthetic valves. Mortality and sudden death, however, have rarely been reported in these trials.

Table 13-2 *Clinical Trials of Sulfinpyrazone in Patients With a Myocardial Infarction*

	Sulfinpyrazone			Control		
Study (Reference No.)	Number Enrolled	Number of Sudden Deaths	Percentage (%)	Number Enrolled	Number of Sudden Deaths	Percentage (%)
30,31	813			816		
TOTAL		29	3.6		39	4.8
<6 months		10	1.2		24	2.9
32	365	11	3.0	362	9	2.5

Table 13-3 *Clinical Trials of Dipyridamole in Patients With a Myocardial Infarction*

	Dipyridamole				Control		
Study (Reference No.)	Daily Dosage (mg)	Number Enrolled	Number of Sudden Deaths	Percentage (%)	Number Enrolled	Number of Sudden Deaths	Percentage (%)
34*	400	51	3	5.9	52	0	0
24	225 (plus aspirin, 972)						
TOTAL		810	30	3.7	406	18	4.4
<6 months		179	5	2.8	95	4	4.2

* Deaths due to ventricular fibrillation and asystole are included as sudden death.

SUMMARY

There is considerable evidence that platelet aggregates or products of the aggregation process are involved in sudden death. This is supported by work in animals and humans. Several platelet-active agents have successfully reduced sudden death in animal models. Unfortunately, clinical trials in humans have not provided a clear picture. Several studies, notably one using sulfinpyrazone[30] in post-MI patients, and two using aspirin in people with unstable angina have been encouraging. Others, however, have yielded disappointing results. Differences in drug selection, drug dosage, and patient population may account for the discrepancies. More work in this field needs to be done before we can say if platelet-active agents have a role in prevention of sudden cardiac death.

REFERENCES

1. Schwartz CJ, Gerrity RG: Anatomical pathology of sudden unexpected cardiac death. Circulation 52(suppl 3):18, 1975
2. Harker LA, Ritchie JL: The role of platelets in acute vascular events. Circulation 62(suppl 5):13, 1980
3. Jorgensen L, Rowsell HC, Hovig T, et al: Adenosine diphosphate-induced platelet aggregation and myocardial infarction in swine. Lab Invest 17:616, 1967
4. Haerem JW: Myocardial lesions in sudden, unexpected coronary death. Am Heart J 90:562, 1975
5. Haerem JW: Sudden, unexpected coronary death: the occurrence of platelet aggregates in the epicardial and myocardial vessels of man. Acta Pathol Microbiol Scand 265(suppl 1):1A, 1978
6. Silver MJ, Hoch W, Kocsis JJ, et al: Arachidonic acid causes sudden death in rabbits. Science 183:1085, 1974
7. Smith JB, Araki H, Lefer AM: Thromboxane A_2, prostacyclin and aspirin: Effects on vascular tone and platelet aggregation. Circulation 62(suppl 5):19, 1980
8. Needleman P, Raz A, Ferrendelli JA, et al: Application of imidazole as a selective inhibitor of thromboxane synthetase in human platelets. Proc Natl Acad Sci USA 74:1716, 1977
9. Puig-Parellada P, Planas JM: Action of selective inhibitor of thromboxane synthetase on experimental thrombosis induced by arachidonic adic in rabbits. (letter) Lancet 2:40, 1977
10. Lefer AM, Smith EF III, Araki H, et al: Dissociation of vasoconstrictor and platelet aggregatory activities of thromboxane by carbocyclic thromboxane A_2, a stable analog of thromboxane A_2. Proc Natl Acad Sci USA 77:1706, 1980
11. Folts JD, Crowell EB Jr, Rowe GG: Platelet aggregation in partially obstructed vessels and its elimination with aspirin. Circulation 54:365, 1976
12. Moschos CB, Haider B, DeLa Cruz C Jr, et al: Antiarrhythmic effects of aspirin during nonthrombotic coronary occlusions. Circulation 57:681, 1978
13. Haft JI, Gershengorn K, Kranz PD, et al: Protection against epinephrine-induced myocardial necrosis by drugs that inhibit platelet aggregation. Am J Cardiol 30:838, 1972
14. Povalski HJ, Olson R, Kopia S, et al: Comparative effects of sulfinpyrazone and aspirin in the coronary occlusion-reperfusion dog model, in McGregor M, Mustard JF, Oliver MF, et al (Eds): Cardiovascular Actions of Sulfinpyrazone: Basic and Clinical Research. Miami, Symposium Specialists, Inc, 1980, p 153

15. Moschos CB, Escobinas AJ, Jorgensen OB, Jr. et al: Effect of sulfinpyrazone on ventricular fibrillation during acute myocardial ischemia. Circulation 64:13, 1981
16. Kelliher GJ, Dix RK, Jurkiewicz N, et al: Effect of sulfinpyrazone on arrhythmia and death following coronary occlusion in cats, in McGregor M, Mustard JF, Oliver MF, et al (Eds): Cardiovascular Actions of Sulfinpyrazone: Basic and Clinical Research. Miami, Symposium Specialists, Inc, 1980, p 193
17. Kelliher GJ, Fasolak W, Jurkiewicz N, et al: The effect of sulfinpyrazone on the response to sympathetic nervous system stimulation. Prostaglandins Leukotrienes Med 8:63, 1982
18. Raeder EA, Verrier RL, Lown B: Effects of sulfinpyrazone on ventricular vulnerability in the normal and the ischemic heart. Am J Cardiol 50:271, 1982
19. May GS, Eberlein KA, Furberg CD, et al: Secondary prevention after myocardial infarction: A review of long-term trials. Prog Cardiovasc Dis 24:331, 1982
20. May GS, Furberg CD, Eberlein KA, et al: Secondary prevention after myocardial infarction: A review of short-term acute phase trials. Prog Cardiovasc Dis 25:335, 1983
21. The Coronary Drug Project Research Group: Aspirin in coronary heart disease. J. Chronic Dis 29:625, 1976
22. Breddin K, Loew, D, Lechner K, et al: Secondary prevention of myocardial infarction: Comparison of acetylsalicyclic acid, phenprocoumon and placebo. A multicenter two-year prospective study. Thromb Haemost 40:225, 1979
23. Aspirin Myocardial Infarction Study Research Group: A randomized, controlled trial of aspirin in persons recovered from myocardial infarction. JAMA 243:661, 1980
24. The Persantine-Aspirin Reinfarction Study Research Group: Persantine and aspirin in coronary heart disease. Circulation 62:449, 1980
25. The EPSIM Research Group: A controlled comparison of aspirin and oral anticoagulants in prevention of death after myocardial infarction. N Engl J Med 307:701, 1982
26. Lewis HD Jr., Davis JW, Archibald DG, et al: Protective effects of aspirin against acute myocardial infarction and death in men with unstable angina: Results of a Veterans Administration cooperative study *N Engl J Med* 309:396, 1983
27. Cairns J, Gent M, Singer J, et al: A study of aspirin (ASA) and/or sulfinpyrazone(s) in unstable angina (UA). *Circulation* 70(Suppl II):II-415, 1984
28. Heikinheimo R, Jarvinen K: Acetylsalicyclic acid and arteriosclerotic-thromboembolic diseases in the aged. J Am Geriatr Soc 19:403, 1971
29. Wilcox RG, Richardson D, Hampton JR, et al: Sulphinpyrazone in acute myocardial infarction: Studies on cardiac rhythm and renal function. Br Med J 281:531, 1980
30. The Anturane Reinfarction Trial Research Group: Sulfinpyrazone in the prevention of sudden death after myocardial infarction. N Engl J Med 302:250, 1980
31. Anturane Reinfarction Trial Policy Committee: The Anturane Reinfarction Trial: Reevaluation of outcome. N Engl J Med 306:1005, 1982
32. Report from the Anturan Reinfarction Italian Study: Sulphinpyrazone in post-myocardial infarction. Lancet 1:237, 1982
33. Blakely JA, Gent M: Platelets, drugs and longevity in a geriatric population, in Hirsh J, Cade JF, Gallus AS, et al (Eds): Platelets, Drugs and Thrombosis. Basel, Switzerland, S Karger, 1975, p 284
34. Gent AE, Brook CGD, Foley TH, et al: Dipyridamole: A controlled trial of its effect in acute myocardial infarction. Br Med J 4:366, 1968
35. Klimt CR, Stamler J, Persantine-Aspirin Reinfarction Study Research Group: Secondary coronary prevention with Persantine and aspirin. *JACC* 5:505, 1985

William B. Kannel
Daniel L. McGee

14

MODIFIABLE RISK FACTORS FOR SUDDEN CORONARY DEATH

Sudden deaths continue to occur with appalling frequency among residents of populations where coronary artery disease is highly prevalent despite a dramatic decline in coronary artery disease mortality over the past decade.[1] More than 500,000 coronary artery disease deaths occur annually and half occur suddenly, in a matter of minutes; consequently, there is great interest in possible modifiable risk factors for sudden death both in the general population and in the high-risk subgroup that already exhibits clinically overt manifestations of coronary artery disease.

Sudden death may be preventable. There is a growing conviction that coronary artery disease results at least in part from a life-style that includes a diet too high in fat, too many cigarettes, too little exercise, and obesity.

THE SUDDEN DEATH ENTITY

Evidence from patients monitored in CCUs and in subjects undergoing ambulatory monitoring indicates that in most sudden deaths the underlying mechanism is ventricular fibrillation and, less commonly, asystole.[2] It is not clear how often this occurs in the course of an evolving myocardial infarction and how often it is a mishap in a reversible ischemic episode. Analysis of data from patients resuscitated from cardiac arrest indicates that less than a third are developing myocardial infarctions.[3] Since this estimate may apply only to those who can be resuscitated, it may be an underestimate. It is also not clear how often the sudden death occurs

Supported in part by Contract Nos. NIH-NO1-HV-92922 and NIH-NO1-HV-52971.

SUDDEN CARDIAC DEATH
0-8089-1725-0

on the basis of an acute occlusive thrombus. Although the data suggest that many are not, fibrinolysis in the agonal state may cause dissolution, again resulting in an underestimate.

The diagnosis of sudden death due to a coronary etiology is generally a process of assuming guilt by association. Few diseases can kill in a matter of minutes, and if dissection of the thoracic aorta, ruptured aorta, and pulmonary embolism are excluded clinically or on postmortem examination, a coronary etiology is assumed.

Death within minutes in persons not presently ill with a potentially lethal illness permits classification as coronary sudden deaths with considerable certainty. The 24-hour definition adopted by the World Health Organization, however, allows many other possible causes (e.g., intracerebral hemorrhage) to be included.

THE FRAMINGHAM STUDY

The present review of the epidemiology of sudden death relies heavily on data from the Framingham Study. This prospective epidemiologic study has amassed more information on sudden death than is available elsewhere. In the course of over 61,000 person-years of medical examinations, comprising 26 years of follow-up, 197 sudden deaths occurred, 147 among men and 50 among women.

Sudden death in the Framingham Study is defined as a death occurring within 1 hour of onset of symptoms. Less rigorous temporal definitions have been adopted, such as those by the World Health Organization, which recommends that deaths occurring within 24 hours of onset of symptoms be classified as sudden deaths. In the Framingham Heart Study, a more rigorous definition was adopted to assure a more homogeneous sudden death entity. Data using this definition provide the basis for this chapter.

The Framingham Heart Study is a long-term prospective study of cardiovascular disease. It began with an initial examination of 5209 men and women during the years 1948 and 1952.[4] The cohort has been reexamined every 2 years since the initial examination. A standard cardiovascular examination was performed at each biennial examination and data on personal and environmental characteristics obtained. Information of cardiovascular endpoints was obtained through the biennial examinations and by daily surveillance of admissions to the only hospital in the town of Framingham, Massachusetts. The present report uses information on characteristics collected at the first 13 biennial examinations and during follow-up for endpoints through 26 years after the initial examination.

In this chapter, data presented use a "person-examination" analysis. Incidence of sudden death is defined as that which occurs 2 years after an examination, with each participant characterized according to status at the examination. Using this analysis a person may be included many times, depending on whether the criteria for being at risk are met at a particular examination. At any examination, roughly 20% of those eligible do not respond. The data for persons not responding are derived by extrapolating earlier data. For example, if a person were known to be at risk at the seventh examination cycle but did not take that examination, then information from the preceding examination for which data were available would be used (usually examination 6).

MULTIVARIATE ANALYSIS

Several methods are available for a multivariate analysis that assesses the joint and net effect of risk factors on the incidence of sudden death. All of the methods assume that the probability of sudden death depends on a set of risk factors. This dependency is expressed as a mathematical relationship.

The simplest mathematical relationship is a linear relationship. Least squares analysis is used to fit the linear model:

$$Y = a + b_1x_1 + \ldots + b_px_p$$

where Y is a dichotomous random variable that is 0 for those individuals who do not die suddenly and is 1 for those who do. This model has been used by some investigators[5] because it is intuitively appealing and is computationally simple. The model has the unappealing feature that the predicted value may take values less than 0 or greater than 1, and assumptions about the joint distribution of the risk factors $x_1, \ldots\ldots, x_p$ must be made in order to draw valid statistical inferences. A model that can be used without the noted distributional assumptions and that never takes values below 0 or above 1 is the logistic function. The logistic model assumes that the risk of disease, given the value of several characteristics say, $X_1, X_2, \ldots\ldots X_p$, is:

$$P = \frac{1}{1 + e - \alpha - \beta_1X_1 - \ldots\ldots - \beta_pX_p}$$

where α and $\beta_1, \beta_2 \ldots \beta_p$ are unknown parameters. Given the value of the characteristics and knowledge as to which individuals subsequently develop disease, estimates of the unknown parameters may be derived. In the present analyses estimates were obtained using an iterative maximum likelihood approach.[6]

To evaluate the ability of the estimated logistic function to discern high-risk individuals, a quantile of risk approach is used. Using the logistic model a risk of sudden death is assigned to each person in the population at risk. The population is then ordered into increasing risk and split into groups of equal size (quantiles). How well the logistic model has functioned is then judged by the comparison of incidence in the different quantiles.

NATURAL HISTORY

Sudden death is a prominent clinical expression of coronary artery disease. One in every five patients with coronary artery disease has sudden death as the first, last, and only clinical manifestation. More than half of all deaths attributed to coronary artery disease are sudden deaths. Among those with prior coronary artery disease, sudden deaths occur at eight to ten times the rate of those of

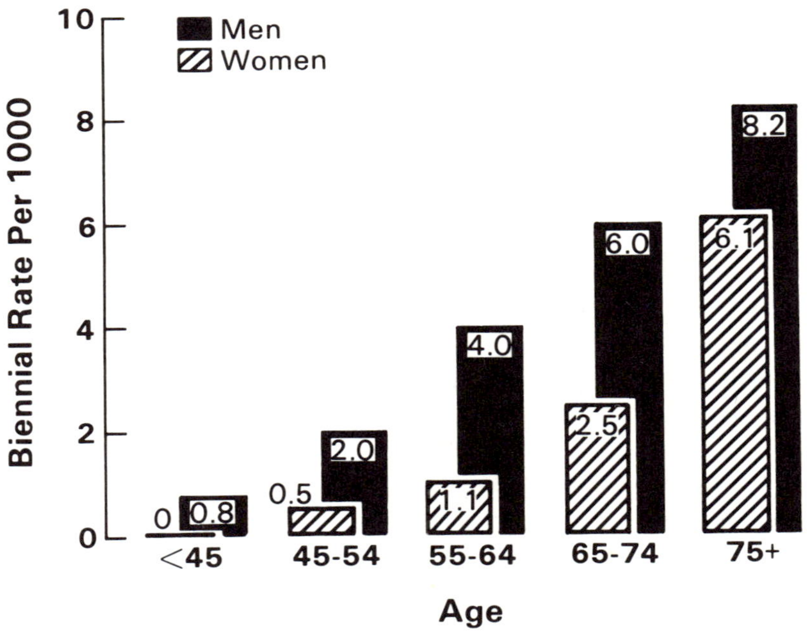

Fig. 14-1. Incidence of sudden death by age and sex in persons free of coronary artery disease.

comparable age and free of coronary artery disease. Nevertheless, 50% of the men who died suddenly had no prior documented coronary artery disease and only 30% of the women who died suddenly had prior evidence of coronary artery disease.

The incidence of sudden death increases with age in both sexes, and women lag behind men by 20 years. The 3:1 male predominance is greater than the 3:2 sex ratio for all clinical manifestations of coronary artery disease combined. With advancing age, the gap in incidence of sudden death between the sexes closes (Figure 14-1).

RISK FACTORS

The risk factors for sudden unexpected death are essentially those related tc development of coronary heart disease in general. None is capable of clearly distinguishing a potential sudden death victim from those subject to coronary heart disease in general.

Hypertension

Elevated blood pressure, whether systolic or diastolic, labile or fixed, at any age, or in either sex, is a powerful contributor to the incidence of coronary hear disease.[7] Either an elevated systolic or diastolic pressure is associated with a

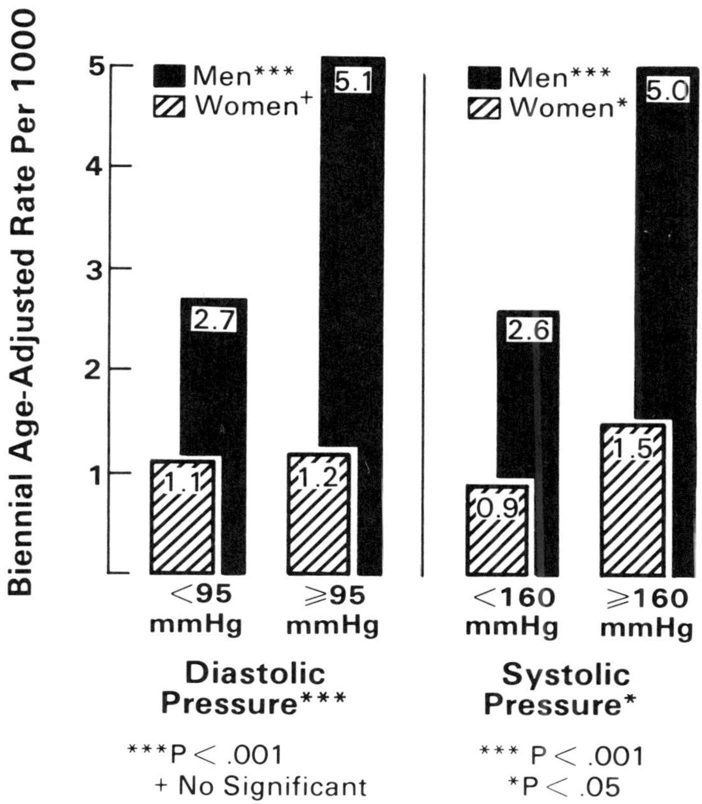

Fig. 14-2. Risk of sudden death by systolic and diastolic pressure.

increased risk of unexpected sudden death (Figure 14-2). This association is more pronounced in men than women. There is no indication of a closer association of sudden death with the diastolic than the systolic pressure.

When the two components of the pressure are combined jointly into the commonly accepted definition of "hypertension" (i.e., > 160/95), a clear trend of increasing sudden death risk by severity of hypertension is demonstrated for men in the Framingham cohort but not for women (Figure 14-3). Even a mild degree of hypertension (140–160/90–94) doubled the risk of a sudden death. Antihypertensive medication is also associated with a significantly increased risk of sudden death in either sex (Figure 14-3). This possibly reflects higher pretreatment blood pressures than a side effect of the medication and may also explain the attenuated association of blood pressure with sudden death incidence in women.

Heart Rate

For reasons that are not clear, the risk of coronary artery disease and mortality increases with the resting heart rate. In the Framingham cohort this is noted for men, but not for women.[8] This could reflect associated blood pressure, since there

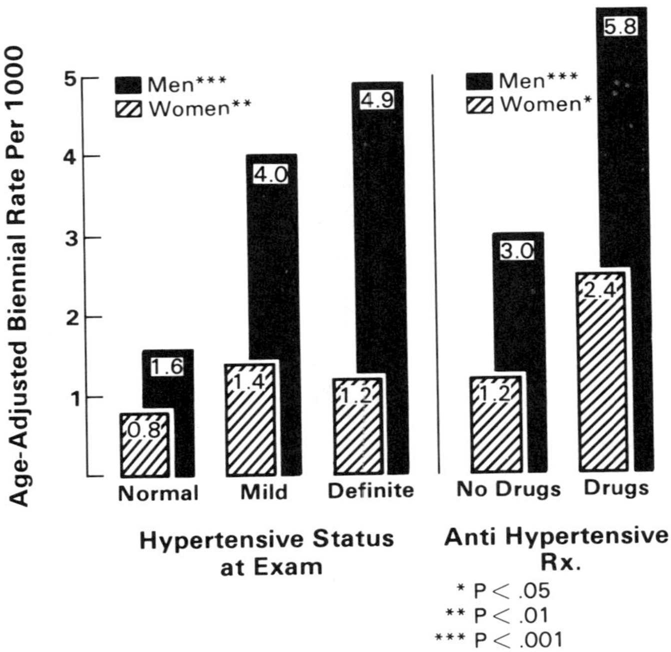

Fig. 14-3. Risk of sudden death by hypertensive status and therapy.

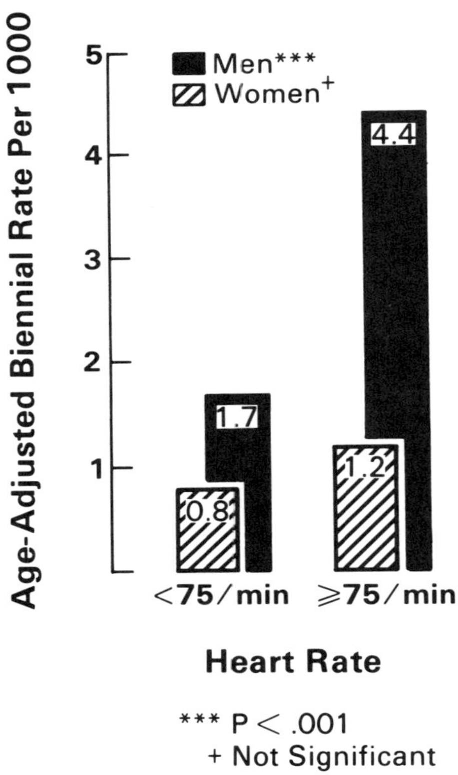

Fig. 14-4. Risk of sudden death by heart rate.

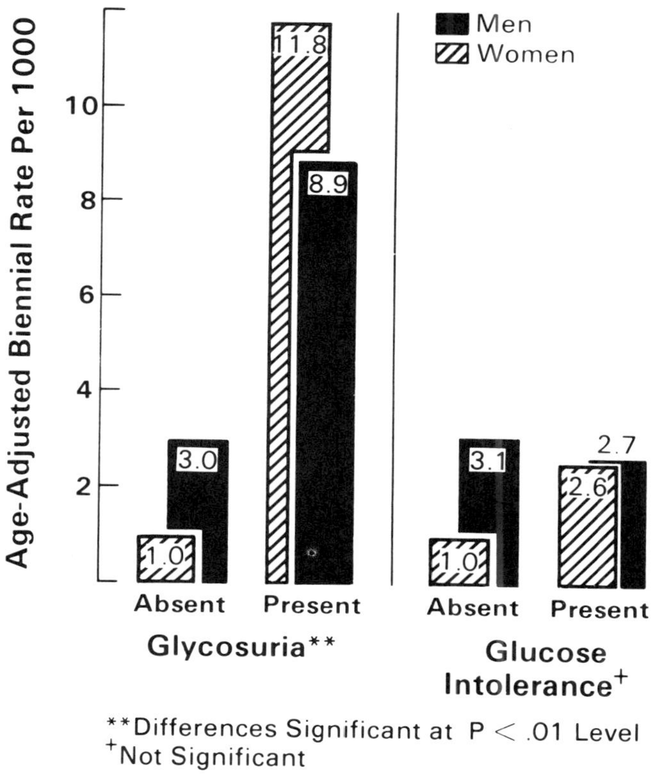

Fig. 14-5. risk of sudden death by evidence of impaired glucose tolerance.

is a significant but modest correlation of heart rate with blood pressure. It could also reflect physical fitness, which is associated both with a lower heart rate and a reduced risk of coronary events. It is of interest that an elevated heart rate is associated with an increased risk of sudden unexpected death in men, but not women (Figure 14-4).

Glucose Intolerance

The clinical observation of an association between diabetes and accelerated atherogenesis and coronary artery disease has been confirmed by prospective epidemiologic data.[9] The impact of diabetes decreases with advancing age in women and is greater in women than men. There is also some unique contribution of diabetes over and above its association with a higher level of other risk factors. This independent effect may be related to blood-clotting aberrations noted in the diabetic, including diminished fibrinolytic activity, increased platelet adhesiveness, and increased fibrinogen, factor VII, or factor VIII.[10,11]

In the Framingham Study glucose intolerance was associated with an increased risk of sudden death (Figure 14-5). This excess was confined to women. Glycosuria was associated with sudden death in both sexes, but again was more pronounced in women.

Obesity

Obesity poses a major metabolic and cardiovascular hazard to health. An excess of cardiovascular morbidity and mortality proportional to the degree of overweight is found in obese persons. Because of its high prevalence, atherogenic metabolic concomitants, and cardiovascular consequences, obesity constitutes a powerful contributor to cardiovascular morbidity and mortality. Despite often expressed uncertainty about the determinants, hazards, pathogenetic mechanism, and efficacy of correcting it, many regard obesity control to be a major hygienic means for controlling cardiovascular risk factors. No other single measure can simultaneously improve such major atherogenic precursors as hypertension, impaired glucose tolerance, low density/high density lipoprotein ratio, and hyperuricemia.

It is noteworthy that obesity is associated with an increased risk of sudden death in both sexes in the Framingham cohort (Figure 14-6). Framingham Study data also suggest that the proportion of coronary artery disease deaths which are sudden also increases with the degree of adiposity, suggesting a more specific relationship to sudden death.[8] Also, taking other major risk factors into account, relative weight makes as strong a contribution to risk of sudden death as to any other clinical manifestation of coronary artery disease (Table 14-1). The mechanism of this possibly unique contribution of obesity to sudden death is obscure.

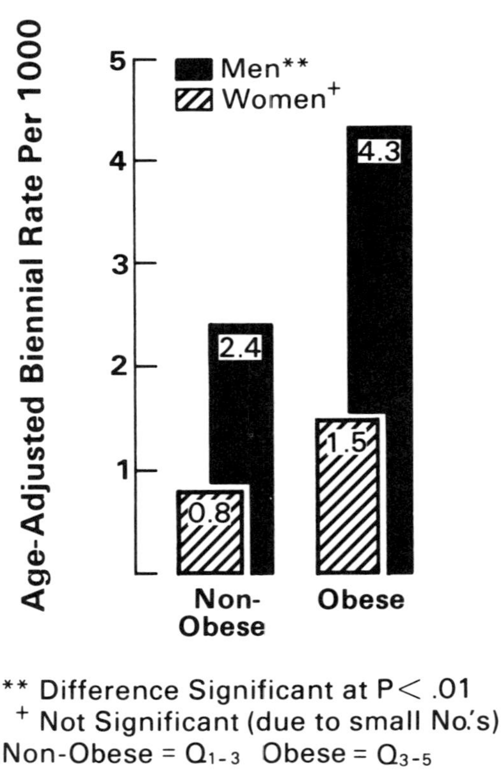

Fig. 14-6. Risk of sudden death by obesity status.

Table 14-1 *The Association between Weight at Entry and Cardiovascular Disease in the Framingham Study*

	Multivariant Logistic Regression Coefficients for Weight*			
Event	Men	Number of events	Women	Number of events
Coronary artery disease	.012†	636	.008‡	437
Angina pectoris	.014†	336	.007§	276
Coronary artery disease other than angina pectoris	.009‡	514	.010†	261
Myocardial infarction	.006	372	.010‡	161
Death from coronary artery disease	.009§	266	.010‡	132
Sudden death from coronary artery disease	.016‡	120	.010	45
TOTAL	2197		2714	

* Regressions include adjustments for age, systolic blood pressure, serum cholesterol level, cigarettes smoked each day, glucose intolerance, and ECG left ventricular hypertrophy in the first examination. Based on data from the Framingham Heart Study.[4]
† $P < .001$.
‡ $P < .01$.
§ $P < .05$.

Cigarette Smoking

Virtually all the major clinical manifestations of atherosclerosis are more common in cigarette smokers. Cigarette smoking is only a modest contributor to atherothrombotic brain infarction, is only one of several equally predisposing factors for coronary artery disease, and is the most important factor for occlusive peripheral arterial disease. The impact of cigarette smoking also varies for specific clinical manifestations of coronary artery disease, exhibiting only a weak relationship to uncomplicated angina compared with the powerful relationship to sudden death and myocardial infarction.[12] In the Framingham cohort cigarette smoking was associated with an increased risk of sudden death among men, but not women (Figure 14-7).

Physical Activity

Transformation of humans from active agrarians to sedentary industrial people may have occurred at the expense of cardiovascular health. Epidemiologic studies have generally indicated a protective effect of physically active occupa-

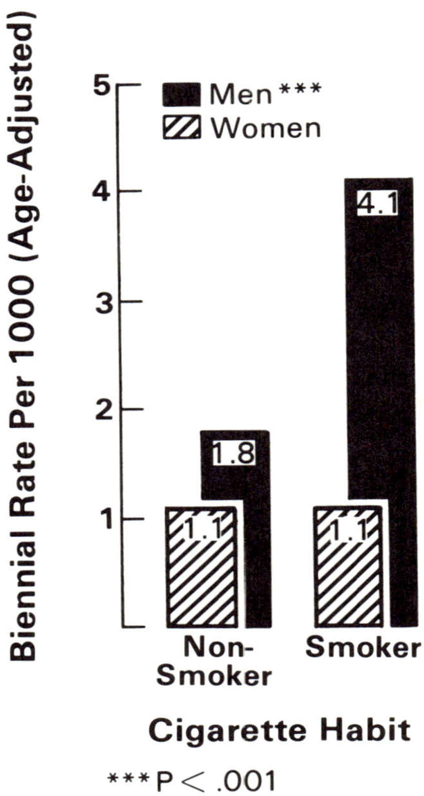

Fig. 14-7. Risk of sudden death by cigarette smoking status.

tions and leisure exercise.[13] Lack of exercise appears to shorten the life span and predisposes individuals to lethal coronary attacks. Inactivity may adversely affect various cardiovascular risk factors or impair the efficiency of operation of the cardiovascular system. Overall mortality, cardiovascular mortality, and coronary artery disease mortality are inversely related to the level of physical activity. Thus far, the evidence of protection conferred by activity seems confined to men.[14] The effect of inactivity is also modest compared to other cardiovascular risk factors, but persists even when these are taken into account. The protection in men can be demonstrated into advanced age.

Although the apparent protection against coronary mortality seems reasonably convincing, the role of physical activity in sudden death is more speculative. The direct relationship of sudden death incidence to heart rate (figure 14-4) may indicate a benefit from physical fitness. The excess risk in the obese may also reflect, in part, poor physical fitness (Figure 14-6).

On the other hand, the fraction of coronary deaths attributed to sudden death appears to *increase* with physical activity.[8,14] It would thus appear that physical activity may protect against coronary attacks and possibly even coronary death, but death, when it comes, may more often be sudden.

Friedman et al.,[2] who found that most sudden victims had a type A personality, also noted that a significant number of the sudden deaths they observed occurred when the patient was engaged in either moderate or strenuous exercise shortly before collapsing. In the Harvard College Alumni Study Paffenbarger, Wing, and Hyde[15] were unable to show any relationship of exercise to the incidence of sudden death. Siskovick et al.[16] concluded that vigorous exercise may be protective against sudden coronary death. These data fall short of either proving or disproving that a high level of physical activity can reduce the risk of sudden death.

Electrocardiogram Precursors

In those persons who have an unfavorable cardiovascular risk profile and who presumably have accelerated atherogenesis, a compromised coronary circulation can often be identified by abnormalities on the resting ECG. Left ventricular hypertrophy, intraventricular conduction disturbances, and even nonspecific repolarization abnormalities (Figure 14-8) are all associated with an increased risk of sudden death. The excess risk associated with left ventricular hypertrophy and intraventricular block is comparable to that for overt coronary heart disease. Unless otherwise explained, persons with such ECG abnormalities deserve the same preventive care and attention as the recovered victim of a myocardial infarction.

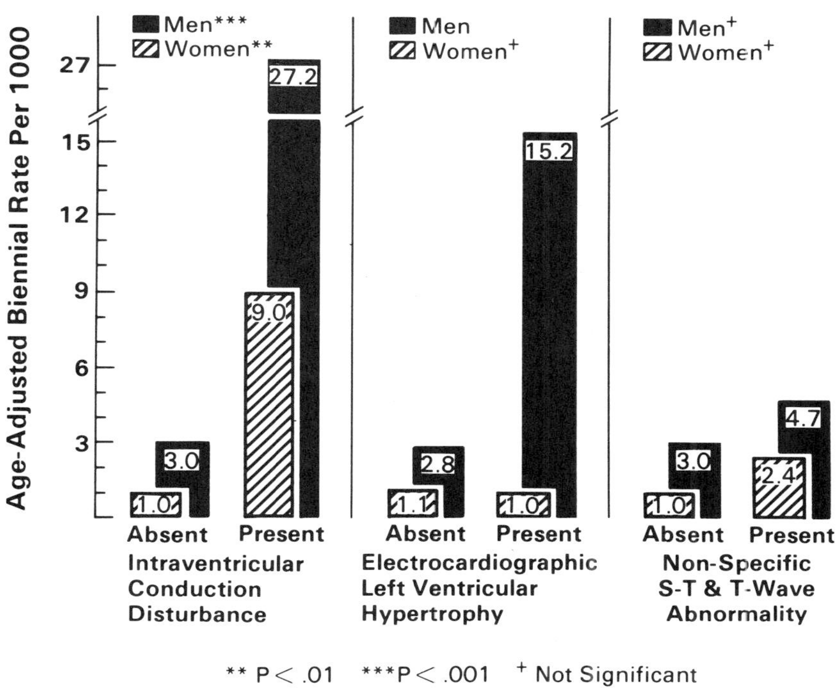

Fig. 14-8. Risk of sudden death by ECG abnormality.

Ventricular Ectopy

Ventricular ectopic activity in the recovered myocardial infarction victim may indicate extensive ventricular dysfunction, particularly if it is frequent. Although its occurrence in normal persons does not indicate an increased risk of sudden death, in the patient with stable coronary artery disease it may signify left ventricular ischemia and an increased risk of death due to pump failure.[8]

In patients with known and documented coronary artery disease, frequent and complex ventricular ectopic activity, whether discovered on routine ECGs, with Holter monitoring, or with exercise testing, indicates significant ventricular dysfunction. Holter monitoring appears to be the most sensitive method for detecting ventricular ectopic activity. There is disagreement about the nature of hazardous ventricular ectopic activity in patients recovered from a myocardial infarction. Critera based on frequency are the most widely endorsed, with less than 10 PVCs/hr considered innocuous and more than 30 PVCs/hr regarded as dangerous. Grading of risk based on multiformity and degree of prematurity is more controversial. Ruberman et al.[17] found that early cycle, runs of PVCs, and multiform bigeminy were associated with a threefold increased risk of sudden coronary death, whereas Moss et al.[18] found only bigeminy and multiformity to be dangerous. Exercise ECGs suggest that multiformity or PVCs at low heart rates may indicate coronary artery disease.[19] The underlying status of the myocardium seems to determine the lethality of PVCs. Their occurrence anywhere in the cardiac cycle may be dangerous in the diseased, irritable myocardium. It is suggested that the Lown grading system for ectopic activity can be improved by giving greater weight to the *frequency* of the multiform, early cycle, and repetitive beats.

Ventricular ectopy demonstrated either on exercise or 1-hour monitoring during convalescence appears to be associated with an increased risk of sudden death. However, 90% of patients with coronary artery disease exhibit ventricular ectopic activity on 24-hour monitoring. Hence, the mere presence of ventricular ectopic activity has little significance. Exercise or monitoring in patients with coronary artery disease are effective ways of demonstrating PVCs and the dangerous, advanced, repetitive forms that may be missed in the resting ECG.[20] These occur not only at peak exercise, but may also emerge during the recovery period. The latter may be especially significant, since experience indicates that ventricular fibrillation is most likely to occur at the termination of exercise. When PVCs are elicited by minimum exertion at low heart rates and are frequent, complex, and persistent, they are likely to be hazardous, particularly when accompanied by associated ST segment changes.

Resting Ventricular Ectopy

Although exercise testing and ambulatory monitoring are more sensitive, the finding of frequent or multifocal PVCs on the resting ECG may be more specific for sudden death risk in the patient with established coronary artery disease. In the Coronary Drug Project[21] twice as many coronary artery disease deaths as expected occurred over 3 years in the placebo group having PVCs in their resting

ECG as in those without them. This excess risk of death, including sudden death, was found to be independent of the level of other risk factors. Since the fraction of coronary artery disease deaths that were sudden was no greater in those with PVCs than in those without PVCs, it seems likely that ventricular ectopic activity may be chiefly a sign of an irritable, damaged myocardium with a lowered fibrillation threshold than a direct inciting cause.

Advanced grades of PVCs are found most frequently in coronary artery disease patients with ejection fractions under 40%, but sudden deaths are less frequent in patients who have had cardiac failure without advanced grades of PVCs.[22] Although extensive coronary artery involvement is usually present in those with ventricular ectopy leading to sudden death, those who are resuscitated sometimes survive for long periods, which suggests such that PVCs are not inevitably a consequence of terminally extensive myocardial damage. However, 30% of patients who experience primary ventricular fibrillation can expect a recurrence within 1 year.[20]

Multivariate Risk

Multivariate logistic analysis, incorporating all the significantly related risk factors for sudden death, indicates that for men, age, systolic pressure, cigarette smoking, and relative weight (Table 14-1) are all independently related to the incidence of sudden unexpected death. For women, in addition to age, serum cholesterol levels and vital capacity are independently related to risk of sudden unexpected death (Table 14-2). Using the indicated set of variables, the risk varies over a wide range (Table 14-3). Some 42% and 53% of the sudden deaths in men and women, respectively, arise from the tenth of the population in the top decile of multivariate risk.

Table 14-2 *Logistic Coefficients for Relating the Risk Characteristics of Sudden Death Among Perons Free of Coronary Artery Disease**

	Males	Females
Age	.0655†	.0713†
Systolic blood pressure	.0151‡	.0011
VC/HT	.1233	−.4954‡
Cigarettes smoked each day	.0129§	−.0161
FRW	.0191§	.0036
α	−15.5270	−11,4763

* Based on data from the Framingham Heart Study.[4]
† $P < .001$.
‡ $P < .01$.
§ $P < .05$.

Table 14-3 *Risk of Sudden Death According to Decile of Multivariate Risk**

Decile of Multivariate Risk†	Probability of Sudden Death per 1000	
	Men	Women
1	.43	.07
2	.75	.14
3	1.04	.21
4	1.35	.30
5	1.70	.42
6	2.14	.59
7	2.71	.83
8	3.57	1.21
9	5.24	1.94
10	13.01	5.34
Percentage of cases in top decile	42%	53%

* Based on data from the Framingham Heart Study.[4]

† Risk variables include age, ECG abnormalities, systolic blood pressure, serum cholesterol level, vital capacity, cigarette smoking, weight, and heart rate.

Risk Factors for Sudden Death in Subjects with Established Coronary Artery Disease

Among men and women with established coronary heart disease, sudden deaths were eight to ten times more frequent than among persons of the same age who do not have overt coronary heart disease in the Framingham Study. Those with established coronary heart disease have been found on angiographic study to have advanced two- and three-vessel occlusive coronary artery disease. With disease this advanced, the standard risk factors no longer appear to have much predictive value for sudden death. An examination of the mean level of risk factors shows few significant differences between those who subsequently experienced sudden death and those who did not (Table 14-4). Only two variables appear to identify potential sudden deaths: LVH and antihypertensive medication. It is likely that these variables, which also emerge from a multivariate analysis, reflect the severity of the underlying disease.

It is possible that risk factor levels before the appearance of coronary heart disease may be more predictive of sudden death than those measured after the coronary heart disease becomes clinically manifest. With an interim infarction, the blood pressure often falls, and those who exhibit a reduction in pressure have an increased cardiovascular mortality.[23] Preliminary data suggest that the same is true for serum cholesterol level and weight. Reductions in all of these parameters and myocardial infarction interim may be associated with excessive mortality.

Preventive Implications

Prospective and retrospective studies indicate that sudden death victims share most of the major risk factors for coronary artery disease, but none of these factors thus far identified can be used to distinguish sudden death victims from those whose deaths are less precipitous. Since the same factors that predispose to sudden death also occur with coronary artery disease, the key to prevention

Table 14-4 *Mean Level of Specified Characteristics According to Coronary Artery Disease Status at Examination and Sudden Death Status in the 2 Years after the Examination**

	Sudden deaths			
	Free of Coronary artery diseases Population at Risk		Prevalent Coronary artery disease Population at Risk	
	(*N* = 23847)‡	(*N* = 73)	(*N* = 2487)	(*N* = 74)
Age	53.5	60.3	62.1	62.6
Systolic blood pressure	135.7	148.6	142.4	144.6
Diastolic blood pressure	83.6	88.2	83.7	84.3
Serum cholesterol level	229.6	239.2	236.1	234.9
Cigarettes smoked each day	14.3	17.9	15.0	16.6
Vital capacity	343.1	311.0	292.3	290.3
Hematocrit value	46.9	47.6	46.8	46.4
Left ventricular hypertrophy†	1.7	12.3	7.3	27.4
Pulse rate	75.1	81.9	76.0	78.1
Hypotensive medication†	8.4	20.0	18.3	33.9
FRW	102.7	106.7	103.3	100.0

* Based on data from the Framingham Heart Study[4]; the statistics are for men only.
† Percentage prevalence.
‡ *N* varies because some characteristics were not measured at particular examinations.

appears to be the reduction of risk of coronary attacks, all of which are potentially lethal. After all, the first prolonged attack of ischemic chest pain carries a 33% case fatality rate!

Evidence that many risk factors for coronary artery disease are correctable is accumulating. It is possible to quit cigarette smoking, reduce obesity, lower cholesterol levels through diet, lower elevated blood pressure with drugs or hygienic measures, and exercise more. Evidence that these same measures will reduce the incidence of sudden death is meager. Those who quit smoking, however, have been shown to have only half the coronary mortality of those who continue to smoke. Use of beta-blockers seems to reduce sudden death rates.[24,25] Reduction of overweight has been shown to improve all elements of the cardiovascular risk profile, including blood pressure, LDL/HDL cholesterol ratio, glucose tolerance, and uric acid values.[26-28] No evidence exists to show a reduced sudden death incidence, and an improvement in coronary attack rates is unproven.

Control of complex and frequent PVCs by drugs has been disappointing. The association of PVCs with sudden death seems to apply mainly in persons with an ischemic, irritable myocardium. It may well be this underlying disease that must be addressed rather than the PVCs.

Most proponents of physical exercise for the prevention of coronary artery disease advocate vigorous, endurance exercise, sufficient to produce a training effect on the cardiovascular system. No data are available yet that prospectively test the relationship of physical fitness to subsequent coronary artery disease in general or to sudden death in particular. Thus far only physical exercise has been examined. Although moderate noncompetitive exercise appears to be safe, sudden deaths have been reported in persons engaged in jogging, marathons, and other vigorous exercise events.[2,12-14] Uncertainty prevails concerning the amount of exercise needed to achieve the cardiovascular benefits of exercise. Some investigations show a substantial amount of protection at less than high-intensity leisure-time activity.[12,13]

Subgroups of convalescent myocardial infarction patients who have a risk of death as high as 50% within the first year can be identified. Low-risk patients are usually asymptomatic, have had a benign acute course, normal creatinine level, normal postmyocardial infarction ECG, no tachycardia, a normal exercise ECG before discharge, and few PVCs on ambulatory monitoring. They are normotensive without a fall in blood pressure from premorbid values and show no evidence of cardiac failure. For those at high risk of sudden death and reinfarction based on the foregoing profile, measures such as anticoagulants, platelet inhibitors, and antiarrhythmic agents, particularly beta-blockers, have been advocated.

Attention to the standard coronary artery disease risk factors assumes greater importance for the recovered myocardial infarction patient once the early high mortality period has passed. At this point, consideration should be given to long-term preventive management designed to retard further progression of the underlying disease.

The key to prevention of sudden death appears to be prevention of either the initial or recurrent coronary attacks. This requires comprehensive multifactorial risk-factor intervention. No single measure can be relied on to prevent either coronary attacks or resultant sudden deaths.

REFERENCES

1. Kannel WB, Thom TJ: Implications of the recent decline in cardiovascular mortality. Cardiovasc Med 4:983, 1979
2. Friedman M, Manwaring JH, Rosenman RH, et al: Instantaneous and sudden deaths: Clinical and pathological differentiation in coronary artery disease. JAMA 225:1319, 1973
3. Baum RS, Alvarez H, Cobb LA: Survival after resuscitation from out-of-hospital ventricular fibrillation. Circulation 50:1231, 1974
4. Dawber TR, Meadors GF, Moore FE: Epidemiologic approaches to heart disease: The Framingham Study. Am J Public Health 41:279, 1951
5. Feldstein M: A binary variable multiple regression method of analyzing factors affecting perinatal mortality and other outcomes of pregnancy. J R Statist Soc A:61, 1966
6. Walker SH, Duncan DB: Estimation of the probability of an event as a function of several independent variables. Biometrika 54:167, 1967
7. Kannel WB, Dawber TR, McGee DL: Perspectives on systolic hypertension: The Framingham Study. Circulation 61:1179, 1980
8. Kannel EB, Thomas HE Jr: Sudden coronary death: The Framingham Study. Ann NY Acad Sci 382:3, 1982
9. Kannel WB, McGee DL: Diabetes and glucose tolerance as risk factors for cardiovascular disease: The Framingham Study. Diabetes Care 2:120, 1979
10. Chakabarti R, Meade TW: Clotting factors, platelet function and fibrinolytic activity in diabetics and in a comparison group. Diabetologia 12:383, 1976
11. Wayne EC, Bridges JM, Weaver JA: Platelet adhesiveness, plasma fibrinogen and factor levels in diabetes mellitus. Diabetologia 6:436, 1970
12. Kannel WB: Update on the role of cigarette smoking in coronary heart disease. Am Heart J 101:319, 1981
13. Froelicher VF, Brown P: Exercise and coronary heart disease. J Cardiac Rehab 1:277, 1981
14. Kannel WB, Sorlie PD: Some health benefits of physical activity: The Framingham Study. Arch Intern Med 139:857, 1979
15. Paffenbarger RS, Wing AL, Hyde RT: Physical activity as an index of heart attack risk in college alumni. Am J Epidemiol 108:161, 1978
16. Siscovick DS, Weiss NS, Hallstrom AP, et al: Physical activity and primary cardiac arrest. N Engl J Med 248:3113, 1982
17. Ruberman W, Weinblatt E, Goldberg JD, et al: Ventricular premature beats and mortality after myocardial infarction. N Engl J Med 279:750, 1977
18. Moss AJ, Henry DT, DeCamilla J, et al: Ventricular ectopic beats and their relation to sudden and non-sudden cardiac death after myocardial infarction. Circulation 60:998, 1979
19. McHenry PL, Morris SN, Kavalier M, et al: Comparative study of exercise-induced ventricular arrhythmias in normal subjects and patients with documented coronary artery disease. Am J Cardiol 37:609, 1976
20. Markiewicz W, Houston N, DeBusk RF: Exercise testing soon after myocardial infarction. Circulation 56:26, 1978
21. Coronary Drug Project Research Group: Factors influencing long-term prognosis after recovery from myocardial infarction—3-year findings of the CDP. J Chronic Dis 27:267, 1974
22. Calvert A, Lown B, Gorlin R: Ventricular premature beats and anatomically defined coronary disease. Am J Cardiol 39:627, 1977
23. Kannel WB, Sorlie PD, Castelli WP, et al: Blood pressure and survival after myocardial infarction: The Framingham Study. Am J Cardiol 45:326, 1980
24. Multicenter International Study: Reduction in mortality after myocardial infarction with long-term β-adrenergic blockade. Br Med J 2:419, 1977

25. The Norwegian Multicenter Study Group: Timolol reduction in mortality and reinfarction in patients surviving acute myocardial infarction. N Engl J Med 304:801, 1981
26. Kannel WB, Gordon T, Castelli WP: Obesity, lipids and glucose intolerance: The Framingham Study. Am J Clin Nutr 32:1238, 1979
27. Garrison RJ, Wilson PW, Castelli WP, et al: Obesity and lipoprotein cholesterol in the Framingham Offspring Study. Metabolism 29:1053, 1980
28. Kannel WB, Gordon T: Physiological and medical concomitants of obesity: The Framingham Study, in Bray GA (Ed): Department of Health, Education, and Welfare, Obesity in America. NIH Publication No. 79-359, 1979, p 125

Douglas P. Zipes
James J. Heger
Eric N. Prystowsky

15

SYNCHRONIZED LOW-ENERGY TRANSVENOUS CARDIOVERSION

For many years electrical transthoracic cardioversion and defibrillation have been used successfully and safely to terminate most tachyarrhythmias. Recently, Mirowski et al.[1,2] after more than decade of research and development, perfected an implantable defibrillator that delivers 25–30 joules to terminate ventricular fibrillation. Based on these concepts, we reasoned that the principles of transthoracic cardioversion could be adapted for use with an intracardiac device that could deliver synchronized cardioversion shocks of low energies via a catheter electrode to successfully and safely terminate sustained ventricular tachyarrhythmias.[3-6] This system might also terminate supraventricular tachyarrhythmias. In the subsequent discussion we present our developmental animal studies and initial clinical experience with this concept.

ANIMAL STUDIES

Mongrel dogs underwent a 2-hour occlusion of the left anterior descending coronary artery proximal to the main diagonal branches supplying the apical region using a Harris two-stage procedure.[3,7] Arterial flow was reestablished 2 hours after complete occlusion. Three to eight days after myocardial infarction, the dogs were anesthetized and a median sternotomy was performed. A No. 10

Supported in part by the Herman C. Krannert Fund; by Grants HL-06308, HL-07182 from the National Heart, Lung, and Blood Institute of the National Institutes of Health, Bethesda, Md.; and by the American Heart Association, Indiana Affiliate, Inc.

SUDDEN CARDIAC DEATH
0-8089-1725-0

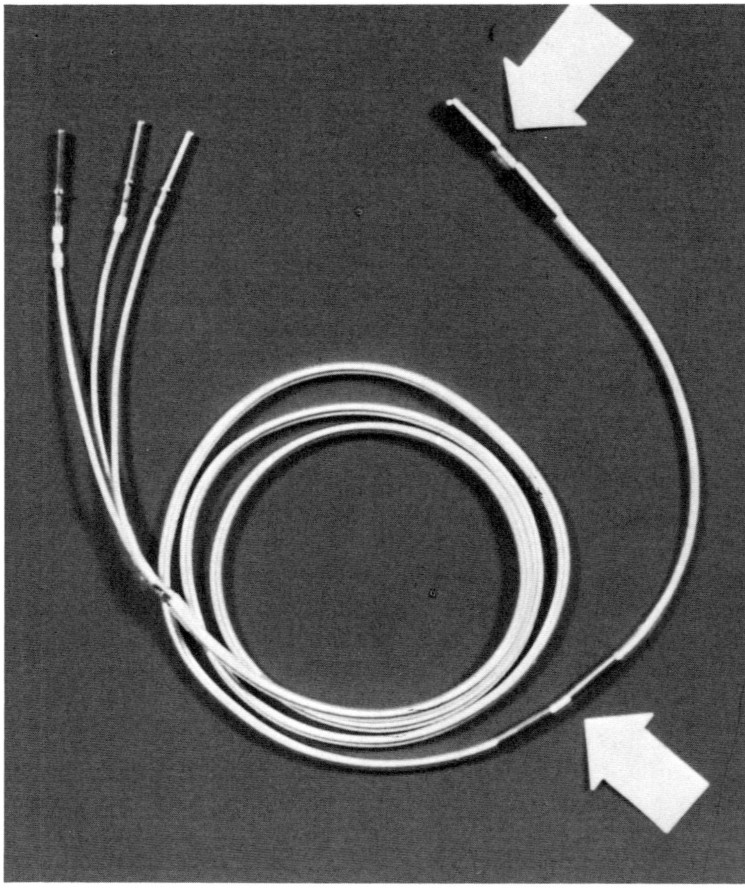

Fig. 15-1. Electrode catheter. Arrows point to pairs of electrodes. From Zipes DP, Jackman WM, Heger JJ, et al: Clinical transvenous cardioversion of recurrent life-threatening ventricular tachyarrhythmias: Low-energy synchronized cardioversion of ventricular tachycardia and termination of ventricular fibrillation in patients using a catheter electrode. Am Heart J 103:789, 1982. With permission.

French electrode catheter, specially designed for cardioversion (Medtronic model 6880), was inserted through the right external jugular vein and advanced to the right ventricular apex (Figure 15-1). The catheter consisted of four stainless steel electrodes: two electrodes at the tip separated by 5 mm and two similarly spaced electrodes 13 cm from the tip. Each electrode had a surface area of 1.25 cm^2. The distal bipolar pair of electrodes located in the right ventricular apex monitored R waves to time cardioversion shocks. On delivery of a shock, the distal pair of electrodes was coupled together to form the cathode and the proximal pair of electrodes (located in the superior vena cava) was coupled together for the anode. In five dogs, a second 6880 electrode catheter was inserted into the left external jugular vein and advanced into the distal coronary sinus. The distal pair of electrodes on this catheter was used as the anode, with the cathode being the two electrodes of the first catheter located in the right ventricular apex. Finally, in three dogs, a 5 cm diameter cone electrode,[8] composed of two stainless steel wire mesh sheets separated by a 5 mm Silastic band, was sutured onto the apex of the heart. The apex cone electrode was the cathode and the superior vena cava electrode formed the anode. Shocks were timed from the bipolar R wave recorded between the two wire mesh sheets. The cardioverter (Medtronic model 2316) delivered a truncated exponential waveform,[9] 6 msec in duration, at nine energy levels of: 0.0005, 0.001, 0.008, 0.025, 0.09, 0.5, 1.0, 2.0, and 2.5 joules. A programmable stimulator (Medtronic model 5325) was interfaced with the pulse generator to provide the sensing function and timing for the cardioversion shocks.

Programmed electrical stimulation (1.8 msec rectangular stimuli at twice the late diastolic current threshold) of the epicardial sites near the infarction border zone was used to induce sustained ventricular tachycardia.[10-12] After induction of sustained ventricular tachycardia, shocks between the right ventricular apex and superior vena cava were introduced at a fixed time within the QRS complex. Beginning with 0.0005 joule, shocks of progressively increasing energy were delivered until ventricular tachycardia was terminated. Ventricular tachycardia was reinitiated, and the same sequence repeated two to five times to determine the minimum energy required to reproducibly terminate the tachycardia at that time in the cycle. Shocks of greater energy (up to 2.5 joules) were applied to determine the safety of higher energy pulses.

Similar testing was done at 5–20 msec intervals throughout the tachycardia cycle. This protocol was repeated with shocks delivered between the right ventricular apex and coronary sinus in five dogs and between the epicardial apex cone electrode and superior vena cava electrodes in three.

All dogs had sinus rhythm at the onset of the study. Programmed electrical stimulation induced sustained ventricular tachycardia with constant cycle length, ventricular activation sequence, and QRS morphology in 14 dogs. Two or more morphologically different forms of sustained ventricular tachycardia, each with a distinct cycle length and ventricular activation sequence, were induced in 12 of the 14 dogs, for a total of 35 different ventricular tachycardias. A mean of 17.9 ± 29.7 (± SD) episodes of each tachycardia was induced, for a total of 627 episodes of sustained ventricular tachycardia tested by intracardiac direct current shock. The mean ventricular tachycardia cycle length was 257 ± 63 msec.

Figure 15-2 shows the analog record of a successful termination of ventricular tachycardia by a shock delivered between the right ventricular apex and superior vena cava. Between 20 and 40 msec from the onset of ventricular activation, shocks of 0.09 joule reproducibly terminated the ventricular tachycardia.

The maximum required termination energy (shocks between the right ventricular apex and superior vena cava) for each of the 35 ventricular tachycardias is plotted as a function of tachycardia cycle length in Figure 15-3. Of the 30 sustained ventricular tachycardias with a cycle length greater than or equal to 200 msec (mean, 275 ± 46 msec), 25 (83%) were reproducibly terminated by shocks of less than or equal to 1 joule and 20 (67%) by shocks of less than or equal to 0.5 joule. Only one of the five tachycardias with a cycle length less than 200 msec (mean, 145 ± 25 msec) was terminated reproducibly by shocks of less than or equal to 1 joule. There was no significant linear or log-linear relationship between the maximum required termination energy and the tachycardia cycle length.

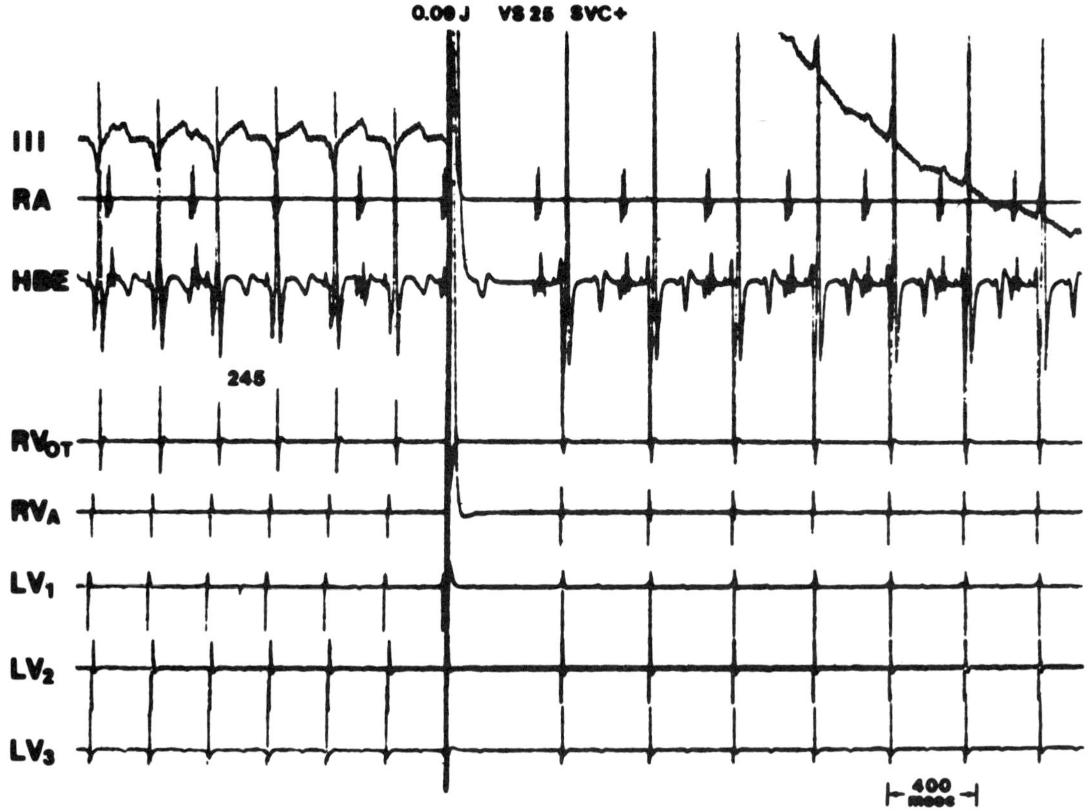

Fig. 15-2. Termination of sustained ventricular tachycardia (cycle length, 245 msec) by a shock of 0.09 joule delivered between the right ventricular apex and superior vena cava. ECG lead III, right atria (*RA*), bundle of His (*HBE*), and epicardial electrograms were recorded from the right ventricular outflow track (RV_{OT}), right ventricular apex (RV_A), and left ventricle (*LV*) around the border of the anteroapical infarction. The shock was introduced 25 msec after the onset of ventricular activation (*VS 25*), which is recorded earliest in lead III. The shock restored sinus rhythm, evidenced by the narrow QRS complexes preceding His bundle potentials at a normal HV interval and fixed association with atrial depolarization. From Jackman WM, Zipes DP: Low-energy synchronous cardioversion of ventricular tachycardia using a

The maximum required termination energy for shocks delivered between the right ventricular apex (cathode) and coronary sinus (anode) was not significantly different from that of shocks between the right ventricular apex (cathode) and superior vena cava (anode) for the seven tachycardias in the five dogs tested. For shocks delivered between the epicardial apex cone electrode (cathode) and the superior vena cava electrodes (anode), the maximum required termination energy was decreased by a factor of 20–250 for all six tachycardias in the three dogs tested (Figure 15-3). Shocks of 0.008 joule terminated five of six ventricular tachycardias using this electrode arrangement.

Of the 748 shocks of 0.008–1 joule introduced within the first 80% of the QRS interval, only 12 (1.6%) produced repetitive ventricular responses and none accelerated the ventricular tachycardia or precipitated ventricular fibrillation (Figure 15-4). For shocks of 2 and 2.5 joules, there was an 11% incidence of RVRs of four or more complexes. However these RVRs began more than 400 msec after the shock, had a cycle length longer than that of the original tachycardia, slowed progressively, and terminated spontaneously.

Shocks introduced during the last 20% of the QRS interval and within the ST-T interval resulted in RVRs. As the energy was increased progressively, multiple-beat repetitive ventricular responses or ventricular fibrillation occurred.

In the ventricular tachycardias with cycle lengths less than 200 msec, the safety of shocks introduced during the QRS interval was inconsistent. Two of seventeen shocks greater than or equal to 0.5 joule, placed within the first 80% of the QRS interval resulted in ventricular fibrillation.

Atrioventricular dissociation occurred frequently during ventricular tachycardia. Therefore, shocks synchronized to the QRS interval fell randomly in the atrial cycle. Shocks introduced during the second quarter of the atrial cycle occasionally resulted in repetitive atrial responses, including atrial flutter or fibrillation. When induced, atrial flutter or fibrillation usually terminated spontaneously within 2–3 seconds after onset.

This study demonstrated that shocks of 1 joule or less, delivered through transvenous intracardiac catheter electrodes and synchronized to the QRS complex, reproducibly terminated 83% of the sustained ventricular tachycardias with cycle lengths greater than or equal to 200 msec that were induced in dogs 3–8 days after myocardial infarction. For shocks introduced within the first 80% of the QRS interval, RVRs were rare and acceleration of the ventricular tachycardia or degeneration to ventricular fibrillation never occurred. For shocks introduced during the ST-T interval, corresponding to the vulnerable period of the ventricular cycle,[13] energies as low as 0.008 joule accelerated the ventricular tachycardia or produced ventricular fibrillation. Since shocks were not synchronized to the atrial cycle due to the presence of atrioventricular dissociation, atrial flutter or fibrillation was precipitated in 9% of shocks greater than or equal to 0.5 joule, but usually terminated spontaneously within 3 seconds.

Only one of five ventricular tachycardias with a cycle length less than 200 msec (greater than 300 beats/min) was terminated by shocks less than or equal to 2.5 joules. Also, in these more rapid tachycardias, shocks greater than or equal to 0.5 joule introduced within the QRS interval occasionally produced ventricular fibrillation. Since ventricular activation extended through most of the cycle length in these tachycardias, repolarization of some part of the ventricular myocardium

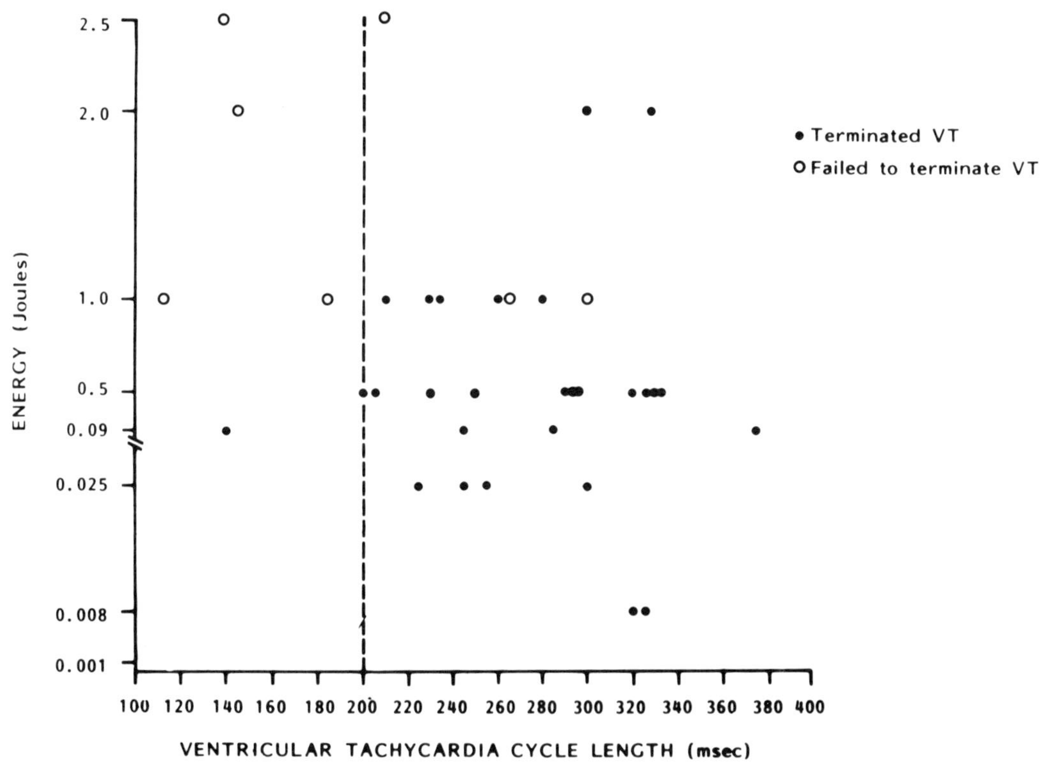

Fig. 15-3. Maximum required termination energy for shocks delivered between the right ventricular apex and superior vena cava for each of the 35 ventricular tachycardias (*VT*), plotted as a function of tachycardia cycle length. Open circles indicate ventricular tachycardias that were not reproducibly terminated by shocks applied within the QRS interval, plotted at the highest energy level at which shocks failed to terminate ventricular tachycardia. From Jackman WM, Zipes DP: Low-energy synchronous cardioversion of ventricular tachycardia using a catheter electrode in a canine model of subacute myocardial infarction. Circulation 66:187, 1982. With permission.

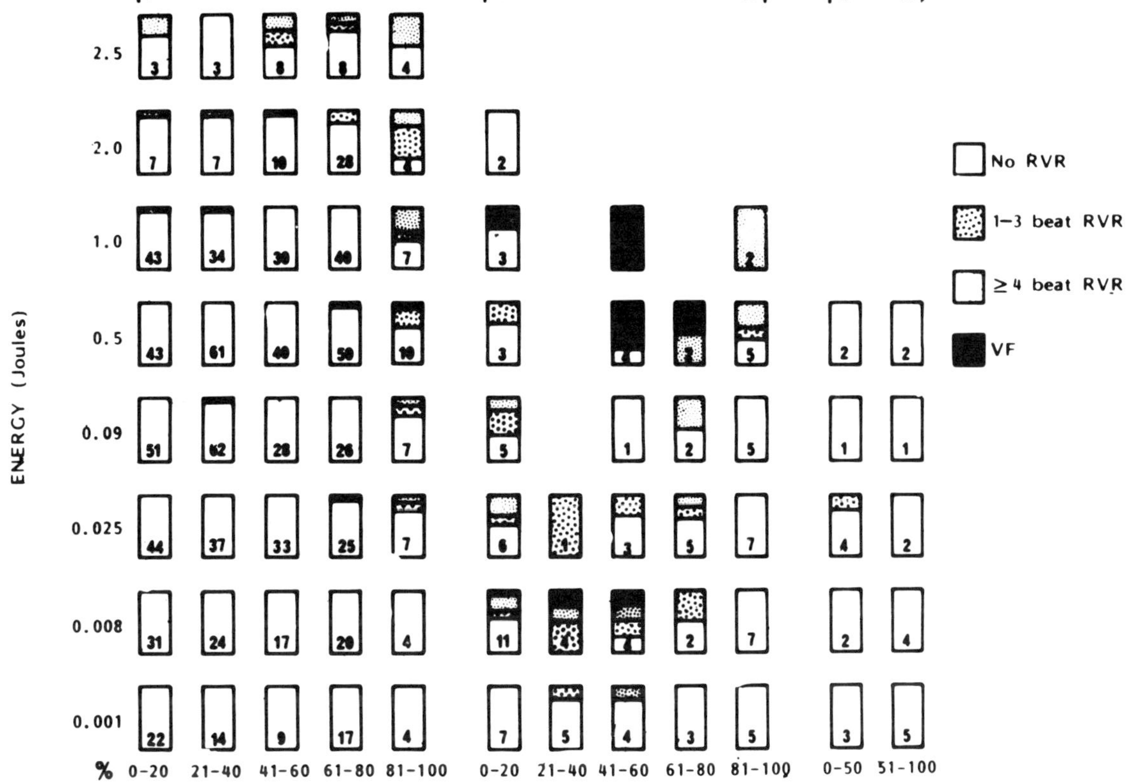

Fig. 15-4. Incidence of RVRs produced by shocks delivered between the right ventricular apex and superior vena cava, plotted as a function of energy level and timed within the tachycardia cycle at which shocks were applied. Data are cumulative for all tachycardias with cycle lengths exceeding 200 msec. Time is normalized to percentage of the QRS, ST-T, and TQ intervals. Numbers inside boxes indicate the number of shocks tested. The percentage of each box that is unfilled represents the percentage of shocks that produced no RVR. The percentage of each box that is coarsely stippled, finely stippled, or solid black represents the percentage of shocks that produced RVRs of one to three complexes, four or more complexes (including acceleration of ventricular tachycardia and ventricular flutter) or ventricular fibrillation (VF), respectively. From Jackman WM, Zipes DP: Low-energy synchronous cardioversion of ventricular tachycardia using a catheter electrode in a canine model of subacute myocardial infarction. Circulation 66:187, 1982. With permission.

(and therefore the vulnerable period) probably extended into the next QRS interval. There may exist no discrete period in the QRS interval during which a low-energy shock can safely terminate these rapid tachycardias.

Placing the anode in the coronary sinus did not significantly decrease the energy requirement to terminate ventricular tachycardia or decrease the incidence of atrial fibrillation, and therefore appeared to offer no advantage over the single catheter electrode configuration. This result may be explained by a ''short-circuiting'' effect of the blood pool. Since the resistivity of blood is approximately one third that of the total biologic media (blood, interstitial fluid, and muscle),[14] much of the current was probably lost to the blood pool between the right ventricular apex and coronary sinus. In contrast, the large epicardial apex cone electrode reduced dramatically (20 to 250 times) the maximum required termination energy. The decrease in energy requirement may relate in part to the pathway traveled by the current, so that shocks of less energy depolarized a region critical to the maintenance of tachycardia. More likely, the large surface area of the cone electrode reduced electrical resistance and the epicardial location minimized loss of current to the blood pool.

HUMAN STUDIES

After written informed consent was obtained, the catheter was inserted in 13 patients percutaneously through an antecubital jugular or subclavian vein, and its tip was positioned using fluoroscopic guidance at the right ventricular apex.[5,6] The patients were men, 55–72 years old (mean, 61 years), who had a history of a remote myocardial infarction. All patients were referred for evaluation and therapy of recurrent sustained ventricular tachycardia. Twelve patients were awake and nonsedated during all cardioversion attempts of ventricular tachycardia. One patient requested an anesthetic when the energy of the shocks exceeded 0.5 joule during the first two cardioversion procedures. For the third cardioversion procedure, the patient remained awake and unsedated. All patients received cardioactive drugs.

Transvenous cardioversion terminated ventricular tachycardia in 11 of 13 patients on one or more occasions with energies of 0.025–2 joules using a truncated exponential waveform (Figure 15-5) and 4–20 joules using a damped sine wave (Table 15-1). In two patients ventricular tachycardia was not terminated by shocks of up to 0.75 and 2 joules, respectively. Ventricular tachycardia resulted in profound hypotension, with loss of consciousness in these two patients, and testing was therefore discontinued. The tachycardia was terminated by transthoracic cardioversion (320 joules) in one patient and in the other, burst right ventricular pacing (six stimuli, cycle length, 260 msec) produced a chaotic ventricular tachycardia (cycle length, 280 msec) that spontaneously terminated after five complexes. Shocks of 25 joules terminated three episodes of ventricular fibrillation in one patient (Figure 15-6).

Including subthreshold attempts, a total of 196 shocks ranging from 0.0075–2 joules was delivered. On several occasions, repetitive ventricular activity occurred. One patient who had undergone 18 consecutive successful transvenous

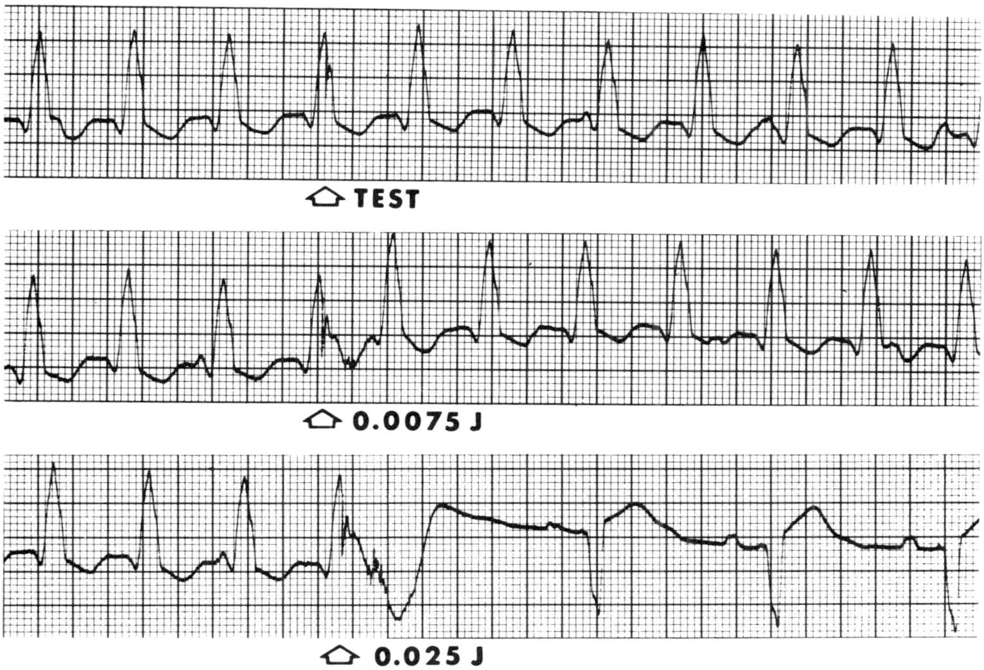

Fig. 15-5. Transvenous cardioversion in lead II. *Top panel,* Test stimulus delivered into QRS complex; *middle panel,* subthreshold shock shortened RR interval of ventricular tachycardia but did not terminate tachycardia; *bottom panel,* threshold shock terminated ventricular tachycardia. From Zipes DP, Jackman WM, Heger JJ, et al: Clinical transvenous cardioversion of recurrent life-threatening ventricular tachyarrhythmias: Low-energy synchronized cardioversion of ventricular tachycardia and termination of ventricular fibrillation in patients using a catheter electrode. Am Heart J 103:426, 1982. With permission.

cardioversions without incident deteriorated clinically. Rapid ventricular tachycardia (200 beats/min) with hypotension was present almost continuously for 72 hours. During that time he received intravenous or oral bretylium, amiodarone, lidocaine, and digoxin. Balloon counterpulsation was begun to provide hemodynamic support. Synchronized transvenous cardioversion (0.075 joule) in this setting transformed the ventricular tachycardia (cycle length, 315 msec) to ventricular flutter (cycle length, 190 msec) that was terminated by a transthoracic shock of 320 joules. Shortly thereafter, a conventional synchronized transthoracic shock of 50 joules precipitated ventricular fibrillation that was then defibrillated with a 320-joule transthoracic shock. Because the cardioverter has a maximum output of 3 joules, termination of ventricular flutter or ventricular fibrillation was not attempted transvenously during these episodes. Subsequently, the catheter electrode was connected to a standard cardioverter/defibrillator, and the next three episodes of spontaneous ventricular fibrillation were terminated by a 25-joule shock delivered transvenously (Figure 15-6).

Another patient had six episodes of sustained ventricular tachycardia successfully terminated by 0.1 (one episode), 0.25 (one episode), 0.5 (two episodes),

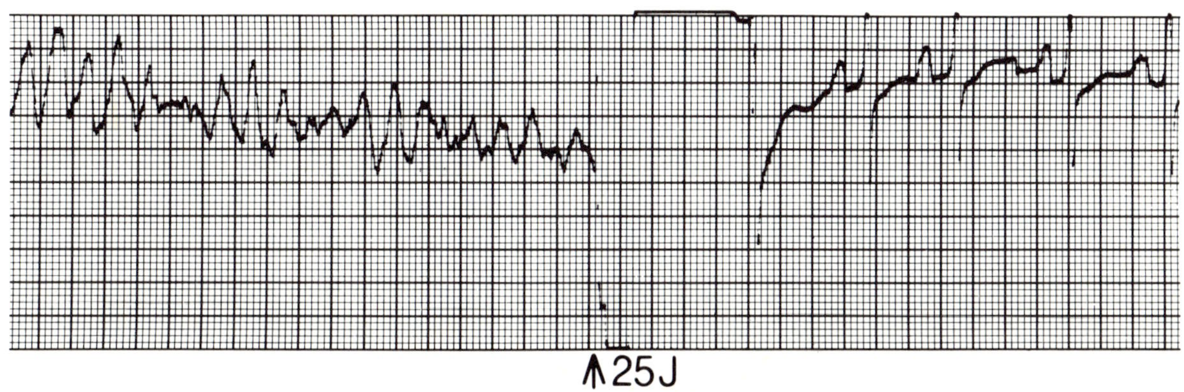

Fig. 15-6. Transvenous defibrillation. A 25-joule shock (*arrow*) terminated ventricular fibrillation. From Zipes, DP, Jackman WM, Heger JJ, et al: Clinical transvenous cardioversion of recurrent life-threatening ventricular tachyarrhythmias: Low-energy synchronized cardioversion of ventricular tachycardia and termination of ventricular fibrillation in patients using a catheter electrode. Am Heart J 103:426, 1982. With permission.

Table 15-1

Patient	Ventricular tachycardia Episodes Terminated	Cardioversion Threshold Joules mean	Range
1	18	0.13	0.075–0.25
2	20	0.06	0.025–0.1
3	6	1.17	0.75–2.0
4	2	0.16	0.075–0.25
5	1	2.0	
6	6	0.68	0.1–2.0
7	1	1.25	
8*	311	5.7	4–20
9	0	>0.75	
10	0	>2.0	
11	1	1.5	
12	1	0.25	
13	5	0.008	0.05–0.1

* American Optical Cardioverter.

0.75 (one episode), and 2 (one episode) joules. The catheter position was probably not stable (accounting for the changing thresholds) and the shock was synchronized at different points in the QRS complex (Figure 15-7). Shocks in the midportion of the QRS complex terminated the ventricular tachycardia with none or one repetitive response (*panel A*). Shocks of equal intensity in the latter portion of the QRS complex (*panel B*) sometimes failed to terminate the ventricular tachycardia. A shock delivered slightly later in the QRS complex, after termination of the absolute ventricular refractory period and during the early portion of the vulnerable period (*panel C*), initiated ventricular flutter/ventricular fibrillation that was promptly terminated by transthoracic cardioversion (*panel D*).

Despite the presence of atrioventricular dissociation during ventricular tachycardia in all patients and the resultant random delivery of the shocks in relation to atrial systole, repetitive atrial activity occurred after only 5 of the 196 shocks. A shock of 0.25 joule did not terminate the ventricular tachycardia in one patient and produced atrial fibrillation that was then terminated, along with the ventricular tachycardia, by a subsequent shock of 1 joule a few minutes later (Figure 15-8).

One patient deserves special note. He was referred for treatment of drug-refractory recurrent ventricular tachycardia that occurred on the precise day that

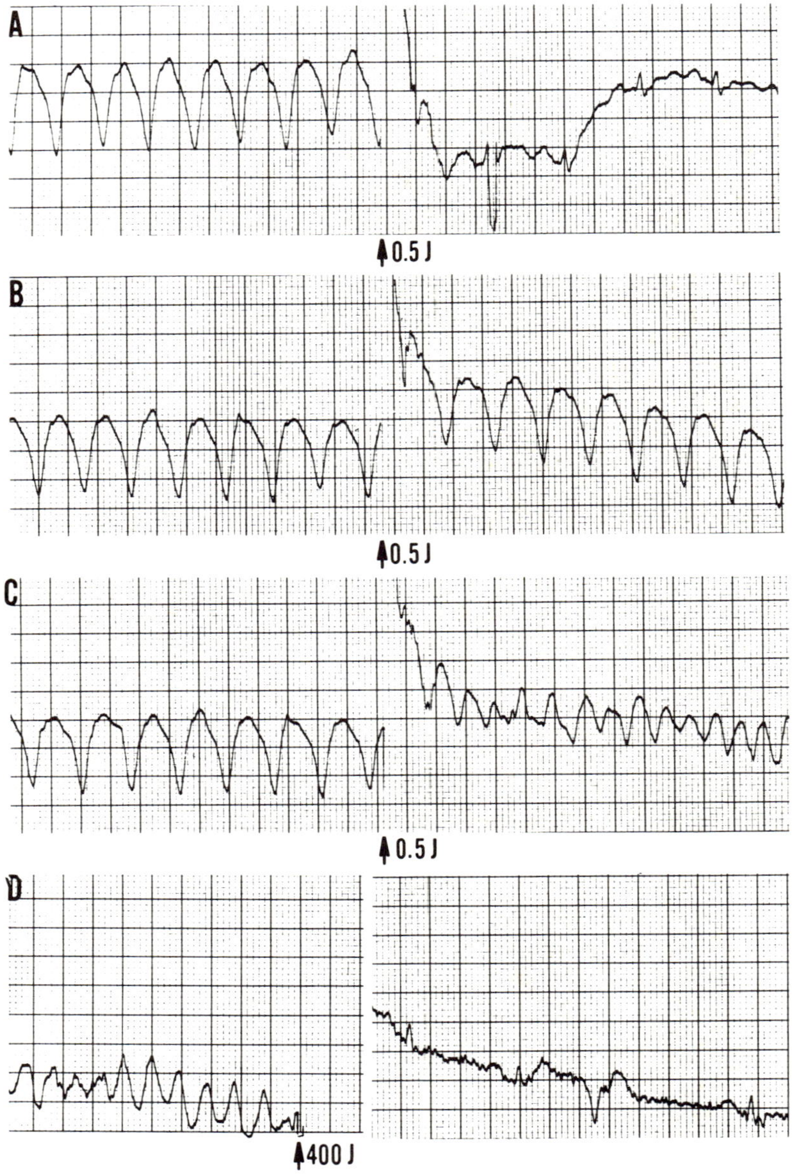

Fig. 15-7. ECG rhythm recordings from a patient showing termination of ventricular tachycardia with 0.5 joule (A), failure to terminate ventricular tachycardia with a slightly greater shock (B), initiation of ventricular fibrillation with a still greater shock (C), and termination of ventricular fibrillation with an external shock of 400 joules (D). From Zipes DP, Prystowsky EN, Browne KF, et al: Additional observations on transvenous cardioversion of recurrent ventricular tachycardia. Am Heart J 104:163, 1982. With permission.

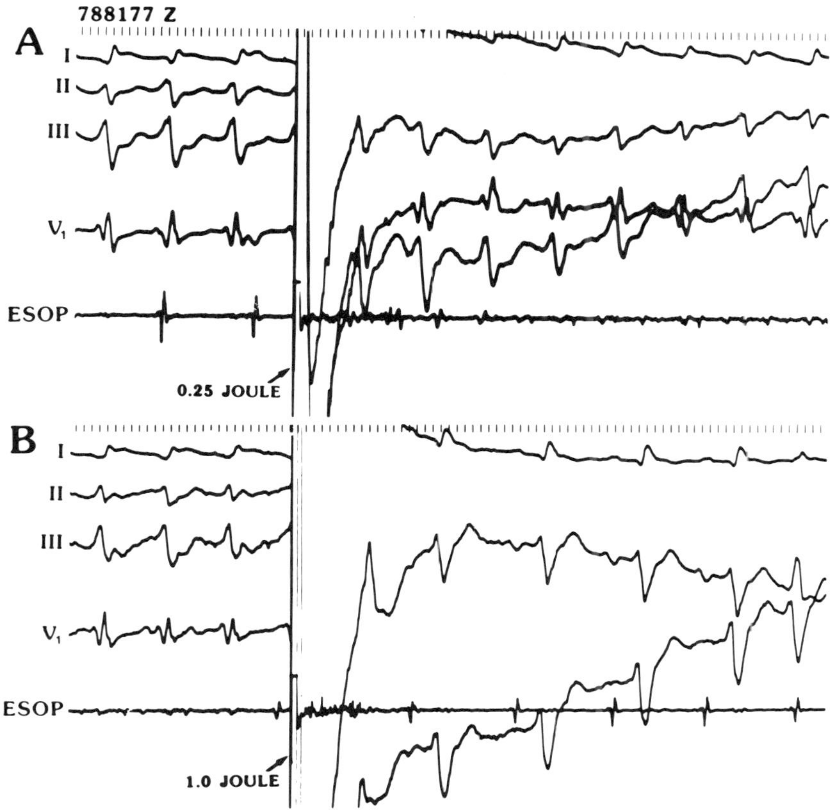

Fig. 15-8. Termination of atrial fibrillation. A 0.25 joule shock is delivered synchronously into the QRS complex through a transvenous catheter. The stimulus fails to convert the ventricular rhythm but induces atrial fibrillation. **B,** A shock of 1 joule is delivered synchronously into the QRS complex and the atrial fibrillation and ventricular tachycardia are both terminated to restore sinus rhythm.

another patient presented. We connected the catheter electrode to a conventional external American Optical cardioverter through a junction box we had built previously, just in case we needed to treat two patients at the same time. He ultimately died with refractory cardiogenic shock in an agonal slow ventricular rhythm with electromechanical dissociation. Before his hemodynamic collapse, he had received 311 cardioversions in a 12-hour period. We synchronized the shock from skin electrodes through the American Optical cardioverter and delivered the shocks from the standard American Optical cardioverter through the transvenous catheter electrode. Naturally the precise voltage setting on the meter of the American Optical cardioverter cannot be determined with the degree of accuracy we were able to achieve using our specially made cardioverter. However, 245 episodes of ventricular tachycardia were terminated with 4 joules, 45 episodes with 8 joules, and 21 episodes with 20 joules. One shock in the latter range accelerated the ventricular tachycardia from 140–210 beats/min, but otherwise there were no problems.

Awake, unsedated patients tolerated shocks of less than 0.5 joule without difficulty. Shocks in this range were described as a "giant hiccough" or a light blow to the chest due to diaphragmatic or intercostal muscle contraction. Shocks exceeding 0.5 joule were less well tolerated and produced moderate skeletal muscle stimulation.

CONCLUSIONS

Conventional synchronous transthoracic cardioversion is the most effective and safest form of electrical therapy to terminate ventricular tachycardia,[15] but has obvious limitations for long-term application. The impetus for this study was to develop a therapeutic approach that was as safe and as effective as synchronous transthoracic cardioversion but could be used long-term, eventually as a totally implanted system.

Transvenous cardioversion terminates ventricular tachycardia in patients with very small amounts of energy. It is possible that antiarrhythmic drugs in these patients influenced the cardioversion thresholds to some degree. Ventricular tachycardia that failed to terminate in two patients with intracardiac shocks of 0.75 and 2 joules possibly would have been terminated by higher energies, had they been tried. Thresholds may be influenced by the size of the heart, origin of the ventricular tachycardia in relation to electrode position, and other factors. Future developments in catheter electrode design and the waveform of the shock may reduce energy requirements further.

Perhaps transvenous cardioversion may be used for some patients who have recurrent episodes of supraventricular tachycardia as well. In the animal study, [3] we terminated several episodes of atrial flutter or atrial fibrillation by delivering a transvenous shock of 1 joule. In the present study, 1 joule terminated atrial fibrillation.

Transvenous cardioversion is not without some risk, but that is not surprising in light of the known potential arrhythmic complications of transthoracic cardioversion.[16] Transvenous cardioversion may not be any different from transthoracic cardioversion regarding safety. All the precautions used with transthoracic cardioversion regarding a precisely synchronized shock should be employed. Delivering electricity to the ventricle is not totally without risk, regardless of how the technique is carried out.

Transvenous cardioversion has multiple potential applications. For example, the catheter electrode connected to an external unit can be used on a temporary basis for the patient who has frequent recurrences of ventricular tachycardia or ventricular fibrillation, thereby avoiding repeated chest trauma and the need for anesthesia if thresholds are low. The catheter electrode can be used also to pace the heart. During electrophysiologic studies in patients, pacing-induced ventricular tachycardia or ventricular fibrillation can be terminated with the same catheter electrode. As a permanent implant, the size of the generator could be relatively small and longevity relatively long, compared to the automatic implantable defibrillator,[1] because of the reduced energy requirements. A transvenous cardioversion system will have the additional advantage of not requiring a thoracotomy for implantation. It is also possible that transvenous cardioversion may be easier to test and use than pacing modalities. The latter generally require in-depth electrophysiologic evaluation of the patient to determine precise electrophysiologic parameters—number of stimuli, intervals, adjustment of cycle length, and other factors necessary to terminate ventricular tachycardia by pacing. Also, cardioversion may be less influenced by physiologic changes or drugs that may alter the parameters of pacing-induced termination. Since episodes of spontaneous ventricular fibrillation are preceded by ventricular tachycardia in many patients,[17] the former may be prevented entirely by cardioverting the latter. Conceivably in the future the ideal implantable device will be capable of transvenous cardioversion and, if that fails or if ventricular fibrillation is precipitated, it will then deliver a defibrillating shock.

Since submission of this manuscript, twenty-eight patients have received implantation of a permanent transvenous cardioverter.

Acknowledgment

The authors thank Drs. W. Jackman, K. Browne, D. Chilson, G. Naccarelli, and G. T. Rahilly,† B. Skale, and Elizabeth Darling, R.N., for their contributions to this study.

REFERENCES

1. Mirowski M, Reid PR, Mower M, et al: Termination of malignant ventricular arrhythmias with an implanted automatic defibrillator in human beings. N Engl J Med 303:322, 1980
2. Mirowski M, Reid PR, Watkins L, et al: Clinical treatment of life-threatening ventricular tachyarrhythmias with the automatic implantable defibrillator. Am Heart J 102:265, 1981
3. Jackman WM, Zipes DP: Low-energy synchronous cardioversion of ventricular tachycardia using a catheter electrode in a canine model of subacute myocardial infarction. Circulation 66:187, 1982
4. Yee R, Zipes DP, Gulamhusein S, et al: Countershock using an intravascular catheter in an acute care setting. Am J Cardiol 50:1124, 1982
5. Zipes DP, Jackman W, Heger JJ, et al: Clinical transvenous cardioversion of recurrent life-threatening ventricular tachyarrhythmias: Low-energy synchronized cardioversion of ventricular tachycardia and termination of ventricular fibrillation in patients using a catheter electrode. Am Heart J 103:789, 1982
6. Zipes DP, Prystowsky EN, Browne K, et al: Additional observations on transvenous cardioversion of recurrent ventricular tachycardia. Am Heart J 104:163, 1982
7. Harris AS: Delayed development of ventricular ectopic rhythms following experimental coronary occlusion. Circulation 1:1318, 1950
8. Rubin L, Hudson P, Snively S, et al: Defibrillation threshold energy and ep-

† Deceased.

icardial electrode size (abstract). Med Instrum 14:58, 1980
9. Schuder JC, Rahmoeller GA, Stoeckle H: Transthoracic ventricular defibrillation with triangular and trapezoidal waveforms. Circ Res 19:689, 1966
10. Garan H, Fallon JT, Ruskin JN: Sustained ventricular tachycardia in recent canine myocardial infarction. Circulation 62:980, 1980
11. Karagueuzian HS, Fenoglio JJ Jr, Weiss MB, et al: Protracted ventricular tachycardia induced by premature stimulation of the canine heart after coronary artery occlusion and reperfusion. Circ Res 44:833, 1979
12. Michaelson EL, Spear JF, Moore EN: Initiation of sustained ventricular tachyarrhythmias in a canine model of chronic myocardial infarction: Importance of the site of stimulation. Circulation 63:776, 1981
13. Wiggers CJ, Wegria R: Ventricular fibrillation due to single, localized induction and condenser shocks applied during the vulnerable phase of ventricular systole. Am J Physiol 128:500, 1940
14. Lesigne C, Levy B, Saumont R, et al: An energy-time analysis of ventricular fibrillation and defibrillation thresholds with internal electrodes. Med Biol Eng 14:617, 1976
15. Kerber RE, Martins JB, Gascho JA, et al: Effect of direct-current countershocks on regional myocardial contractility and perfusion. Circulation 63:323, 1981
16. Lown B: Electrical reversion of cardiac arrhythmias. Br Heart J 29:469, 1967
17. Ruskin JN, DiMarco JP, Garan H: Out-of-hospital cardiac arrest. Electrophysiologic observations and selection of long-term antiarrhythmic therapy. N Engl J Med 303:607, 1980

Harold R. Kay

16

CARDIAC SURGERY FOR THE TREATMENT OF VENTRICULAR TACHYARRHYTHMIAS

The role of cardiac surgery in the management of ventricular tachyarrhythmias has evolved as a direct extension of laboratory investigations that elucidated the physiology, etiology, and mechanism of these arrhythmias. Before the development of invasive electrophysiologic studies, surgical approaches were based on unproven theories about the pathogenesis of these arrhythmias, and the results of antiarrhythmia operations were unsatisfactory. In the past 5 years sufficient data have been collected from long-term studies to delineate those areas in which a surgical approach may be beneficial. In addition, analysis of carefully controlled studies has identified those areas in which surgical intervention is either contraindicated or not efficacious.

Because the term ventricular arrhythmia includes a wide variety of arrhythmias ranging from isolated premature ventricular depolarizations to recurrent ventricular fibrillation, it is helpful to divide patients with ventricular arrhythmias into three categories: (1) ventricular premature depolarizations, (2) sustained ventricular tachycardia, and (3) ventricular fibrillation.

Ventricular premature depolarizations include premature depolarizations, bigeminy, couplets, and nonsustained (self-terminating) ventricular tachycardia. These lower forms of ventricular arrhythmias have in common the fact that the primary rhythm is supraventricular.

Sustained ventricular tachycardia is defined as a rhythm that arises either de novo or as the result of programmed premature stimulation, which lasts for more than 4 beats or 30 seconds. Drugs, electrical stimulation, or cardioversion are required to terminate the arrhythmia. Unless treated, this arrhythmia tends to recur, hence the term recurrent sustained ventricular tachycardia.

Ventricular fibrillation is the most dangerous arrhythmia, since it almost invariably leads to hemodynamic deterioration. It is characterized by uncoordinated

SUDDEN CARDIAC DEATH
0-8089-1725-0

ventricular depolarizations and usually requires cardioversion to terminate. Recurrent ventricular fibrillation is frequently seen in the setting of severe myocardial ischemia.

All three types of arrhythmia may coexist in the same patient. Since effective surgical therapy requires precise identification of the underlying pathophysiologic mechanism, the first step in surgical treatment is determining which arrhythmia represents the most serious threat to the patient's life. Electrophysiologic testing, including introduction of premature extrastimuli, is the most effective means to classify the patient's arrhythmia.

Once the mechanism of the arrhythmia is identified, attempts are made to control the arrhythmia medically. Surgery is usually indicated only when the arrhythmia is refractory to maximum medical therapy. Although surgical results may not appear to be effective, they are significantly better than the results of any other treatment.

VENTRICULAR PREMATURE DEPOLARIZATIONS

The high correlation between the extent of coronary artery disease and the complexity of ventricular ectopic activity[1] raised the possibility that ischemia was the common etiologic factor in the pathogenesis of these arrhythmias. With the introduction of coronary artery bypass surgery in 1968,[2] surgeons could provide immediate relief of the ischemia for the first time. It was initially believed that relieving the ischemia would eliminate the coexistent ventricular arrhythmias.

The results of coronary revascularization, with or without resection of an isolated segment of ischemic myocardium (aneurysmectomy or infarctectomy), have been disappointing.[3-8] Even in the best reported series, coronary bypass operations have only been successful in obliterating complex ventricular ectopic activity in 55% of patients. Other authors have reported persistent ventricular premature depolarizations in 100% of patients. Even more distressing is the finding in some series[5,6,9] that coronary revascularization may increase ectopic activity in 25% of patients. Although the mechanism responsible for this increase in ectopic activity is not clear and may be due to the fact that patients who have had bypass operations do not receive antiarrhythmic medications postoperatively, there are no data to suggest that the increase in ectopic activity is due to incomplete revascularization or postoperative graft closure.

Myocardial revascularization operations alone are not adequate treatment for ventricular premature depolarizations, bigeminy, and nonsustained ventricular tachycardia. Although ischemia or postischemic myocardial damage may be the mechanism responsible for the arrhythmia, myocardial revascularization is not sufficient to reverse the underlying pathophysiologic process. Patients with ventricular ectopy who are otherwise candidates for coronary bypass operations should still have bypass operations. Amelioration of the arrhythmia should not be anticipated, however. Patients who have any sign of ventricular ectopic activity postoperatively should be treated for their arrhythmia in the same protocol as patients who have not had surgery. Conversely, patients with ventricular ectopy who are *not* otherwise candidates for coronary bypass operations should not be sent for operation with the anticipation that myocardial revascularization will eliminate the arrhythmia.

VENTRICULAR FIBRILLATION

In contrast to ventricular premature depolarizations that probably arise from microscopic areas of ischemic or anatomically disrupted myocardium, recurrent ventricular fibrillation usually occurs in the setting of global ischemia and severely diminished myocardial perfusion. Inadequate myocardial perfusion causes further depression of cardiac performance and establishes a vicious cycle of further reduction in myocardial blood flow and worsening of cardiac performance. Ventricular fibrillation usually results if this vicious cycle cannot be broken.

The earliest surgical attempts at control of recurrent ventricular fibrillation were directed at altering the physiologic milieu that propagated the arrhythmia. Two approaches have been advocated to treat recurrent ventricular fibrillation: cervical sympathectomy and myocardial revascularization with or without resection.

Cervical Sympathectomy

Because increased sympathetic tone was shown to increase myocardial susceptibility to ventricular irritability[10] and several experimental studies had shown that lowering of sympathetic tone after experimental myocardial infarction will decrease myocardial vulnerability,[11,12] Sealy and Oldham[13] advocated left cervical sympathectomy for patients with coronary artery disease and ventricular arrhythmias. Sympathectomy abolished the arrhythmia in 3 of 6 patients in this series, but the remaining 3 patients died.

Recent work[14] has shown that transmural infarction may interrupt epicardial neural pathways and thus create a heterogeneous zone of sympathetic innervation distal to an area of transmural infarction. These experiments may explain the genesis of postinfarction arrhythmias in areas of the myocardium not involved in the infarct. The rationale of cervical sympathectomy is to create total sympathectomy and eliminate the areas of heterogenicity. Although this concept has not been proven in humans, it does provide a physiologic explanation of the mechanism by which surgical sympathectomy may be effective in some patients.

Despite the results of Sealy and Oldham, the importance of sympathectomy in the treatment of ventricular fibrillation remains an interesting laboratory finding that has not gained widespread clinical application; the preferred approach is myocardial revascularization.

Myocardial Revascularization and/or Resection

Patients with ventricular fibrillation and coronary artery disease can be classified into two subsets: those with an acute exacerbation of chronic coronary artery disease without recent myocardial infarction and those with recent infarction.

In patients without recent infarction, when ventricular fibrillation is precipitated by exercise[15,16] or associated with severe ischemia and unstable angina,[17-21] direct myocardial revascularization with or without an aneurysmectomy or infarctectomy has usually abolished the arrhythmia. The relative efficacy of medical treatment in these patients is unknown, since they usually have clinical indications for bypass operation and therefore have not received an adequate medical trial.

Aggressive, early operative intervention has been advocated for patients with ventricular fibrillation after myocardial infarction. Unless the severe myocardial oxygen supply/demand imbalance can be corrected with drugs or intraaortic balloon counterpulsation, the mortality with medical management approaches 100%. These patients typically have poor left ventricular function, triple-vessel coronary artery disease (usually with total occlusion or high-grade stenosis of the left anterior descending coronary artery, and large areas of myocardial infarction or aneurysm.[22-29]

The operative approach in patients with recurrent ventricular fibrillation after myocardial infarction has been hemodynamic stabilization with intraaortic balloon counterpulsation followed by urgent cardiac catheterization and surgery. Overall results have been encouraging[22,25-29] (Table 16-1). Although the operative mortality is 27%, arrhythmias have been controlled in 60%–90% of the survivors. Ventricular ectopic activity persists in 50% of the survivors; however, these arrhythmias usually can be controlled with appropriate antiarrhythmic agents and the late (3–96 months) mortality is 5%–6%. Most of these late deaths are sudden and presumably due to recurrence of arrhythmia.

The prerequisite of a successful surgical approach to recurrent ventricular fibrillation appears to be the presence of reversible myocardial ischemia. The high

Table 16-1 *Results of Coronary Revascularization and Myocardial Resection for Recurrent Ventricular Fibrillation*

References Numbers	Number of Patients	Number of Operative Deaths	Number of Late Deaths	Arrhythmias Controlled*	Follow-Up (months)
25	10	3	1	6	3–24
26	11	0	2	9	3–57
27	23	6	1	15	4–32
22	16	5	1	10	8–39
28	5	0	0	5	12–96
29	15	8	0	7	9–92
23	10	2	0	8	2–21
TOTAL	90	24 (27%)	5	60 (67%)	

From Horowitz LN, Harken AH, Josephson ME, et al: Surgical treatment of ventricular arrhythmias in coronary artery disease. Ann Intern Med 95:88, 1981. With permission.
*Includes patients who are controlled postoperatively with or without drugs.

operative mortality probably reflects the risk of operation in the setting of an acute myocardial infarction, but the overall patient salvage rate after operation is much better than that of medical treatment in patients with recurrent ventricular fibrillation, which is refractory to antiarrhythmic agents.

RECURRENT SUSTAINED VENTRICULAR TACHYCARDIA

Surgical approaches to ventricular arrhythmias have been most successful in the treatment of medically refractory recurrent sustained ventricular tachycardia. This arrhythmia seems to be particularly amenable to surgical treatment. Two new operations, direct endocardial excision and encircling endocardial ventriculotomy, have proven successful in its treatment.

Three major technologic advances have contributed to the success of operations directed at the treatment of recurrent sustained ventricular tachycardia:

1. As advanced life-support and resuscitation equipment become available to a larger segment of the population, more patients are being resuscitated from their initial episode of ventricular tachycardia. This early salvage increases the pool of patients who are at high risk for recurrent ventricular tachycardia. Similarly, the increased availability of more effective pharmacologic agents has allowed patients to survive long enough to undergo electrophysiologic evaluation and operation.
2. The increased availability of Holter monitoring and electrophysiologic studies has helped identify more patients with ventricular arrhythmias and has allowed more precise electrophysiologic mapping of the arrhythmogenic focus.
3. Improvements in operative technique, including new concepts of intraoperative myocardial preservation, cardiac anesthesia, perioperative support, and intraoperative mapping, have decreased the operative mortality in these high-risk patients.

Equally important has been the recognition that medical treatment is successful in controlling only 25%–50% of patients with sustained ventricular tachycardia.[30,31]

Unlike recurrent ventricular fibrillation, which is usually seen in the setting of global ischemia after acute myocardial infarction, and premature ventricular depolarizations, which probably represent microscopic areas of ischemia or anatomic abnormality, recurrent sustained ventricular tachycardia is probably a reentrant phenomenon,[32,33] that does not appear to require the presence of acute ischemia. Rather, it results from fixed anatomic and electrophysiologic abnormalities that are the sequelae of previous myocardial infarction.[34,35]

Surgical approaches to sustained ventricular tachycardia have included sympathectomy, coronary revascularization, myocardial resection, encircling endocardial ventriculotomy, and electrophysiologically guided resection or ablation of the endocardial site of origin of the arrhythmia.

Older Techniques

Sympathectomy had been proposed as a treatment for recurrent sustained ventricular tachycardia as early as 1961.[30] The successful application of bilateral cervical sympathectomy is documented only in a few case reports and small series.[36-40] The physiologic rationale for sympathectomy is similar for recurrent ventricular fibrillation and recurrent sustained ventricular tachycardia, namely, that certain ventricular arrhythmias may be induced by exercise or sympathomimetic drugs and terminated by parasympathetic stimulation.[41-43] The 25% cure rate[40] and significant morbidity (Horner's syndrome) make it unlikely that sympathectomy will attain any clinical prominence, except as an adjunct to other treatment modalities.

Because recurrent sustained ventricular tachycardia is most frequently seen in coronary artery disease and ventricular aneurysm, early operative approaches to this arrhythmia usually included myocardial revascularization, with or without left ventricular aneurysmectomy. This association between recurrent sustained ventricular tachycardia and left ventricular aneurysm was noted in 1938, but the first successful aneurysmectomy for recurrent ventricular tachycardia was not reported until 1956.[44] With the advent of coronary bypass surgery in 1968, interest in aneurysmectomy, with or without concurrent coronary revascularization, for recurrent sustained ventricular tachycardia was rekindled.

Between 1968 and 1974 17 publications reported the results of aneurysmectomy in 55 patients.[40,45-60] The arrhythmia was ablated in 70%–90% of the patients, and the operative mortality was 15%. The small number of patients and the absence of a rigid definition for aneurysm excision has raised some question about the general applicability of these results.

In better-controlled, larger series,[27,61-65] both operative mortality and arrhythmia cure rates were disappointing. In these series, encompassing 118 patients, the operative mortality was 26%, late mortality was 21%, and arrhythmia cure rate (including patients who are controlled postoperatively with antiarrhythmic agents) was only 28%.

These recent series probably more accurately reflect the results of ventricular aneurysm resection because they represent the results of consecutive series of patients who have not responded to a maximum medical regimen. Despite the dismal mortality and inconsistent cure rate, the results of routine aneurysmectomy still compare favorably to the very high mortality in patients with medically refractory ventricular tachycardia who are treated nonoperatively. If it is the only procedure available, routine aneurysmectomy can be considered potentially beneficial, although not remarkably effective.

Because aneurysmectomy and coronary revascularization were frequently done simultaneously in these patients, the question has always arisen as to whether the aneurysmectomy, the myocardial revascularization, or a combination was the effective part of the therapy. In the reported series, 10%–15% of the patients had coronary bypass alone. This subset of patients had a higher operative mortality than for the group as a whole; most operative survivors succumb to persistent recurrent sustained ventricular tachycardia or die suddenly in the early follow-up period.[64-66] In contrast, patients who had aneurysmectomy without a coronary artery bypass had results no different from the group as a whole.

These findings refocused the attention of investigators on the left ventricular aneurysm as a possible arrhythmogenic factor. Although the operative results are not impressive by today's standards, they did serve as a helpful preliminary step in the evolution both of a better physiologic understanding of the etiology of this arrhythmia and in defining the limitations of surgery.

Encircling Endocardiac Ventriculotomy

In the early 1970s numerous experimental and pathologic studies had postulated that ventricular tachycardia arose from the border zone along the subendocardial periphery of an infarction.[67-70] Subsequent work in humans[71] has confirmed this hypothesis.

Guiraudon et al.[71-74] designed an operation that they called an encircling endocardial ventriculotomy in an attempt to electrically isolate this subendocardial border zone from the rest of the myocardium. Theoretically, electrical isolation would eliminate the possibility of electrical stimuli entering the diseased area or, if ventricular tachycardia were initiated within the diseased area, it could be contained and not spread to the entire myocardium.

During an encircling endocardial ventriculotomy the aneurysm is opened and a transmural incision (sparing only the epicardium) is made around the entire infarct. The early and late results in Guiraudon's experience were excellent. Of 23 patients,[17] (69%) had successful outcomes. The operative mortality was low (4%), and only 20% of the survivors had recurrent arrhythmias in a follow-up of 1–55 months. The procedure is not difficult and the results seemed very attractive.

Unfortunately, other investigators could not reproduce Guiraudon's results.[75,76] The operative mortality was 17% and left ventricular power failure accounted for 2 of 4 (50%) late deaths. There is now increasing experimental evidence that encircling endocardial ventriculotomy causes a decrease in regional myocardial blood flow[77] and causes regional disturbances in diastolic compliance,[78,79] which may account both for the high operative mortality[73,74] and the high incidence of left ventricular power failure.

The effectiveness of the encircling endocardial ventriculotomy has not been questioned, but for most centers the high operative and late mortality have outweighed any potential antiarrhythmic benefit.

Ventriculotomy and Epicardial Mapping

Another alternative to encircling endocardial ventriculotomy is the use of electrophysiologic mapping techniques to precisely identify the site of earliest activation of the arrhythmia. The rationale of this approach is that, if the site of earliest activation can be identified, the arrhythmogenic focus can be resected.

There was initially great enthusiasm for this technique because it was believed that intraoperative epicardial mapping could guide the surgeon to the arrhythmogenic focus. Once the focus was identified, the surgeon could perform either a simple ventriculotomy to isolate the area or a transmural excision of the involved myocardium.

This procedure is moderately effective (72% arrhythmia cure) in patients with cardiomyopathy and normal coronary arteries[73,80,81]; however, except for one center,[82,83] the majority of surgeons have had little or no success controlling arrhythmias using epicardial mapping techniques in patients with ischemic heart disease.[62,72,84]

The reason for the poor results with epicardial mapping has subsequently been elucidated in a canine model.[85] Spielman et al. showed that when the tachycardia originates in the endocardium, the earliest epicardial activation may occur 0.5–10 cm from the site of origin. Resecting the epicardially mapped focus therefore may not resect the true focus.

Other investigators[71,84] have confirmed the concept of an endocardial or intramural site of origin in humans. Recurrent sustained ventricular tachycardia after myocardial infarction usually arises in the left ventricular endocardium along the border of the infarction or aneurysm. The earliest epicardial activity may occur as far as 10 cm from the origin or may even appear on the right ventricle. Epicardial mapping is not currently used in the surgical approach to recurrent sustained ventricular tachycardia.

Endocardial Mapping and Excision or Cryoablation

Poor results with other techniques led to the development of a new operative procedure for recurrent sustained ventricular tachycardia. The operation was conceived and developed by Harken, Josephson, and Horowitz at the University of Pennsylvania in 1977.[86-89] The physiologic basis for the operation rests on the principles of precise intraoperative identification of the arrhythmogenic focus during the ventricular tachycardia and resection of the identified abnormal region of the endocardium.

In the operating room the patient is placed on cardiopulmonary bypass, and the body temperature is maintained at normothermic levels. The aneurysm is opened and ventricular tachycardia is induced by programmed stimulation. Once ventricular tachycardia is induced, a probe is used to identify (map) the site of earliest activation. The site is almost invariably found in the endocardium 1–6 cm from the margin of the aneurysm. The entire aneurysm is then resected and an extended endocardial excision is performed to include the area that was identified as the site of earliest activation.

Results from this operation have been encouraging. An operative mortality of 9%–12% has been reported from many centers.[35,76,86-93] This mortality is similar to that of aneurysmectomy alone. Considering that these patients have an average LVEF of 20%, the mortality is not significantly higher than the operative mortality for coronary artery bypass operations in patients with severely compromised left ventricular function.

The late mortality is 13%, which is not surprising in this very sick group of patients, and the postoperative recurrence rate in patients who are not receiving drug therapy is approximately 5%. Fortunately, recurrence of the arrhythmia postoperatively usually can be controlled with appropriate antiarrhythmic agents, and the recurrence rate (subtracting patients who are controlled with drugs) is 2%. This means that the overall success rate (patients alive with arrhythmia controlled) is 81%–89%. There is also good evidence of improvement in global ventricular function (as a result of the aneurysmectomy) in most patients[92] (Table 16-2).

Table 16-2 *Results of Indirect and Direct Surgical Procedures for the Treatment of Refractory Ischemic Ventricular Tachycardia*

Procedure	Number of Patients	Number of Operative Deaths (%)	Number of Late Deaths (%)	Postoperative recurrence Without Drug Therapy (%)	Refractory Postoperative recurrence With Drug Therapy (%)	Overall Success Rate * (%)
Indirect procedures	179	47 (26)	? (?)	29 (16)	29 (16)	103 (58)
Encircling endocardial ventriculotomy	47	8 (17)	4† (9)	3 (7)	(0)	37 (79)
Endocardial resection	76	7 (9)	10‡ (13)	4 (5)	1 (1)	68 (89)

From Cox JL, Gallagher JJ, Ungerleider RM: Encircling endocardial ventriculotomy for refractory ischemic ventricular tachycardia. IV. Clinical indications, surgical technique, mechanism of action, and results. J Thorac Cardiovasc Surg 83:865, 1982. With permission.

* Includes the total number of patients (column 1) minus the operative deaths (column 2), late deaths related to operation of recurrent ventricular tachycardia, and postoperative recurrences with medical therapy (column 5).

† Two late deaths.

‡ No late deaths.

Although the extended endocardial resection provides the best results of any current antiarrhythmic operation, there are still several problems with the procedure:

1. The procedure is not applicable in patients with posterior aneurysms. It is technically difficult or impossible to induce sustained ventricular tachycardia and perform intraoperative mapping because the location of the aneurysm requires that the heart be lifted for surgical access. Lifting the heart frequently terminates the tachycardia. Fortunately, the vast majority of aneurysms are anterior or apical and are thus accessible for mapping. In those patients with posterior aneurysms, the arrhythmogenic focus is identified by preoperative catheter mapping in the electrophysiology laboratory, and the approximate site of earliest activation is subsequently excised during surgery.
2. When the arrhythmogenic focus occurs at the base of a papillary muscle, excision of the focus will create a dysfunctional papillary muscle and mitral regurgitation. Three approaches have been advocated if the arrhythmogenic focus is identified at the base of the papillary muscle: excision of the papillary muscle and mitral valve replacement, encircling endocardial ventriculotomy around the papillary muscle, and cryoablation of the base of the papillary muscle. There are insufficient data to predict which of these approaches will ultimately prove to be the most successful.
3. Another problem with the procedure arises when the tachycardia arises from multiple sites. The length of time that it takes to map each of 5 or 6 different sites makes its application difficult; in this situation most surgeons would recommend preoperative catheter mapping in the electrophysiology laboratory followed by extensive resection of all visibly involved endocardial scar. Results from this "extended aneurysmectomy" have been better than those following routine aneurysmectomy.
4. Electrophysiologic mapping requires that the arrhythmia can be induced by programmed stimulation in the operating room on cardiopulmonary bypass. It may be difficult to reproduce the arrhythmia under the temperature and anesthetic conditions in the operating room, and interpretation of the findings may be difficult in patients with multiple origins or in whom the tachycardia is very rapid.

Cryoablation, application of a cold (−60° C) probe to the involved area of the endocardium, has been proposed as an alternative to endocardial excision.[94-97] This technique holds great promise, but there is as yet insufficient experience to predict long-term results.

Current Concepts

Although the concept of a surgical approach to ventricular arrhythmias is effective in many patients, the operative mortality, postoperative morbidity, and arrhythmia recurrence rate still limit its application in all ventricular arrhythmias. Effective pharmacologic treatment of the early arrhythmia, confirmed by electrophysiologic testing, is still the first line of treatment.

Operation is indicated when the arrhythmia is refractory to a medical regimen or when surgery is otherwise indicated (e.g., patients with coronary artery disease and recurrent sustained ventricular tachycardia who require a coronary bypass operation should have simultaneous antiarrhythmia operations). Because patients with left ventricular aneurysms are prone to develop ventricular arrhythmias, the current tendency is to recommend extended endocardial resection in patients who are otherwise candidates for aneurysmectomy, even if the patient does not have arrhythmias before aneurysmectomy. There are no data to support this concept, but the extended resection does not significantly add to the morbidity or mortality of the procedure and may prove to be beneficial in long-term follow-up.

SUMMARY

There is no evidence to support the recommendation of surgery to ameliorate or ablate the lower forms of ventricular arrhythmias (ventricular premature depolarizations or nonsustained ventricular tachycardia). Coronary bypass operations are ineffective in controlling these arrhythmias.

Surgery may play an important role in the treatment of recurrent ventricular fibrillation in patients with reversible ischemia. Although the operative mortality is 27% and 50% of the patients require antiarrhythmic agents after the operation, the overall salvage rate compares favorably with medical therapy.

Surgery is definitely indicated in patients with recurrent sustained ventricular tachycardia that is refractory to medical therapy. In these patients precise localization of arrhythmogenic foci allows either resection or ablation of these areas, with a reasonable operative mortality and good long-term arrhythmia cure rates.

The short-term future of surgery for ventricular arrhythmias is promising. As more electrophysiologists and surgeons become familiar with the technique, it will become more available in a greater number of medical centers. Surgery rarely provides a long-term solution to any problem, however, and the ultimate therapy of ventricular arrhythmias will probably lie in the development of more effective pharmacologic agents to either control the arrhythmias or reverse the disease process that causes the arrhythmias.

REFERENCES

1. Amsterdam EA, Vismara L, Brocchini R, et al: Ventricular ectopic beats: Relation to angiographically documented coronary artery disease (abstract). Clin Res 21:399, 1973
2. Favalaro RG: Saphenous vein graft in the surgical treatment of coronary artery disease: Operative technique. J Thorac Cardiovasc Surg 58:178, 1969
3. Gunn GA, Mathur VS: Ambulatory, nocturnal and exercise arrhythmias in coronary artery disease: A prospective randomized study to assess the influence of aorto-coronary bypass surgery (abstract). Am J Cardiol 39:270, 1977
4. Tilkian AG, Pfeifer JF, Barry WH, et al: The effect of coronary bypass surgery on exercise-induced ventricular arrhythmias. Am Heart J 92:707, 1976
5. De Soyza N, Murphy ML, Bissett JK, et al: Ventricular arrhythmias in

chronic stable angina pectoris with surgical or medical treatment. Ann Intern Med 89:10, 1978

6. Leutenegger F, Giger G, Fuhr P, et al: Evaluation of aortocoronary venous bypass for prevention of cardiac arrhythmias. Am Heart J 98:15, 1979
7. Graboys TB, Lown B, Collins JJ, et al: Does coronary revascularization reduce the prevalence of ventricular ectopic activity (abstract)? Am J Cardiol 41:401, 1978
8. Ricks WB, Winkle RA, Shumway NA, et al: Surgical management of life-threatening ventricular arrhythmias in patients with coronary artery disease. Circulation 56:38, 1977
9. Winkle RA: Sudden death and bypass surgery. Prim Cardiol Clin 4:20, 1982
10. Hans J, Garcia De Jalon P, Moe GK: Adrenergic effects on ventricular vulnerability. Circ Res 14:516, 1964
11. Harris AS, Estandia A, Tillotson RF: Ventricular ectopic rhythms and ventricular fibrillation following cardiac sympathectomy and coronary occlusion. Am J Physiol 165:505, 1951
12. Schaal SF, Wallace AG, Sealy WC: Protective influence of cardiac denervation against arrhythmias of myocardial infarction. Cardiovasc Res 3:241, 1969
13. Sealy WC, Oldham HN: Surgical treatment of ventricular arrhythmias by sympathectomy, coronary artery grafts and heart wall resection, in Kelley, DT (Ed): Advances in the Management of Arrhythmias. Lane Cove, Australia, Telectronics Pty, Ltd, 1978, p 218
14. Barber MJ, Mueller TM, Henry DP, et al: Transmural myocardial infarction in the dog produces sympathectomy in noninfarcted myocardium. Circulation 67:787, 1983
15. Cline RE, Armstrong RG, Stanford W: Successful myocardial revascularization after ventricular fibrillation induced by treadmill exercise. J Thorac Cardiovasc Surg 65:802, 1973
16. Bryson AL, Parisi AF, Schechter E, et al: Life-threatening ventricular arrhythmias induced by exercise cessation after coronary bypass surgery. Am J Cardiol 32:995, 1973
17. White M, Hershey JE: Multiple transmyocardial puncture revascularization in refractory ventricular fibrillation due to myocardial ischemia. Ann Thorac Surg 6:557, 1968
18. Lambert CJ, Adam M, Geisler GF, et al: Emergency myocardial revascularization for impending infarctions and arrhythmias. J Thorac Cardiovasc Surg 62:522, 1971
19. Hutchinson JE, Kemp HG, Schwarz MJ: Emergency treatment of cardiac arrest in CHD with coronary bypass graft (letter). JAMA 216:1645, 1971
20. Alexander S, Makar Y, Ellis FH Jr: Recurrent ventricular fibrillation: Treatment by emergency aortocoronary saphenous vein bypass. JAMA 228:70, 1974
21. Nordstrom LA, Lillehei JP, Adicoff A, et al: Coronary artery surgery for recurrent ventricular arrhythmias in patients with variant angina. Am Heart J 89:236, 1975
22. Wald RW, Waxman MB, Corey PN, et al: Management of intractable ventricular tachyarrhythmias after myocardial infarction. Am J Cardiol 44:329, 1979
23. Bar FW, Lie KI, Wellens HJJ: Surgical treatment of ventricular tachyarrhythmias complicating acute myocardial infarction (abstract). Circulation 54(suppl 2):37, 1976
24. Najafi H, Hunter JA, Dye WS, et al: Emergency left ventricular aneurysmectomy for the dying patient (abstract). Am J Cardiol 25:119, 1970
25. Mundth ED, Buckley MJ, DeSanctis RW, et al: Surgical treatment of ventricular irritability. J Thorac Cardiovasc Surg 66:943, 1973
26. Yashar J, Yashar JJ, Witoszka M, et al: The treatment of patients with recurrent ventricular fibrillation. Am J Surg 133:453, 1977
27. Tabry IF, Geha AS, Hammond GL, et al: Effect of surgery on ventricular tachyarrhythmias associated with coro-

nary arterial occlusive disease. Circulation 58(suppl 1):66, 1978
28. Walker WE, Stoney WS, Alford WC Jr, et al: Results of surgical management of acute left ventricular aneurysms. Circulation 62(suppl 1):75, 1980
29. Hanson EC, Levine FH, Kay HR, et al: Control of postinfarction irritability with the intra-aortic balloon pump. Circulation 62(suppl 1):130, 1980
30. Horowitz LN, Josephson ME, Kastor JA: Intracardiac electrophysiologic studies as a method for the optimization of drug therapy in chronic ventricular arrhythmia. Prog Cardiovasc Dis 23:81, 1980
31. Horowitz LN, Josephson ME, Spielman SR, et al: New approaches to diagnosing and treating ventricular tachycardia. J Cardiovasc Med 5:715, 1980
32. Wellens HJJ: Observations on the pathophysiology of ventricular tachycardia in man. Arch Intern Med 135:473, 1975
33. Wellens HJJ, Durken DR, Lie KI: Observations on mechanisms of ventricular tachycardia in man. Circulation 54:237, 1976
34. Spielman SR, Greenspan AM, Horowitz LN, et al: Anatomic substrates of recurrent sustained ventricular tachycardia. Clin Res 27:560A, 1979
35. Harken AH, Horowitz LN, Josephson ME: Ventricular tachycardias, in Glenn WWL, Baue AE, Geha AS, et al (Eds): Thoracic and Cardiovascular Surgery. Norwalk, Conn., Appleton-Century-Crofts, 1983, p 85
36. Estes LH Jr, Izlar HL Jr: Recurrent ventricular tachycardia: a case successfully treated by bilateral cardiac sympathectomy. Am J Med 31:493, 1961
37. Schoonmaker FW, Carey T, Grow JB: Treatment of tachyarrhythmias and bradyarrhythmias by cardiac sympathectomy and permanent ventricular pacing. Ann Thorac Surg 19:80, 1975
38. Lloyd R, Okada R, Stagg J, et al: The treatment of recurrent ventricular tachycardia with bilateral cervicothoracic sympathetic-ganglionectomy: A report of two cases. Circulation 50:382, 1974
39. Zipes DJ, Festoff B, Schaal SF, et al: Treatment of ventricular arrhythmia by permanent atrial pacemaker and cardiac sympathectomy. Ann Intern Med 68:591, 1968
40. Nitter-Hauge S, Storstein O: Surgical treatment of recurrent ventricular tachycardia. Br Heart J 35:1132, 1973
41. Waxman MB, Wald RW: Termination of ventricular tachycardia by an increase in cardiac vagal drive. Circulation 56:385, 1977
42. Reddy CP, Gettes LS: Use of isoproterenol as an aid to electric induction of chronic recurrent ventricular tachycardia. Am J Cardiol 44:705, 1979
43. Demaria AN, Vera Z, Amsterdam EA, et al: Disturbance of cardiac rhythm and conduction induced by exercise: diagnostic, prognostic and therapeutic implications, in Amsterdam EA, Wilmore JH, Demaria AN (Eds): Exercise in Cardiovascular Health and Disease. New York, Yorke Medical Books, 1977, p 209
44. Likoff W, Bailey CP: Problems of myocardial aneurysm: recognition and treatment (abstract). Circulation 14:968, 1956
45. Magidson O: Resection of postmyocardial infarction ventricular aneuryms for cardiac arrhythmias. Dis Chest 56:211, 1969
46. Ritter ER: Intractable ventricular tachycardia due to ventricular aneurysm with surgical cure. Ann Intern Med 7:1155, 1969
47. Favaloro RG, Effler DB, Groves LK, et al: Ventricular aneurysm—clinical experience. Ann Thorac Surg 6:227, 1968
48. Hunt D, Sloman G, Westlake G: Ventricular aneurysmectomy for recurrent tachycardia. Br Heart J 31:264, 1969
49. Thind GS, Blakemore WS, Zinsser HF: Ventricular aneurysmectomy for the treatment of recurrent ventricular

tachyarrhythmia. Am J Cardiol 27:690, 1971

50. Schlesinger Z, Lieberman Y, Neufeld HN: Ventricular aneurysmectomy for severe rhythm disturbances. J Thorac Cardiovasc Surg 61:602, 1971
51. Maloy WC, Arrants JE, Sowell BF, et al: Left ventricular aneurysm of uncertain etiology with recurrent ventricular arrhythmias. N Engl J Med 285:662, 1971
52. Barry WH, Alderman EL, Daily PO, et al: Diagnosis and treatment of a case of recurrent ventricular tachycardia. Am Heart J 84:235, 1972
53. Lull RJ, Dunn BE, Gregoratos G, et al: Ventricular aneurysm due to cardiac sarcoidosis with surgical cure of refractory ventricular tachycardia. Am J Cardiol 30:282, 1972
54. Welch TG, Fontana ME, Vasko JS: Aneurysmectomy for recurrent ventricular tachyarrhythmias. Am Heart J 85:685, 1973
55. Wardekar A, Son B, Gosaynie CD, et al: Recurrent ventricular tachycardia successfully treated by excision of ventricular aneurysm. Chest 62:505, 1972
56. Kenaan G, Mendez AM, Zubiate P, et al: Surgery for ventricular tachycardia unresponsive to medical treatment. Chest 64:574, 1973
57. Ecker RR, Mullins CB, Grammer JC, et al: Control of intractable ventricular tachycardia by coronary revascularization. Circulation 44:666, 1971
58. Basta LL, Takeshita A, Theilen EO, et al: Aneurysmectomy in treatment of ventricular and supraventricular tachyarrhythmias in patients with postinfarction and traumatic ventricular aneurysms. Am J Cardiol 32:693, 1973
59. Graham AF, Miller DC, Stinson EB, et al: Surgical treatment of refractory life-threatening ventricular tachycardia. Am J Cardiol 32:909, 1973
60. Liotta D, Ferrari H, Pinsanu A, et al: Medically uncontrollable recurrent ventricular tachyarrhythmia in association with ventricular aneurysm (letter). Am J Cardiol 33:693, 1974
61. Ricks WB, Winkle RA, Shumway NE, et al: Surgical management of life-threatening ventricular arrhythmias in patients with coronary artery disease. Circulation 56:38, 1977
62. Moran JM, Talano JV, Euler D, et al: Refractory ventricular arrhythmia: The role of intraoperative electrophysiological study. Surgery 82:809, 1977
63. Sami M, Chaitman BR, Bourassa MG, et al: Long-term follow-up of aneurysmectomy for recurrent ventricular tachycardia or fibrillation. Am Heart J 96:303, 1978
64. Buda AJ, Stinson EB, Harrison DC: Surgery for life-threatening ventricular tachyarrhythmias. Am J Cardiol 44:1171, 1979
65. Harken AH, Horowitz LN, Josephson JE: Comparison of standard aneurysmectomy and aneurysmectomy with directed endocardial resection for the treatment of recurrent sustained ventricular tachycardia. J Thorac Cardiovasc Surg 80:257, 1980
66. Winkle RA, Alderman EL, Fitzgerald JW, et al: Treatment of recurrent symptomatic ventricular tachycardia. Ann Intern Med 85:1, 1976
67. Fendelio JJ Jr, Albala A, Silva FG, et al: Structural basis of ventricular arrhythmias in human myocardial infarction: A hypothesis. Hum Pathol 7:547, 1976
68. Daniel TM, Boineu JP, Sabiston DC: Comparison of human ventricular activation with a canine model in chronic myocardial infarction. Circulation 44:74, 1971
69. Horowitz LN, Spear JF, Moore EN: Subendocardial origin of ventricular arrhythmia in 24-hour old experimental myocardial infarction. Circulation 53:56, 1976
70. Friedman PL, Stewart JR, Wit AL: Spontaneous and induced cardiac arrhythmias in sub-endocardial Purkinje fibers surviving extensive myocardial infarction in dogs. Circ Res 33:612, 1973
71. Horowitz LN, Josephson ME, Harken AH: Epicardial and endocardial acti-

vation during sustained ventricular tachycardia in man. Circulation 61:1227, 1980

72. Guiraudon G, Fontaine G, Frank R, et al: Encircling endocardial ventriculotomy: a new surgical treatment for life-threatening ventricular tachycardias resistant to medical treatment following myocardial infarction. Ann Thorac Surg 26:438, 1978
73. Fontaine G, Guiraudon G, Frank R, et al: The surgical management of ventricular tachycardia. Herz 4:276, 1979
74. Guiraudon G, Fontaine G, Frank R, et al: Encircling endocardial ventriculotomy: Late follow-up results (abstract). Circulation 62(suppl 3):320, 1980
75. Arciniegas JG, Klein H, Karp RB, et al: Surgical treatment of life-threatening ventricular tachyarrhythmias (abstract). Circulation 62(suppl 3):42, 1980
76. Cox JL, Gallagher JJ, Ungerleider RM: Encircling endocardial ventriculotomy for refractory ischemic ventricular tachycardia. IV. Clinical indications, surgical technique, mechanism of action, and results. J Thorac Cardiovasc Surg 83:865, 1982
77. Ungerleider RM, Holman WL, Stanley TE III, et al: Encircling endocardial ventriculotomy for refractory ischemic ventricular tachycardia. II. Effects on regional myocardial blood flow. J Thorac Cardiovasc Surg 83:850, 1982
78. Ungerleider RM, Holman WL, Calcagno D, et al: Encircling endocardial ventriculotomy for refractory ischemic ventricular tachycardia. III. Effects on regional left ventricular function. J Thorac Cardiovasc Surg 83:857, 1982
79. Ungerleider RM, Calcagno D, Williams JM, et al: Comparison of the effects of the endocardial resection procedure and the encircling endocardial ventriculotomy. Surg Forum 33:320, 1982
80. Fontaine G, Guiraudon G, Frank R, et al: Stimulation studies and epicardial mapping in ventricular tachycardia: Study of mechanisms and selection for surgery, in Kulbertus HE (Ed): Re-entrant Arrhythmias: Mechanisms and Treatment. Baltimore, University Park Press, 1977, p 334
81. Fontaine G, Guiraudon G, Frank R, et al: Epicardial mapping and surgical treatment in six cases of resistant ventricular tachycardia not related to coronary artery disease, in Wellens HJJ, Lie KI, Janse MJ, (Eds): The Conduction System of the Heart. Leiden, The Netherlands, Kroese B. V., 545:63, 1976
82. Spurrell RAJ, Sowton E, Deuchar DC: Ventricular tachycardia in 4 patients evaluated by programmed electrical stimulation of the heart and treated in 2 patients by surgical division of anterior radiation of left bundle-branch. Br Heart J 35:1014, 1973
83. Spurrell RAJ, Yates AK, Thorburn CW, et al: Surgical treatment of ventricular tachycardia after epicardial mapping studies. Br Heart J 37:115, 1975
84. Wittig JH, Boineau JP: Surgical treatment of ventricular arrhythmia using epicardial, transmural and endocardial mapping. Ann Thorac Surg 20:117, 1975
85. Spielman SR, Michelson EL, Horowitz LN, et al: The limitations of epicardial mapping as a guide to the surgical therapy of ventricular tachycardia. Circulation 57:666, 1978
86. Harken AH, Josephson ME, Horowitz LN: Surgical endocardial resection for the treatment of malignant ventricular tachycardia. Ann Surg 190:456, 1979
87. Josephson ME, Harken AH, Horowitz LN: Endocardial excision: A new surgical technique for the treatment of recurrent ventricular tachycardia. Circulation 60:1430, 1979
88. Horowitz LN, Harken AH, Kastor JA, et al: Ventricular resection guided by epicardial and mapping for treatment of recurrent ventricular tachycardia. N Engl J Med 302:589, 1980

89. Horowitz LN, Harken AH, Josephson ME: Electrophysiologically directed ventricular resection for recurrent sustained ventricular tachycardia: The University of Pennsylvania experience, 1977-1980, in Harrison DC, Winkle RA, Mason JW (Eds): Symposium on Cardiac Arrhythmias—A Decade of Progress, 1980. San Bernardino, Calif., GK Hall & Co, 1981 (in press)
90. Mason JW, Stinson EB, Derby G, et al: Advantages of activation sequence mapping in the treatment of ventricular tachycardia, in Harrison DC, Winkle RA, Mason JW (Eds): Symposium on Cardiac Arrhythmia—A Decade of Progress, 1980. San Bernardino, Calif., GK Hall & Co, 1981 (in press)
91. Horowitz LN, Harken AH, Josephson ME, et al: Surgical treatment of ventricular arrhythmias in coronary artery disease. Ann Intern Med 95:88, 1981
92. Martin JL, Untereker WJ, Harken AH, et al: Aneurysmectomy and endocardial resection for ventricular tachycardia: Favorable hemodynamic and antiarrhythmic results in patients with global ventricular dysfunction. Am Heart J 103:960, 1982
93. Josephson ME, Horowitz LN, Harken AH: Surgery for recurrent sustained ventricular tachycardia associated with coronary artery disease: The role of subendocardial resection. Ann NY Acad Sci 382:381, 1982
94. Gallagher JJ: Surgical treatment of arrhythmias: Current status and future directions. Am J Cardiol 41:1035, 1978
95. Gallagher JJ, Anderson RW, Kasell J, et al: Cryoblation of drug-resistant ventricular tachycardia in a patient with a variant of scleroderma. Circulation 75:190, 1979
96. Camm J, Ward DE, Cory-Pearce R, et al: The successful cryosurgical treatment of paroxysmal ventricular tachycardia. Chest 75:621, 1979
97. Klein GJ, Harrison L, Ideker RF, et al: Reaction of the myocardium to cryosurgery: Electrophysiology and arrhythmogenic potential. Circulation 59:364, 1979

INDEX